The Fundamentals of Healthcare Administration

Navigating Challenges and Coordinating Care

Dorothy Howell | Whitney Hamilton | Melissa Jordan

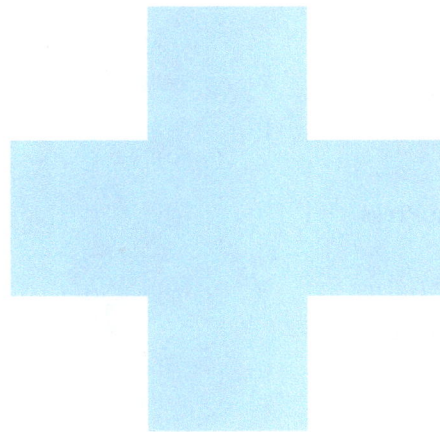

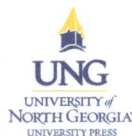

UNG
UNIVERSITY *of*
NORTH GEORGIA™
UNIVERSITY PRESS

Blue Ridge | Cumming | Dahlonega | Gainesville | Oconee

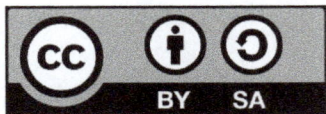

ISBN: 978-1-940771-88-5

Produced by:
University System of Georgia

Published by:
University of North Georgia Press
Dahlonega, Georgia

Cover Design and Layout Design:
Corey Parson

For more information, please visit http://ung.edu/university-press
Or email ungpress@ung.edu
Instructor Resources available upon request.

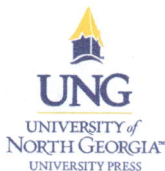

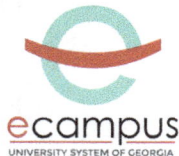

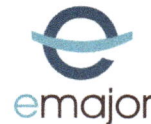

TABLE OF CONTENTS

Part I: Overview of Healthcare Organizations

CHAPTER 3: HEALTHCARE TECHNOLOGY AND INFORMATION STRATEGIES   69

CHAPTER 4: EMERGING TRENDS IN HEALTHCARE ORGANIZATIONS AND THEIR MANAGERIAL IMPLICATIONS   97

Part II: Leadership

CHAPTER 5: THE CONVERGENCE OF LEADERS AND MANAGERS 121

CHAPTER 6: BUILDING A FOUNDATION IN LEADERSHIP AND MANAGEMENT THEORY — 141

Chapter 7: The Role of Leaders and Managers in Establishing Organizational Ethics 171

Chapter 8: Core Leadership and Managerial Processes 193

Part III: Organizational Behavior and Models

CHAPTER 9: ORGANIZATIONAL THEORY AND BEHAVIOR PRACTICES IN HEALTHCARE: EXAMINING THE THREE LENSES OF THE HEALTHCARE INDUSTRY 213

CHAPTER 10: ANALYSIS OF ORGANIZATIONAL MODELS 232

Part IV: Organizational Culture Performance and Change

CHAPTER 11: ELIMINATING HEALTH DISPARITIES IN HEALTHCARE ORGANIZATIONS THROUGH CULTURAL PROFICIENCY   254

CHAPTER 12: ORGANIZATIONAL CULTURE IN HEALTHCARE   271

CHAPTER 13: ORGANIZATIONAL PERFORMANCE   283

CHAPTER 14: MANAGING ORGANIZATIONAL CHANGE   296

CHAPTER 15: ORGANIZATIONAL CHALLENGES FROM A GLOBAL PERSPECTIVE   307

ABOUT THE AUTHORS

Whitney N. Hamilton, DrPH, MPH is an Assistant Professor of Healthcare Services Administration at Middle Georgia State University. Her research primarily investigates the role of policy on maternal and child health, specifically seeking to further the development of comprehensive policies that will aid in the improvement of healthcare quality and access for vulnerable populations. Her previous research also includes a National Institutes of Health funded project, which sought to identify modifiable risk factors during the transition from care to home that influence the long-term effects of an Acute Coronary Syndrome event.

Dorothy J. Howell, DHA, MSN serves as the Department Chair/Assistant Professor for the Healthcare Services Administration within the School of Business at Middle Georgia State University. Dr. Howell received her Master of Science in Nursing from Georgia College and State University and a Doctor of Health Services Administration from University of Phoenix. Her current research interest includes student perceptions on improving student engagement in academic programs. Her previous research included Evaluating the Relationship of Computer Literacy, Training, Competence and Nursing Experience to CPIS Resistance.

Melissa Jordan, DHSc, EdD is an Assistant Professor of Healthcare Services Administration at Middle Georgia State University in Macon, Georgia. She was awarded her EdD from the Department of Adult and Career Education at Valdosta State University in Valdosta, Georgia. Dr. Jordan has published several scientific articles in peer-reviewed journals, book chapters, and presented her research studies at several major conferences across Georgia and the U.S. Her current research includes the retention strategies of diverse students in undergraduate healthcare administration programs within the University System of Georgia. Previous research includes teen pregnancy with a focus on understanding the problems of teenage motherhood with the development of preventative strategies and interventions to break the cycle of poverty, poor education, and risky behaviors that can lead to health and child welfare issues.

ACKNOWLEDGMENTS

First and foremost, we would like to collectively thank God and our families for enabling and empowering our abilities to complete this work. We also gratefully acknowledge Middle Georgia State University for cultivating the spirit and collegial atmosphere for collaboration that enabled our work on this textbook. We have had the pleasure of teaching this subject and feel privileged to further share our passion- we would like to thank our Dean, Dr. Steve Morse, as well as our students and colleagues here at MGA for the ongoing feedback and valuable insights they have provided over the years that has influenced and shaped our ideas for this text. We also extend our deepest gratitude to Yinning Zhang, our instructional designer, as well as *USG Publishing* and the myriad of USG contributors/editors we have had the pleasure of working with as we developed this text. We also greatly appreciate and honor the brave healthcare leaders who are on the frontline battling the current pandemic- we empathize and are encouraged by their daily sacrifice to facilitate successful healthcare delivery through novel approaches emphasizing collaboration, communication, and innovation in the midst of the challenges stemming from COVID-19.

PREFACE

As the authors of this book, we sincerely thank you for reading this text for instruction and professional leadership development. This textbook expresses our collective hope to support the advancement of rising healthcare leaders. The material is ideal for undergraduate students in healthcare administration and students in nursing or allied health programs. The book is written for those interested in acquiring a thorough knowledge base relative to the intricacies of the organizational theories, customs, and insights significant to the management of health service organizations. An explanation of the premise of leadership and management as it relates to establishing and maintaining the principles and practices within healthcare organizations is also examined.

The book opens with a discussion on the differences between health, healthcare and health care and provides an overview of healthcare management and organizational trends. And it culminates in discussions of leadership, management, motivation, and organizational behavior and management thinking. Additionally, the topics of information technology, teamwork, health disparities, organizational culture, performance, and change are included in the discussions.

The text contains a logical sequence of chapters with content that builds from the previous chapter. The first four chapters of the text provide an overview of healthcare management and establishes the basis of understanding the healthcare delivery system. Chapter One describes the differences between health, health care, and healthcare systems. Chapter Two then provides an overview of the healthcare management profession and discusses the major responsibilities of healthcare managers. Chapter Three illustrates the integration of information technology in healthcare and illustrates the use of health information technology to improve healthcare quality and efficiency. Chapter Four presents the emerging trends and challenges faced by healthcare administrators and issues such as the growth of strategic alliances in the health sector, the expansion and complexity of health law and regulation, health information technology, the rise of consumerism in health care, and the global interconnectedness of health systems.

Following the overview of healthcare management, the next three chapters describes the practices and core principles of healthcare leadership. Chapter Five explores the most common leadership theories and demonstrates the contribution of organizational theories to the healthcare management industry. Chapter Six differentiates between the functions, roles, and responsibilities of healthcare managers and leaders. Chapter Seven expands on the distinction of leadership and management skills by delineating the roles of leaders and managers in influencing organizational culture, performance, and change.

The next section of the book explores critical managerial functions relative to organizational behavior. Chapter Eight provides an overview of leadership and managerial processes including motivation, effective communication, team coordination, team management, influence exertion, performance improvement, negotiation and conflict resolution. Chapter Nine illustrates the incorporation of well-known theories and design strategies into the management of the healthcare environment. Chapter Ten analyzes various perspectives related to the management of a healthcare organization.

The next five chapters reflect on the environment of the healthcare organization illustrating how the organization's leadership and processes shape the culture. Chapter Eleven describes culturally competent strategies that address health disparities in healthcare organizations. Chapter Twelve demonstrates how the organizational culture influences the organization's performance. The principles and processes of healthcare performance, improvement, and quality assurance will be discussed in Chapter Thirteen, and providing strategies to manage organizational change will be the focus of Chapter Fourteen. Finally, Chapter Fifteen presents global organizational challenges such as aging populations, health care accessibility, healthcare provider shortages, changing demographics, and rising healthcare costs.

The book is filled with learning aids including introductions, chapter objectives, on-page definitions, key points, real-world examples, case studies, practical applications, discussion questions, and chapter summaries. This text is meant to enable students to critically analyze real-world healthcare management scenarios. The book is equipped with a case study and critical thinking questions that are used throughout the chapters to help the reader put the contents into action. This textbook will utilize one major case study called "Managing the Case of Mr. Rodriquez." Leadership examples, critical thinking exercises and/or questions have been added into each chapter to help the reader apply what he/she has read in efforts to aid in an understanding of the content. The case is laid out here in its entirety and will be referenced using a sidebar within or as a caption at the beginning of the chapters.

COMMENTS FOR CONSIDERATION

This book is written for those interested in acquiring a thorough knowledge base relative to the intricacies of the organizational theories, customs, and insights significant to the management of health service organizations. It examines the foundational aspects of leadership and management as they relate to establishing and maintaining the principles and practices within healthcare organizations. The book opens with a discussion on the differences between health, healthcare, and health care while providing an overview of healthcare management and organizational trends. It culminates in discussions of leadership, management, motivation, organizational behavior, and management thinking. Additionally, it discusses topics of information technology, teamwork, health disparities, organizational culture, performance, and change.

The book's chapters logically and sequentially progress with content that builds from the previous chapter. The first four chapters of the text provide an overview of healthcare management and establish the basis of understanding the healthcare delivery system. Chapter one describes the differences between health, health care, and healthcare systems. Chapter two then provides an overview of the healthcare management profession and discusses the major responsibilities of healthcare managers. Chapter three illustrates the integration of information technology in healthcare and illustrates the use of health information technology to improve healthcare quality and efficiency. Chapter four presents the emerging trends and challenges faced by healthcare administrators as well as such issues as the growth of strategic alliances in the health sector, the expansion and complexity of health law and regulation, health information technology, the rise of consumerism in health care, and the global interconnectedness of health systems.

Following the overview of healthcare management, the next three chapters describe the practices and core principles of healthcare leadership. Chapter five explores the most common leadership theories and demonstrates the contribution of organizational theories to the healthcare management industry. Chapter six differentiates between the functions, roles, and responsibilities of healthcare managers and leaders. Chapter seven expands on the distinction of leadership and management skills by delineating the roles of leaders and managers in influencing organizational culture, performance, and change.

The next section of the book explores critical managerial functions relative to organizational behavior. Chapter eight provides an overview of leadership and managerial processes, including motivation, effective communication, team coordination, team management, influence exertion, performance improvement, negotiation, and conflict resolution. Chapter nine illustrates the incorporation of well-known theories and design strategies into the management of the healthcare environment. Chapter ten analyzes various perspectives related to the management of a healthcare organization.

The next five chapters reflect on the environment of the healthcare organization, illustrating how the organization's leadership and processes shape the culture. Chapter eleven describes culturally-competent strategies that address health disparities in healthcare organizations. Chapter twelve demonstrates how the organizational culture influences the organization's performance. Chapter thirteen discusses principles and processes of healthcare performance, improvement, and quality assurance; also, chapter fourteen focuses on providing strategies to manage organizational change. Finally, chapter fifteen presents such global organizational challenges as aging populations, health care accessibility, healthcare provider shortages, changing demographics, and rising healthcare costs.

Throughout all of these chapters, the book provides learning aids, including introductions, chapter objectives, on-page definitions, key points, real-world examples, case studies, practical applications, discussion questions, and chapter summaries. This book intends to enable students to critically analyze real-world healthcare management scenarios. Leadership examples, critical thinking exercises and/or questions have been added into each chapter to help the reader apply what they have read in efforts to aid in an understanding of the content. And throughout all of its chapters, the book uses a case study and critical thinking questions to help the reader put the contents into action. This book uses one major case study called "Managing the Case of Mr. Rodriquez"; it lays out the case in its entirety and references it within or as a caption at the beginning of the chapters.

The book is ideal for undergraduate students in healthcare administration and students in nursing or allied health programs.

MANAGING THE CASE OF MR. RODRIQUEZ

Mr. Rodriquez is married with 2 adult children. He lives in a predominantly Hispanic-speaking community. He has retired after 35 years as a high-pressure sales representative. Mr. Rodriquez worked long hours and usually slept in. He did not regularly eat breakfast and obtained most of his lunch and dinner meals from local fast food restaurants. His work schedule left him little time to engage in physical activity. He is 5'10" and weighs 206 pounds. His body mass index (BMI) is 32. He has smoked 1 pack of cigarettes daily for the past 30 years. At his 50-year annual physical with his primary care physician, he was diagnosed with hypertension and placed on an antihypertensive. On a subsequent visit, his blood pressure remained elevated and his healthcare provider (HCP) noticed swelling in his legs and ankles. A second antihypertensive was added to his medical regimen along with a diuretic. On his 55th birthday, Mr. Rodriquez developed shortness of breath and chest pain and collapsed at work. He was taken to the hospital by ambulance. He underwent a cardiac catheterization and was diagnosed with coronary artery disease. He was treated while in the hospital and sent home with medications, dietary modifications, and an exercise regimen. At the age of 65, Mr. Rodriquez retired due to memory loss, inability to perform tasks, confusion, and misplacing things. He was taken to his primary care provider (PCP) and diagnosed with Alzheimer's disease.

Because of his history of coronary artery disease, hypertension, and worsening Alzheimer's disease, Mr. Rodriquez was admitted to Southern Healthcare Hospice Center at age 80. On day 2 following admission, he had sudden onset of confusion, bradycardia, and hypotension. He lost consciousness, requiring the initiation of a medical emergency.

The hospice care facility is adjacent to a major academic medical center. Thus, the "code team" (comprising a senior medical resident, medical intern, anesthesia resident, anesthesia attending, and critical care nurse) within the main hospital was activated. The message blared through the overhead speaker system: "Code blue, fourth floor Hospice Center. Code blue, fourth floor Hospice Center."

The senior resident and intern had never been to the Hospice facility. "How do we get to Hospice?" the senior resident asked a few other residents in a panic. "I don't know how to get there except to go outside and through the front door," a colleague answered. So, the senior resident and intern ran down numerous flights of stairs, outside the front of the hospital, down the block, into the Hospice facility, and up four flights of stairs (the two buildings are actually connected on the fourth floor).

Upon arrival, they found the patient apneic and pulseless. The nurses on the inpatient Hospice unit had placed an oxygen mask on the patient, but the patient was not receiving ventilatory support or chest compressions. The resident and intern began basic life support (CPR with chest compressions) with the bag-valve-mask. When the critical care nurse and the rest of the code team arrived, they attempted to hook the patient up to their portable monitor. Unfortunately, the leads on the monitor were incompatible with the stickers on the patient, which were from the Hospice floor (the stickers were more than 10 years old). The team did not have appropriate leads to connect the monitor and sent a nurse back to the main hospital to obtain compatible stickers. In the meantime, the patient remained pulseless with an uncertain rhythm. Moreover, despite ventilation with the bag-valve-mask, the patient's saturations remained less than 80%. After minutes of trying to determine the cause, it was discovered that the mask had been attached to the oxygen nozzle on the wall, but the oxygen had not initially been turned on by the nursing staff. The oxygen was turned on, the patient's saturations started to rise, and the anesthesiologist prepared to intubate the patient. Chest compressions continued.

At this point, a staff nurse on the Hospice floor came into the room, recognized the patient, and shouted, "Stop! Stop! He's a no code!" Confusion ensued—some team members stopped while others continued the resuscitation. A review of the chart showed no documentation of a "Do Not Resuscitate" order, and the resuscitation continued. However, the intern on the team called the patient's son, who confirmed the patient's desire to not be resuscitated. The efforts were stopped, and the patient died moments later.

PART I

OVERVIEW OF HEALTHCARE ORGANIZATIONS

1

Healthcare Organizations

1.1 LEARNING OBJECTIVES

- To explain the basic principles of healthcare organizations
- To discuss key concepts associated with healthcare organizations
- To demonstrate the various types of healthcare organizations
- To identify the various parts of the healthcare system
- To describe the structure of healthcare organizations
- To explain the various types of healthcare facilities

1.2 INTRODUCTION

This chapter will address the potential differences between health, healthcare, and health care while also providing an overview of healthcare organizations. Because readers need a reasonable understanding of the types of healthcare organizations and the components of the healthcare system, the chapter also discusses managed care organizations, preferred provider organizations, and health maintenance organizations. These organizations include health care organizations and hospitals, ambulatory care centers, public health, long term care, home health, hospice, emergency/urgent care services, orthopedic and rehabilitation centers, clinics and physician practices, and telehealth. This chapter also covers financing, insurance, delivery, and payment as components of the healthcare system.

1.3 KEY CONCEPTS OF HEALTH

1.3.1 Overview

Access to healthcare is significant to the overall wellbeing of individuals within the United States and globally. Patients' access to healthcare can be deprived by such barriers as the following: lack of transportation; limited office hours causing limited appointment availability; lack of physicians, clinics, pharmacies, and hospitals in rural areas; and the lack of insurance coverage or finances to afford healthcare. The provision of healthcare takes on many forms based on population needs. For example, chronically-ill patients are at risk for poor healthcare outcomes; chronic illnesses include heart disease, such as with Mr. Rodriquez; cancer, diabetes, asthma, etc. If a chronically-ill patient is also disabled, this condition further exacerbates the problem. A disability is any physical or mental impairment that significantly limits one or more major life activities; individuals with disabilities, therefore, require medical care and assistance in making and keeping an appointment as well as following through with the treatment regimen. Based on the extent of the illness, individual patients may require long term care or home health, as with the case of Mr. Rodriquez. Many types of healthcare organizations have been established to respond to these various possible needs. For example, there are both private (owned and governed by a person, many people, or an organization) and publicly funded hospitals that care for the sick and injured in various locations (Kisacky, 2017).

Health policy plays a major role in health care organizations within the United States. They are a collection of rules or laws that illustrate the distribution of resources, services, and political influences on the health of the population, and they were developed to govern how health systems operate and function. One policy with which most people are familiar is the Social Security Act that led to the creation of public health insurance, such as Medicare and Medicaid in the 1940's, the Children's Health Insurance Program (CHIP) in 1997 and the Affordable Care Act developed under the Obama Administration. Another outgrowth of health policy was the requirement that employers provide health insurance as part of their benefit package. Health policies also promote biomedical research and the growth of medical technology. Indeed, they affect health maintenance organizations (HMOs), hospitals, medical schools, nursing homes, manufacturers of medical technology and pharmaceuticals, and employers (Shi & Singh, 2015). Health policy, therefore, is crucial in improving factors that affect our health risks and outcomes. These factors, known as social determinants of health, include income levels, housing, access to healthy food, education, exercise, tobacco, illicit drug, or alcohol usage, practicing preventive health measures, etc. Because of these determinants, the government must develop and maintain health policy to intervene in health-related issues.

1.3.2 Health Defined

Health should be a comparatively easy term to define by individuals as we all have a perception of what health means to us. However, we all have various perceptions of health, making the definition of health more difficult. Is it the absence of disease or a feeling of wellness? Does it encompass the entire being (body, mind, spirit) from a holistic perspective? Do we view health as an entity experienced by children and young adults, with illness occurring as we age? Many words are used to convey health, such as wellness, soundness, well-being, healthy, fit, whole, etc. So, what is health?

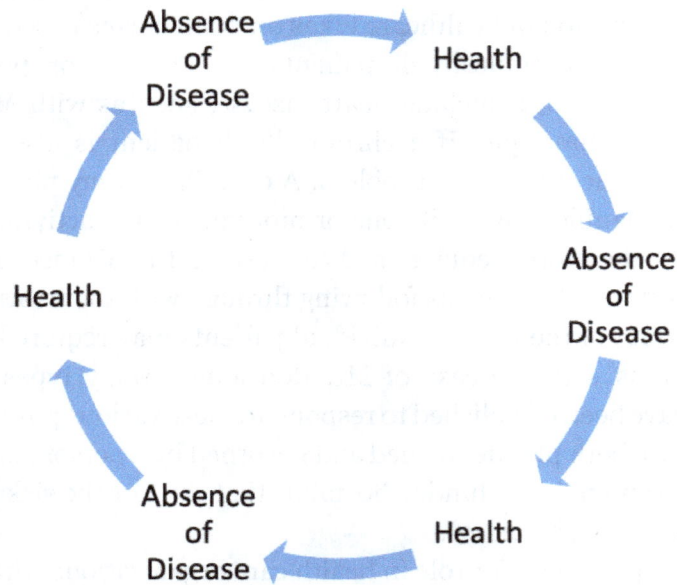

Figure 1.1: Health

Source: Original Work
Attribution: Dorothy Howell
License: CC BY-SA 4.0

When performing a search on the MEDLINE database, a platform of references and abstracts on life sciences and biomedical topics, located on PUBMED.gov, the term "health" does not exist unaccompanied by other terms. For instance, terminology such as health literacy, health system, health behavior, and health policy appear. Neither does the National Institutes of Health have a distinct definition of health. To obtain a clear-cut definition, we must rely on internet or dictionary sources. For example, Merriam-Webster defines health as a "condition of sound mind, body, and spirit" (Merriam Webster, s.v.). The World Health Organization (WHO) defines health as:

> a state of complete physical, mental and social well-being and not merely the absence of disease or infirmity. With this definition, a person with mental or physical disabilities would not be in a state of health. The enjoyment of the highest attainable standard of health is one of the fundamental rights of every human being without distinction of race, religion, political belief, economic or social condition.

Even with the WHO's definition, one must still break down words within it to understand health, words such as well-being, disease, or infirmity.

Additionally, what is the highest attainable standard of health? The National Academy of Medicine defines health as a state of well-being and the ability to function in various situations. It considers social and personal resources and physical ability (Niles, 2018). As you think about all the definitions of health, ask yourself where you fit in. Are you happy? Do you have a social life and get along well with others? Do you feel safe? Is there balance in your life? Do you have mental or physical challenges?

Many authors seek to understand health. One such author, Rattan, describes health as "having physical and mental independence in activities of daily living; and this state may vary widely but can be established objectively" (Rattan, 2013). Based on this observation, individuals function at various levels of health daily, dependent upon their beliefs. Thus, this definition may provide one with a greater perception of health, as health for an individual is whatever that individual believes it to be. For example, Anna has Down's syndrome. However, she has friends, a loving family; she is outgoing and has no other health issues. She views herself as a healthy individual. Moreover, Plugge, Douglas, & Fitzpatrick (2008) conducted a study in the United Kingdom of women prisoners to determine if their perception of health and illness differed from lay people. Many of these women viewed health in relation to behaviors, such as diet, exercise, smoking, drinking or illicit drug use. The women believed that external appearance (i.e., physique or skin glow) revealed an individual's level of health. They denoted a healthy lifestyle as a significant factor in determining one's health and reviewed health as more than the absence of disease.

Health, therefore, is the function of several variables or determinants. Health determinants refer to social, personal, economic, and environmental factors that affect individual and population-based health. Other factors that affect our health include our genetic makeup or biology and our behaviors. Our family history can have a bearing on specific disease risks, both physical and mental. Our health behaviors can alter our biology. For example, smoking, physical activity, aging, stress, use of alcohol or illicit drugs, injury or exposure to violence, or toxic or infectious agents can change our biology and increase the risk for development of such diseases as cancer or heart disease. The social environment includes the individuals we are surround by, including family, friends, or coworkers in such places as places of worship, the workplace, supermarkets, or schools. The physical environment incorporates anything you can see, hear, feel, touch, or taste. And it is in the physical environment where we are exposed to toxic or infectious agents, such as radiation (Longest, 2016).

Stop and Apply

Refer to the case study of the 80-year-old man at Southern Hospice Center. His condition clearly indicates a deterioration in his health status. Based on the case, what led to the change in his condition?

1.3.3 Biomedical or Medical Model

A biomedical model describes the human being as a biological system that may or may not function normally and thus requires therapeutic or preventive intervention to reduce or eradicate disease. Much of what we know about health is based on the biomedical model of health's definition, which describes health as the absence of illness or disease (National Research Council, 1998). Segen's Medical Dictionary considers that all diseases are rooted in biological processes requiring treatment modalities geared toward physical or chemical intervention (Segen's Medical Dictionary, n.d.). This premise is based on the psychiatrist Dr. R. Laing's view of the medical model, a medical model he initially originated in *The Politics of the Family and Other Essays* (1971). His perspective of the medical model was that mental illness was derived from a physical disease process, and a medication was required to treat the disorder. This biological stance suggests that mental disorders stem from the brain's physical structure and functioning (National Research Council, 1998). Regardless of its origination, the term medical model reflects an intent to provide insight on the meaning of health. Health describes a lack of symptoms or a situation where one does not feel ill. The question is, "does this state really exist in human nature?" Let's put this question in perspective. Jane was a 35-year-old African American female who presented to the health care provider for a routine gynecological examination. Two weeks later, Jane was notified to report to the physician's office for a review of her lab results. Jane was told that she had Stage 1 cervical cancer. With early stage cervical cancer, no signs and symptoms of the disease are evident to the individual. Up until that point in time, Jane always viewed herself as healthy or without disease—based on the medical model's presentation of health. Therefore, one can surmise from this story that the absence of illness or disease may not be the most accurate description of health. There are occurrences when an individual is unaware of an existing illness or disease due to the absence of signs and symptoms.

1.3.4 Holistic Health and Holistic Medicine

With holistic health, a person thinks in terms of overall well-being, wherein one is whole and complete. The external and internal environments are an integral part of the person's wellbeing, given the negative influences emanating from these environments (Tomljenovic, 2014). **Holistic health** encompasses the physical, spiritual, mental, and social aspects of a human being, which are interdependent (Zamanzadeh, Jasemi, Valizadeh, Keogh, & Taleghani, 2015). All must work in harmony for the individual to achieve wholeness or optimal health or wellness[7]. Plugge, Douglas, & Fitzpatrick (2008) report women prisoners in the United Kingdom believed mental health status, resilience and inner strength played a role in an individual's wellbeing. In the holistic approach, the patient's beliefs, emotions, cultures, opinions, posture, and attitudes are significant components that influence the healing process and feelings of contentment and gratification[11]. Holistic healthcare provides an avenue for the patient to be treated with dignity and mutual respect while engaging the patient as an equal partner when making healthcare decisions (Zamanzadeh, Jasemi, Valizadeh, Keogh, & Taleghani, 2015). **Holistic Medicine,** then, becomes the practice of holistic health by healthcare professionals. Holistic medicine practitioners take into consideration the interdependent parts of a person that, when not in harmony, adversely affect all the parts and ultimately lead to illness (Mohan, 2017). With this practice, conventional and alternative therapies are used to treat the patient. For example, Johnson, Roberts, & Elkins (2019) conveys the results of two randomized clinical trials initiated to investigate the effects of evening primrose oil on premenopausal and postmenopausal women in treatment of bone mineral density. Results showed that evening primrose oil combined with calcium and marine fish oil revealed clinically significant results (an increase of 1%) in treatment of bone mineral density. One interesting principle regarding holistic medicine is that the individual is treated as a person and not a disease, thereby requiring the person to take ownership of their health and wellbeing. One of the most significant elements is finding and treating the cause of the illness rather than treating the symptoms, as is the case with traditional medical practice (Mohan, 2017). Holistic medicine practitioners treat the patient through such measures as diet, exercise, psychotherapy, relationship and spiritual counseling, acupuncture, chiropractic care, homeopathy, massage therapy, naturopathy, medication, and surgery, if needed (Fritscher, 2019).

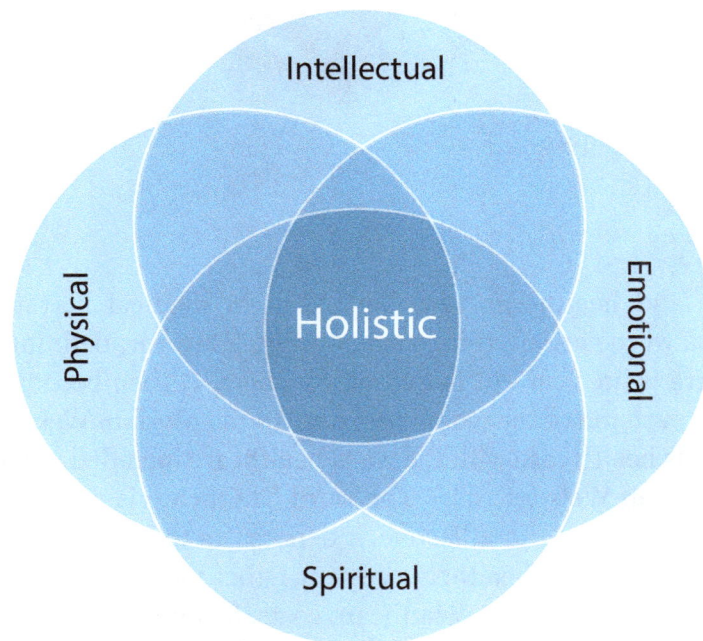

Figure 1.2: Health

Source: Original Work
Attribution: Corey Parson
License: CC BY-SA 4.0

> **Stop and Apply**
>
> How could Mr. Rodriquez have benefited from holistic health care services?

1.3.5 Healthcare versus Health Care

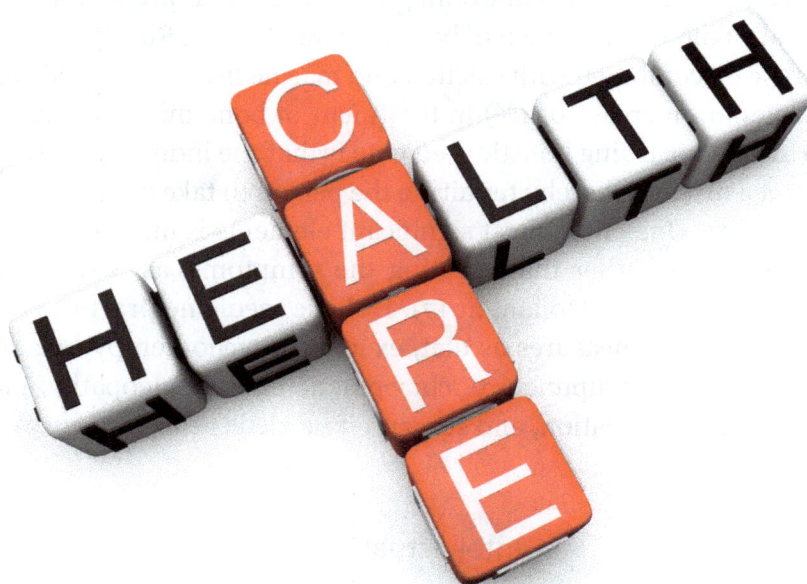

Figure 1.3: Health/Healthcare

Source: Clipart Library
Attribution: Clipart Library
License: © Clipart Library. Used with permission.

Healthcare and health care are both seen in medical literature. In some instances, these words are used interchangeably. However, defining the words is difficult, as there is no clear-cut definition for them. It then becomes a matter of debate on which version of the word is correct. In the Meriam Webster dictionary, we find the words health care with the word healthcare included as a variant of the two words (Merriem Webster, s.v.). The word healthcare is an adjective or noun based on how it is used. As an adjective, it denotes an industry or system, such as the healthcare industry or a healthcare system. Other uses of this term are denoted as follows: healthcare resources, healthcare costs, healthcare provider, healthcare facility or organization. Used as a noun, the word healthcare can be used in the following contexts: "the theme for our discussion this week is healthcare" or performing a search on the healthcare job board (Ruhl, 2013). **Health care** refers to an act or deed between the healthcare provider and the patient to maintain or improve the patient's healthcare status (Ruhl, 2013). Therefore, health care can be used to describe a variety of services to improve an individual's health and well-being.

1.4 OVERVIEW OF HEALTHCARE ORGANIZATIONS

1.4.1 Description of Healthcare Organizations

This section intends to provide only a brief overview of healthcare organizations. An organization is an entity developed for s specific purpose. The organization will usually have a mission, vision, and values supporting the purpose of the organization. Additionally, an organization will employ individuals who can share in the mission and vision and act as advocates to ensure the organization's objectives are met and sustained. The purpose of an organization is to create products or provide services, using people and resources, and to maintain relationships with the external environment consisting of customers, suppliers, competitors and regulatory bodies.

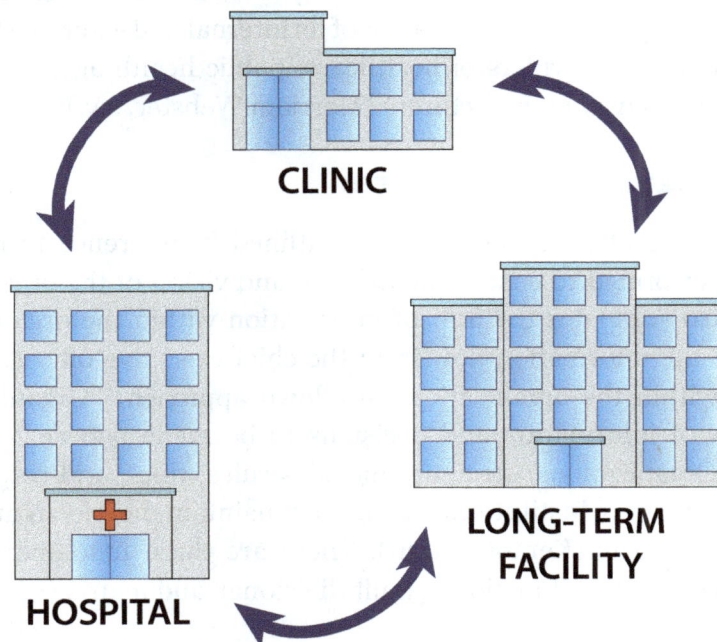

CLINIC

LONG-TERM FACILITY

HOSPITAL

Figure 1.4: Hospital Clinic LTC

Source: Original Work
Attribution: Corey Parson
License: CC BY-SA 4.0

Based on the premise that health care refers to services provided within a health care system to improve the health of an individual, a healthcare organization is an establishment that provides healthcare services. A health care organization can range from a single physician's private practice to a health system to an integrated delivery network of health systems. Examples of healthcare organizations include insurance companies that serve as payors for healthcare services rendered, independent physicians' practices that take care of the mzedical needs of patients, and pharmaceutical companies that provide medicines prescribed to treat various diseases. Other examples include various types of facilities that treat individuals with acute, chronic, rehabilitative, or long-term health care needs or issues, such as hospitals; nursing homes; home health agencies; outpatient medical, imaging, and surgical centers; and manufacturers of medical devices. Public health agencies seek to promote optimum health for the society as a whole (Shi & Singh, 2015). Highly integrated health care systems include a hospital, a physician component, and some type of payer, such as insurance or Medicare. Integrated delivery systems or networks, accountable care organizations, and payer-provider integration are three types of integrated health care systems (Walston, 2017).

Healthcare organizations rely on health policies, the healthcare market, organizational governing bodies, and the overall desire to improve patient satisfaction to dictate how work is structured and completed. Internal policies, external governing bodies, and various levels of authority govern organizations and thereby assist the organization in making decisions. Each has its own set of challenges that will influence the behavior of its internal and external stakeholders, including payers and providers of healthcare, public health agencies, providers, and services provided by manufacturers (Merriam Webster, s.v.).

1.4.2 Organizational Structure

The **structure** of an organization is outlined in reference to how specific activities are performed to ensure the mission and vision of the organization are achieved. It also stipulates the flow of information within the organization. For example, does the information flow from the chief executive officer to the lower subordinates within the organization (top-down approach)? Organizations also allow the flow of information and decisions to be made between levels of the organization. Organizational structure includes rules, roles, and responsibilities. Organizations that have instituted structure can maintain their focus and efficiency in meeting their goals (Kenton, 2020). There are three fundamental types of organizational structures: functional, multidivisional, and matrix (Walston, 2017).

Functional Organizations

The **functional organization structure** (also called bureaucratic organizational structure) splits the organization into departments based on the expertise of employees. Therefore, a health care organization may have various departments, such as the manager or chief executive officer, commercial and marketing, finance, accounting, managerial, facilities, operations, maintenance, safety, or environment, housekeeping, nursing, laboratory, pharmacy, etc. This type of structure works best in small to medium size organizations wherein the business environment is stable and predictable and routine tasks are emphasized and practiced to improve quality. Healthcare delivery is usually structured based on functionality, with unit level divisions established according to roles, services, tasks, etc. Examples of this type of structure include admissions, pharmacy, accounting, business office, maintenance, food service, housekeeping, nursing, laboratory, radiology, and emergency services, among others. The structure of an organization also encompasses higher levels of supervision comprising a chief executive officer, chief financial officer, chief nursing officer, chief information officer, and other specialized officers.

Several advantages and disadvantages of functional organizations exist. One significant advantage is the incorporation of personnel with specialized skill sets, which increases quality and efficiency within the organization. Units can then be developed based on specialization, such as oncology, maternity, pediatrics, renal, medical, surgical, cardiology, orthopedic, ears, nose and throat (ENT), etc. Other advantages include reduction in duplication of services and an increase in communication within departments. Specialized tasks, such as finance, marketing, or purchasing, can be placed at centralized locations within the organization. Because of specialization, departments can often operate in silos, which leads to poor communication and coordination of services (Walston, 2017). This situation occurs because of reduced communication between departments, narrowed business perspectives, and a short-term focus on tasks.

Correcting this problem would entail developing key criteria that would define the scope of departmental specialization and devising a means of evaluating outcomes based on the overall purpose of the organization (Bach, 2018). Another method of improving specialization problems is to find out the root cause of the problem by identifying the problem; analyzing it; developing, planning, and implementing the best solutions and finally evaluating the implemented solution to see if changes are warranted (Elsaid, Okasha, & Abdelghaly, 2013). The following chart depicts a simple organization chart with a summary of advantages and disadvantages of the functional structure.

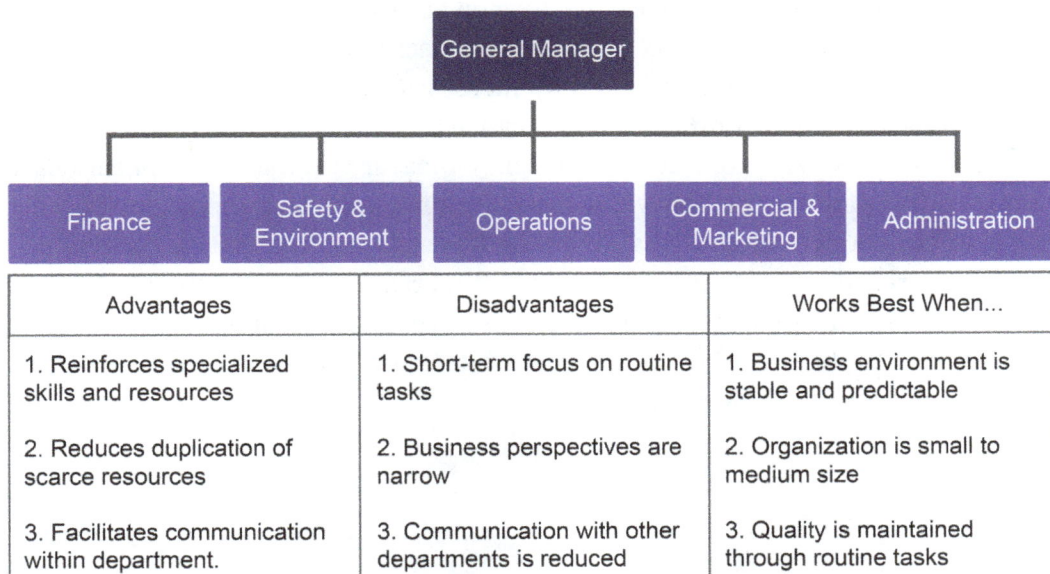

Advantages	Disadvantages	Works Best When...
1. Reinforces specialized skills and resources	1. Short-term focus on routine tasks	1. Business environment is stable and predictable
2. Reduces duplication of scarce resources	2. Business perspectives are narrow	2. Organization is small to medium size
3. Facilitates communication within department.	3. Communication with other departments is reduced	3. Quality is maintained through routine tasks

Figure 1.5: The Functional Structure

Multidivisional Organizations

Walston describes a multidivisional organization as one wherein the chief corporation comprises several smaller business units or divisions, which are based on geographic locations, products or services so that the daily processes or functions occur at the unit or divisional level, thus allowing the separate units or divisions to operate independently. In this structure, tasks are duplicated by each division, fostering innovation and receptiveness to their specific requirements. This process allows executives at the corporate level to use statistics from each unit to focus on strategies that will propel overall organizational performance through the successful allocating of people and resources (Walston, 2017). When organizations create divisions based on geography or products, cultures, markets, or laws will vary significantly. Because of this, healthcare organizations, such as Hospital Corporation of America (HCA), established an international division to manage its ventures in other countries more effectively and efficiently. This is also true for pharmaceutical and medical device companies. Examples of multidivisional structures in healthcare include cardiology, orthopedics, pediatrics, neurology, and women's services. There are also specialty hospitals geared towards cardiology, such as with Heart Tower at Navicent Health, spine surgery, sports medicine and cancer treatment.

Advantages of the multidivisional structure include the ability to hold corporate executives accountable for the results of local operations that are within their control. Each division monitors shifts in the external environment relative to consumer needs and focuses their operating efforts accordingly. A major issue with the multidivisional level is healthcare costs and quality. With the multidivisional organizational structure, duplication of functions, such as products and services across divisions, place the division at a disadvantage, which threatens quality and costs of healthcare. This process decreases the division's ability to achieve economies of scale and thereby increases the division's operating cost. Additionally, the duplication of functions can also lead to a lack of standardization and inefficiencies (Walston, 2017). Efficiency measures the ability of healthcare resources in attaining the best value for the money invested. Inefficiency occurs as a result of poor resource allocation in the form of spending that can be reduced without decreasing quality and spending that increases overall costs (equipment, labor, capital) and quality of services. Healthcare leaders should review these inefficiencies to determine if the benefits of decentralization exceed the costs of duplication (Delaune & Everett, 2008).

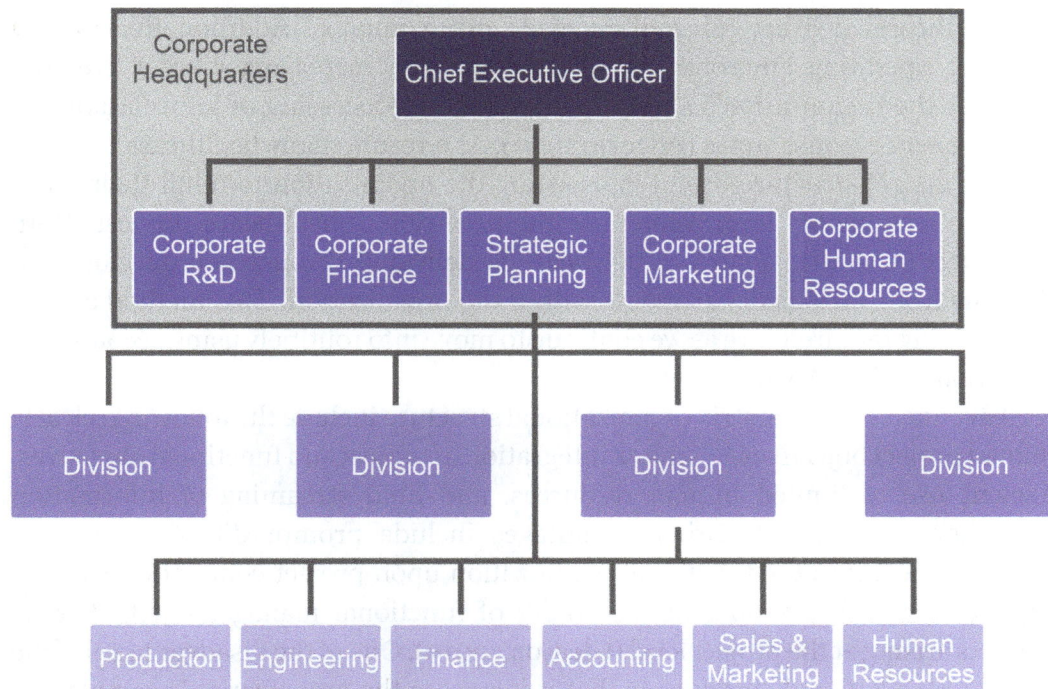

Figure 1.6: Multidivisional Structure

Source: Original Work
Attribution: Corey Parson
License: CC BY-SA 4.0

Matrix Organizations

Many healthcare facilities operate using the **matrix organizational structure**, which is most useful when problems need to be solved. The matrix structure comprises the functional structure, along with a temporary project structure (Gleeson, 2019). One of the characteristics of the matrix organizational structure is the presence of two managers creating multiple reporting relationships. The departmental manager controls vertical relationships, while the project manager handles horizontal relationships. Employees are organized based on their function or services provided. Therefore, they work in their functional departments and on a service line team. This can be noted with hospital clinical areas wherein an administrator or manager is placed on the unit to promote the coordination and integration of department personnel, such as nurses, housekeeping, dining room, and social services. These employees will report to their immediate supervisors and to the unit administrator or manager. Instead of disassembling the functional structure to create this temporary project structure, the matrix structure retains the functional structure and superimposes on it a temporary project structure (Walston, 2017). With a matrix organizational structure, the project manager and their team will complete the project assigned to them independently. The senior manager of each department (finance, operations, HR, marketing, etc.) is responsible for ensuring everything is in accordance with the company's policies and level of services.

Healthcare delivery is multifaceted and complex. Additionally, rapidly changing operating environments created through increasing market pressure increases the organization's ability to improve the processing of information and allows faster response times (Allcorn, 1990). As a result, many healthcare facilities find the matrix structure useful in assisting the organization to fulfill their quest of continuous quality improvement in the provision of healthcare services. With the matrix structure, quality patient care is delivered through the development of teams from various departments within the organization. This method aids in coordinating required care as we continue to move into routinely using accountable care organizations (Walston, 2017).

Advantages of the matrix organizational structure include the following: clearly defined project objectives, seamless integration of project and functional objectives, efficient use of limited human resources, and fluid streaming of information throughout the project. Other advantages include prompt diffusion of team members back into the functional organization upon project completion without organizational disruption and the ability of functional management to handle conflicts arising at the project level (Gleeson,, 2019). One of the disadvantages of the matrix organizational structure is that it increases the organization's complexity. Other disadvantages include problems due to employees having to answer too many bosses and having conflicting managerial directives. Additionally, establishing priorities suitable to both the functional and project management may prove difficult. Another disadvantage is the potential delay in management's reaction to problems when both structures are required to provide solutions. Please review Table 1.1 for a comparison of organizational structure.

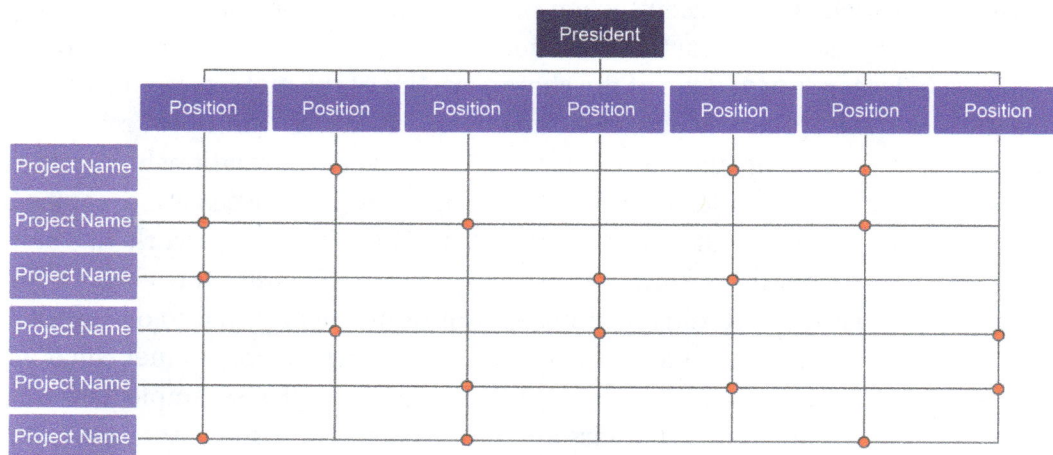

Figure 1.7: Matrix Structure

Source: Original Work
Attribution: Corey Parson
License: CC BY-SA 4.0

Table 1.1 Comparison of Organizational Structures

	Functional	Multidivisional	Matrix
Description	The organization is split into departments based on the employees' expertise, such as the manager or chief executive officer, commercial and marketing, finance, accounting, managerial, facilities, etc.	The chief corporation comprises several smaller business units or divisions which are based on geographic locations, products, or services so that the daily processes or functions occur at the unit or divisional level, allowing the separate units or divisions to operate independently.	The matrix structure comprises the functional structure along with a temporary project structure, which requires using two managers simultaneously.
Advantages	**Efficient** use of skills and resources. **Decreases** duplication. **Facilitates** communication and collaboration.	**Ability** to hold corporate executives accountable for the results of local operations that are within their control.	**Clearly** defined project objectives. **Seamless** integration of project and functional objectives. **Efficient** use of limited human resources. **Fluid** streaming of information throughout the project. **Prompt** diffusion of team members back into the functional organization upon project completion without organizational disruption. **Ability** of functional management to handle conflicts arising at the project level.
Disadvantages	**Specialization** can lead to departments operating in silos. **Potential** for decreased communication. **Narrow** business perspectives.	**Duplication** of functions, such as products and services across divisions, which threatens quality and costs of healthcare. **Increased** operational costs due to inability to achieve economies of scale. **Leads** to lack of standardization and inefficiencies.	**Increases** the complexity of the organization. **Problems** derived from having employees answer to too many bosses and having conflicting managerial directives. **Difficulty** in establishing priorities for functional and project management. **Delay** in management reactions.

Stop and Apply

Think about the size and structure of the hospice center where Mr. Rodriquez resided. Describe how the hospice center can fit into the functional structure described above.

1.5 COMPONENTS OF A HEALTHCARE SYSTEM

The World Health Organization (WHO) indicates that a well-functioning healthcare system operates according to the needs and expectations of the population (2010). The health system performs for the purpose of improving the population's health status; protecting the population from toxic and infectious agents; shielding the population from financial burdens associated with chronic illnesses; providing access to care; and allowing individuals an opportunity to participate in their care, health, and health system. Healthcare systems are subjected to forces that prevent the development of policies. These forces emphasize unequal curative care services, fragmentation of services, and commercialization of healthcare delivery (WHO, 2010).

Healthcare delivery is provided through both private and public institutions where there are various actors that assist in healthcare delivery, such as community, media, and healthcare delivery systems; businesses; academic institutions; local and state health departments, and laboratories (IOM, 2002). As such, healthcare delivery should be an integrated network of components that work together. However, this is not the case in the U.S. Instead, the components of financing, insurance, delivery, and payment represent a combination of public and private sources. In order to participate in governmentally run programs, participants must meet specific eligibility criteria. Additionally, the government runs specific programs geared towards certain populations, such as veterans, military personnel, American Indians and the uninsured. The functions of financing, insurance, payment, and delivery are reserved for the private sector (Shi & Singh, 2015). As such, the focus of this discussion will include MCOs.

1.5.1 Financing

Financing refers to premiums established through negotiations between employers and the MCO. A contract is developed based on negotiated fees for services to be provided. Individuals enrolled in the plan pay a set fee for all services provided by the plan (Shi & Singh, 2015). Providers rely on the patient's insurance to pay for services rendered. Similarly, this function controls how much the provider is paid for services rendered to the insured individual. Additionally, financing plays a major role in access to care, making it easier for individuals with health insurance to gain access and thereby increase the demand for covered services. However, the uninsured can also gain access to care through what is known as charitable care. Financing, additionally, plays a role in factors affecting the amount of services that the private section can provide (Shi & Singh, 2015). Likewise, financing affects the demand side relative to reimbursement and the type and extent of services offered as well as the supply and distribution of health care professionals. Finally, financing influences overall healthcare expenditures (Shi & Singh, 2015). Policy makers can use financing as a mechanism to improve the public's overall health and reduce inequalities related to accessing healthcare, along with eliminating potentially catastrophic costs for patients, by providing universal coverage. This strategy can be achieved by raising funds to cover healthcare, pooling financial resources across population groups to share risks, and developing legislation to govern financing as well as operational rules depicting how funds should be spent (WHO, 2010).

1.5.2 Insurance

The primary purpose of **insurance** is to decrease risk, which is the potential to undergo catastrophic financial loss from an event that has a low probability of occurrence. An example would be purchasing cancer insurance when there is no indication that an individual may develop cancer. The insurance agency or the insurer assumes the risk. Shi & Singh (2015) cite four principles of insurance: (1) the unpredictability of risk for the insured, (2) the predictability of risk for a group or a population, (3) the transferability of risk from the individual to the insurer through pooling of resources, and (4) the equal shareability of actual losses among members of the insured group. Public health insurance includes the Children's Health Insurance Plan (CHIP), Medicare, and Medicaid, whereas private insurance includes plans such as United Health Care, Cigna, Blue Cross Blue Shield, Self-Insurance, and managed care organizations. In the case of a managed care organization, the MCO assumes all risks that would otherwise be experienced by the insurance company. If the cost of the provided services exceeds the profits generated from the fixed premiums, the MCO will absorb the costs (Shi & Singh, 2015).

1.5.3 Delivery

Delivery refers to the provision of healthcare services by various providers in exchange for payment for services rendered. These providers include physicians, hospitals, nursing homes, home health agencies, health departments and clinics, health centers, etc. Most health care services, through MCOs, are contracted and delivered by independent physicians, clinics, and hospitals while others employ their own physicians (Shi & Singh, 2015). Providers render services to individuals with the ability to pay out of pocket, through health insurance plans, Medicare, Medicaid, or private insurance. Service delivery is a significant factor in maintaining or improving population health. Healthcare delivery should be comprehensive in that it meets the needs of the population. Medical care should also be accessible regardless of such barriers as insurance coverage, language, culture, or geographic location. Good health care delivery imparts continuity of care for individuals. It therefore should be centered on the patient, coordinated, and high quality (WHO, 2010).

1.5.4 Payment

The purpose of the **payment** function is to determine fees for services, how much a provider should be paid for services rendered, and the actual payment to the provider after services have been rendered. Each service provided carries a specific fee attached to it called a charge (provider set) or rate (set by third party payer). The following three parties are payers for services rendered: the patient, the provider, and insurance companies. Third party payers include private insurance; insurance companies, such as Aetna, Humana, Blue Cross Blue Shield, United Healthcare, and HMOs; and governmental plans, such as Medicare and Medicaid. MCOs receive payment through capitation, discounted fees, and salaries. Using this type of system allows the MCO to share risk with the provider. With capitation, all health care services are included with one set fee paid by the healthcare plan member to the provider. A discounted fee is a financial reimbursement system whereby a provider agrees to supply services on a Fee for Service basis but with the fees discounted by a certain percentage from the physician's usual and customary charges. Salaries refer to money paid to physicians, including bonuses (Shi & Singh, 2015).

1.5.5 Types of Healthcare Organizations

The many types of healthcare organizations include facilities that provide treatment, tests, rehabilitation, and therapy. We also rely on insurance plans to help us pay for health care. Therefore, to be able to decide which best suits our needs, we must understand the different healthcare organizations, which are managed care organizations (MCOs); preferred provider organizations (PPOs); health maintenance organizations (HMOs); integrated delivery systems (IDS); accountable care organizations (ACOs); payer-provider integration; consumer-driven, point of service (POS), and fee-for-service. Figure 1.8 provides an overview of each type of organization, which we will explore in more detail.

MCO The healthcare provider and insurance company develop an agreement or contract wherein the provider offers services at a reduced cost and the insurance company limits their members' options of providers to only those who participated in the agreement.	**PPO** Type of organization that provides services based on contracts with groups of physicians and hospitals that are referred to as preferred providers.	**HMO** A prepaid medical service wherein members pay monthly or annually for healthcare services.
IDS A network of organizations that provides or arranges to provide an organized variety of services to specific populations and is held accountable for the outcomes and health status of the population	**ACO** An integrated set of providers who assume responsibility for improving the health status, quality, and satisfaction for services delivered to a specific population.	**PPI** A merger between the payers of healthcare and the providers of healthcare to control healthcare costs and improve the delivery of healthcare services provided.
CDHP Combine a savings option (health savings account or HSA) with a high deductible insurance plan.	**FFS** A system wherein health care is provided in individuals units of service such as a magnetic resonance imaging (MRI) or other x-ray, medical examination, flu shot, or other service.	**POS** A combination of HMOs and PPOs

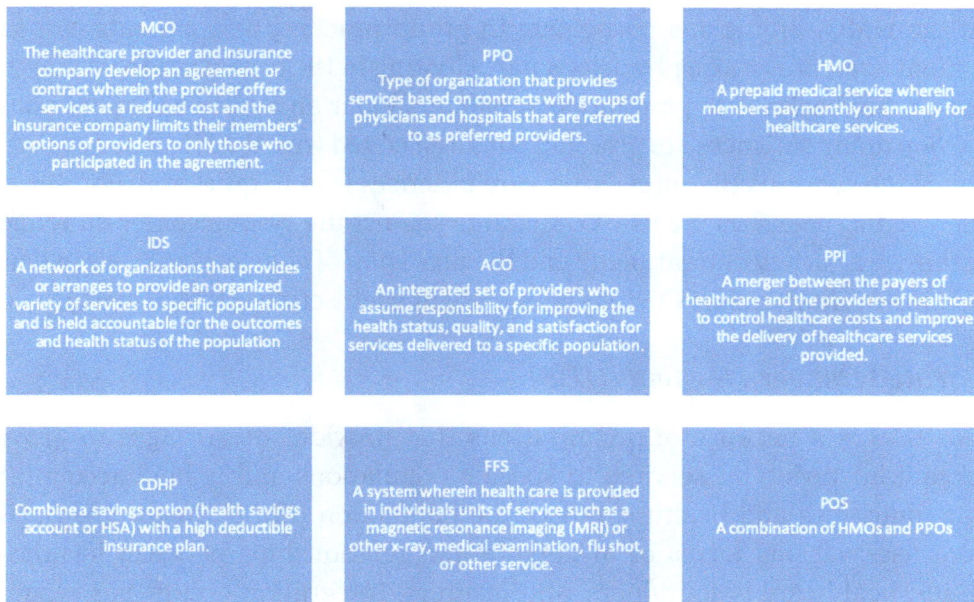

Figure 1.8: Types of Healthcare Organizations

Source: Original Work
Attribution: Dorothy Howell
License: CC BY-SA 4.0

Managed Care Organizations

A **managed care organization** does not require the use of insurance companies to control risk or a third-party administrator to make payments for the provision of health care services (Shi & Singh, 2015). In other words, the healthcare provider and insurance company develop an agreement or contract wherein the provider offers services at a reduced cost, and the insurance company limits their members' options of providers to only those who have participated in the agreement. Alternative forms of MCOs are health maintenance organizations and preferred provider organizations (Shi & Singh, 2015).

Preferred Provider Organization

The **preferred provider** is a type of organization that provides services based on contracts with groups of physicians and hospitals that are referred to as preferred providers. Out of network providers can be used at a higher out of pocket cost to the consumer. Service costs are negotiated between the organization and the provider, allowing the consumer to receive healthcare services at a discounted rate (Shi & Singh, 2015).

Health Maintenance Organizations

A **Health Maintenance Organization** (HMO) is a prepaid medical service wherein members pay monthly or annually for healthcare services. Prevention of illness is a significant factor in an HMO. Therefore, cost of services are fixed.

With the HMO, physicians participate in group practice, and patients can seek treatment from only those physicians participating in the organization. While they can see other health care practitioners, patients incur an additional out of pocket cost when doing so. There are pros and cons associated with the HMO. One positive aspect is the synopsis that preventive care practices lead to quicker diagnoses and thereby reduce healthcare costs. Complaints against the system center on refusals to authorize a variety of treatments and the provision of substandard care in lieu of increasing profit margins. Current laws prevent such actions (HMO, 2019).

Integrated Delivery Systems (IDS)

An **IDS** is a network of organizations that provides or arranges to provide an organized variety of services to specific populations and is held accountable for the outcomes and health status of the population (Shi & Singh, 2015). This system uses various forms of ownership and relationships between healthcare facilities, healthcare practitioners, and insurers. Integration occurs as a result of the domination of managed care markets for three reasons: cost effectiveness; quality of services; and concern to protect the autonomy of hospitals, physicians, and other providers. Although the quality of care has increased with the institution of IDS, costs have not been reduced. Some IDSs lowered usage of healthcare and began experiencing financial distress, thereby causing the number of IDSs to drop while the number of hospitals and physician practices owned or contracted by IDSs grew.

Accountable Care Organization (ACO)

As a result of IDSs' inability to provide quality cost-effective services, Accountable Care Organizations became prominent. An **ACO** is defined as an integrated set of providers who assume responsibility for improving the health status, quality, and satisfaction for services delivered to a specific population. ACOs use such mechanisms as "disease management, care coordination, sharing of cost savings with providers, use of information technology, etc." to achieve cost quality and population health (Shi & Singh, 2015). The same issue remains regarding the provision of quality healthcare at a low cost with ACOs as with other systems. In addition to operating under the laws set up by the Affordable Care Act requiring increased governmental oversight, smaller physician practices and clinics have not been included in ACOs and are not able to experience the benefits. Safety-net providers such as community health centers and public hospitals may also experience exclusion from ACOs. Antitrust laws have been developed to prevent ACOs from dominating geographic markets, reducing competition, increasing prices and decreasing quality of services (Shi & Singh, 2015).

Payer-Provider Integration

The **payer-provider integration** system comprises a merger between the payers of healthcare and the providers of healthcare in order to control healthcare costs and improve the delivery of healthcare services provided. An example of this system is the acquisition of a physician practice group and health system by an insurance company to gain more control over healthcare delivery. This is called an insurance company owned IDS. There is also a hospital owned IDS wherein the hospitals own and employ physicians and ancillary providers and a health insurance plan. The physician owned IDS is one wherein the physician owns or contracts with the hospital for service and an insurance company. The issue of concern is if this type of system will impede access to healthcare while having little impact on healthcare costs (Fine, 2016).

Consumer Driven Health Plans

Consumer driven health plans are also called high deductible health plans. These plans combine a savings option (health savings account or HSA) with a high deductible insurance plan. Premiums are lower for these types of health plans. The HSA is owned and funded by the employee and allows the employee control on how funds are used. Another savings option is the health reimbursement option or HRA, which is owned by the employer. These funds can be sued for deductibles, copayments, insurance premiums, etc. (Shi & Singh, 2015).

Fee for Service

Fee for service describes a system wherein health care is provided as individual units of service, such as a magnetic resonance imaging (MRI) or other x-ray, medical examination, flu shot, or other service. If a patient is admitted to the hospital, their admission kit, supplies, blood draws, etc., are charged separately. The patient will be sent a bill from each service that provided care, such as the physician, pathologist, radiologist, anesthesiologist, surgeon, etc. (Shi & Singh, 2015).

Point of Service

A **point of service plan** combines HMOs and PPOs. They are also called open-ended HMOs. These plans include capitation and a gate keeper to control usage. If they choose to use an out-of-network provider, then the consumer pays the difference in cost. Enrollment in these plans is declining. (Shi & Singh, 2015).

1.5.6 Types of Healthcare Facilities

Prior to the current advancement in treatment facilities, sick individuals who could afford to pay for healthcare services were cared for in their homes or in private health clinics. Those who could not afford healthcare were cared for in poorly run facilities without physicians until they died. Healthcare facilities have evolved over time from just providing housing and custodial care to the sick and underprivileged to technologically advanced, highly specialized facilities that provide cancer treatment, psychiatric services, renal services, obstetrics and gynecology, children's services, cardiovascular services, etc. In addition to the previously mentioned healthcare facilities, healthcare providers also utilize emergency centers, urgent care centers, ambulatory care centers, imaging and radiology centers, medical and/or surgical hospitals, surgery centers, orthopedic and rehabilitation centers, long-term care, hospice, and home health to care for terminally ill individuals (McConnell, 2015).

A **healthcare facility** provides healthcare services regardless of the facility's location. They range from doctors' offices; to clinics; to urgent care centers; to large hospitals with cardiac, pediatric, and mental health wings; emergency rooms; and trauma centers. Many types of health care facilities exist under the umbrella of healthcare organizations. This section will provide a brief description of these facilities.

Ambulatory Care Center

An **ambulatory care center**, also referred to as an outpatient care center, is a medical care facility that provides outpatient services. Examples of ambulatory care centers include private practice; hospitals; free standing clinics; retail clinics, such as Kroger or Walmart; mobile medical services; home health care; hospice; ambulatory long-term care; public health; and community health centers. Their care includes clinics, telephone access, and complementary and alternative medicine as well as diagnosis, treatment, consultation and intervention services. Some ambulatory care centers offer specialized medical services and advanced medical technology that is equal to or higher than successful hospital chains (Shi & Singh, 2015).

Imaging and Radiology Centers

Imaging and Radiology facilities, much like their hospital counterparts, offer diagnostic imaging services to patients. Diagnostic imaging includes CT scans, ultrasounds, X-rays, MRIs, and more. While hospitals and even clinics have imaging centers, outpatient facilities help keep costs lower and allow more convenient scheduling for patients (Falvin, 2018).

Emergency Services and Urgent Care Centers

Many hospitals have an emergency department (ED) in house. The urgent care center is usually located at a different location from the hospital and offers extended hours. Some centers are open 24 hours, seven days a week. Patients can come in without an appointment for basic and acute conditions. The purpose of the **emergency department** is to provide medical services around the clock for patients who are acutely ill or injured, especially those individuals with life threatening illnesses or injuries that require immediate attention. These patients can be admitted directly into the hospital from the emergency department or urgent care center. Physicians and nurses receive specialized training to work in these areas. The emergency department, however, is overused as people seek treatment for nonurgent conditions that are nonacute and minor in severity. There are several reasons for this overuse of the emergency department. For example, people who cannot access their primary care physicians when they need them may use the ED, which is convenient and open every day and after hours. In addition, people use the ED because they misjudge the severity of their ailments or injuries. And lack of insurance coverage or finances to pay for services and psychiatric conditions are other reasons for using the ED.

Hospitals

Hospitals of long ago had a nursing focus in that they were geared toward the provision of nursing care. They were operated by churches or social welfare and, as such, were charitable institutions. Today's hospitals are run more like a business. Now **hospitals** are organizations that focus on preventing illnesses, restoring health, and preserving life (McConnell, 2015). We view hospitals today as facilities that provide medical diagnostic and treatment services. Hospitals are staffed by physicians, nurses, and allied health practitioners, unlike those of the past that were staffed only by nurses. There are different types of hospitals, based on the care provided. They can be public or private. Some hospitals are teaching hospitals because they combine teaching to medical students and nurses with providing people with healthcare services and assistance. Also, a general (or acute care) hospital provides general medical and surgical care to patients. This is typically called a community hospital (Shi & Singh, 2015). Hospitals also provide outpatient services, such as x-rays, bloodwork, colonoscopies, same day surgery, etc.

Business functions that are critical to the delivery of healthcare are present in hospitals and other healthcare organizations. Indeed, over the past few years, the degree of growth in for profit facilities, health maintenance organizations, accountable care organizations, and other healthcare organizations indicates the vast business operations of these facilities (McConnell, 2015). Once the acute medical needs of the patient have been met, the patient may be sent home, to a hospice care facility, to a long-term care, to an orthopedic or rehabilitation center, or to a home health facility (Shi & Singh, 2015).

Long Term Care

Long-term care is designed to meet the needs of a specific population. **Long-term care** is described as a mixture of holistic, patient-centered services that maximizes the independent functioning of individuals with limited ability to perform daily living activities. Long-term care encompasses both inpatient care and ambulatory long-term care services. In Chapter 15, we will discuss long-term care in more detail.

Nursing homes offer a living situation for patients (regardless of age) whose medical needs are not severe enough for hospitalization but are too serious to manage at home. The elderly, though, are the greatest users of these services. Individuals are placed in these settings due to functional deficits originating from cognitive impairment, chronic conditions, serious illnesses, or injuries that prevent the individuals from performing daily self-care tasks. These individuals rely on others to take care of their needs (Shi & Singh, 2015). Some nursing homes offer services for heavier medical needs, such as speech and occupational therapy. Other nursing homes offer a homier atmosphere and might operate like an apartment complex with medical staff on hand (Flavin, 2018).

Ambulatory long-term care also includes case management and adult day care services. Maintaining population health is a major concern for the healthcare system in general. Therefore, healthcare organizations (from acute care to long term care to hospice care) integrate various methods of care delivery to ensure the population receiving care under their auspices receives quality care. One such method of doing so is by using case managers. Case management provides coordination and referrals among a variety of health care services to meet patient needs. The following list of services are offered to meet the needs of the long-term care population: medical, nursing, dementia, rehabilitative, respite and end-of-life care, mental health services, social support, community-based and institutional services, housing, and preventive and therapeutic long-term care.[15] Adult day care assists family members with their loved ones by providing such services as socialization and basic support, including meals; counseling; Alzheimer's and dementia support, such as mental stimulation; and medical support, such as occupational, speech, and physical therapy, for example, during the normal work day (Shi & Singh, 2015).

Home Health

The purpose of a **home health care service** is to bring specific types of services to patients within their homes. Their goal is to slow the decline of disease progression and assist the patient to maintain their independence and become more self-sufficient. Without this service, hospital length of stay would increase. Home health services include the following types of nursing care: dressing changes; medication monitoring; provision of assistance with activities of daily living; short-term rehabilitation, such as physical, occupational and speech therapy; intravenous therapy; patient and caregiver education; and nutrition counseling and monitoring. The patient may also receive homemaker services consisting of meal preparation, housekeeping, transportation, shopping, etc. [15]. Most home health agencies in the U.S. are private for profit. Medicare and Medicaid are the largest payers of home health services (Shi & Singh, 2015).

Hospice Services

The CDC reports that, in 2017, there were more than 4,515 hospice centers in the U.S. treating more than 1.49 million patients (NHPCO, 2018). Patients who have been deemed as terminally ill with a life expectancy of six months or less are placed under hospice care to receive comprehensive services. Over half of the individuals in hospice care have been diagnosed with cancer. Hospice takes into account the patient and the family as a unit of care, including meeting the needs of the patient while focusing on pain management and comfort; meeting the emotional and spiritual needs of the family and patient; providing support for the family before and after the death of the patient; and maintaining quality of life over time. Hospice care can be an extension of home health if the person is cared for in their homes. Patients in nursing homes, retirement centers, or hospitals can also receive hospice services. Hospice is a cost-effective option for private and public payers, such as private insurance, Medicare, and Medicaid (Shi & Singh, 2015).

There are four types of hospice: routine, continuous home care, inpatient respite care, and general inpatient care. Routine hospice care is for individuals electing to receive care at home and is the most common type of hospice used. Continuous Home Care provides patients with nursing care for 8-24 hours a day for pain and acute symptom management. These patients also have access to caregivers and hospice aide services as needed. Inpatient respite care provides temporary relief to the patient's caregiver. The patient is cared for in another setting, such as a hospital, hospice facility, or nursing home. General inpatient care is provided at hospitals or other nursing facilities when the patients' symptoms and pain can no longer be managed at home (NHPCO, 2018).

Orthopedic and Rehabilitation

Orthopedic centers handle everything from athletic injuries to therapy for patients with disabilities. They typically offer evaluation and diagnosis of the problem, as well as prevention, treatment and rehabilitation work involving bone, tendon, ligament, muscle, and joint conditions. There are also **rehabilitation centers** where patients can receive various therapies to help restore their abilities after an illness or injury. Their purpose is to restore function after a person has had a stroke or heart attack, spinal cord or sports injury, major trauma, or brain injury. Physical therapy, occupational therapy, and speech therapy are all processes that help people gain or regain skills they need to move around, work, or speak in daily life (Flavin, 2018).

Public Health

Public health services are provided by local health departments. These services include well-baby care, venereal disease clinics, family planning services, screening and treatment for tuberculosis, and ambulatory mental health services.

School health programs that provide vision and hearing screening and assistance with learning disabilities also fall under public health (Shi & Singh, 2015).

Mental Health and Addiction Treatment Centers

Mental health treatment facilities exist as general institutions for any mental health issue. These institutions are sometimes specialized. Examples of these kinds of facilities are suicidal thoughts (or suicidal ideation) treatment, depression treatment, trauma and post-traumatic stress disorder (PTSD) treatment, treatment for anxiety disorders, behavioral disorders, and more. Addiction treatment centers typically deal with drug and alcohol addictions, as well as problematic behavioral addictions, such as to gambling, work, shopping, or the internet (Flavin, 2018).

Clinics and Physician Practices

Clinics are facilities that provide ambulatory care services ranging from basic primary care to urgent care. Other examples of clinics include sports medicine that care for individuals with acute and chronic sports injuries; walk in urgent care that provides non-emergency medical care; chiropractors that diagnose and treat disorders of the musculoskeletal system; physiotherapy that assists the individual in developing, maintaining, and restoring maximum movement and functioning; immunizations and vaccinations; rehabilitation; and skin care. They offer convenience to consumers due to their location, late, and weekend office hours[15]. Some services are provided in free clinics for those individuals who are poor, homeless, or uninsured. Volunteer staff provide services, and these patients are not charged.

Private practice are facilities wherein physicians provide some ambulatory primary care services. Patients typically receive limited examinations and tests. Although office waits are long, the patient spends little time with the physician[15]. While some physicians prefer to practice by themselves or in small partnerships, others prefer group practices, such as with MCOs, or to work in hospitals. The trend of group practice has occurred for several reasons, including the following: cost associated with operating a solo practice, complex billing issues, ambiguity resulting from shifts in the health care delivery system, MCO agreements, market competition, and technology demands. In addition, patients tend to reap greater benefits from the group practice, such as the latest diagnostic, treatment, pharmaceutical, and surgical services. They can receive labs, x-rays, and other services without leaving the facility (Shi & Singh, 2015). The rise in managed care and consolidation by hospital-centered institutions led to minimizing the physician's control over the delivery of medical care and subsequently to loss of income. To regain control, physicians developed their own specialized care centers, such as orthopedic and rehabilitation centers, cardiac centers, or renal care centers (Shi & Singh, 2015).

In addition to primary care, there is specialty care. Primary and specialty care focus on prevention, diagnosis and treatment, and minor surgical procedures.

However, services provided by specialists are encapsulated within a specific specialty domain, such as optometry, podiatry, orthopedic care, etc. Please review the table below to see differences between primary and specialty care (Shi & Singh, 2015).

Table 1.2 Primary and Specialty Care	
Primary Care	Specialty Care
First contact and is the gateway to the health care system.	Occurs when needed after the patient has been seen at primary care. Patients are referred to a specialist based on their presenting symptoms.
In integrated systems such as managed care, Primary care physicians (PCP) serve as gatekeepers to control cost, usage of services, and allocation of resources.	The patient cannot see the specialist unless they receive a referral from the PCP.
PCPs must follow a specific course of treatment for a diagnosis, including treatment, referrals, monitoring and follow-up—which maintains continuity of care for chronic conditions.	More intense, as it is focused on the current specific need of a patient.
Treats the person holistically.	Treats specific diseases or organ systems of the body. If the patient has multiple health conditions (comorbidity), such as heart disease, diabetes, renal failure, etc., they can be referred to multiple specialists.
Trains in ambulatory care setting to learn how to treat many types of patient conditions and diseases.	Spends a significant amount of time in inpatient hospitals using state of the art technology to diagnose and treat patients' medical conditions.

Source: Original Work
Attribution: Dorothy Howell
License: CC BY-SA 4.0

1.6 CONCLUSION

Physicians work in a variety of health systems, such as hospitals, federal government agencies, public health departments, mental health facilities, community and migrant health centers colleges, and prisons. They can also work in group practices, freestanding ambulatory care clinics, etc. The Affordable Care Act and the quest for low cost, high quality healthcare services led to the development of healthcare systems that were able to coordinate, manage, and provide better health care services. Integrated Delivery Networks (IDN) grew out of this process. An IDN is a group of physicians who have formed an association with hospitals to provide holistic healthcare services to patients. Electronic health records are used so that patient information can be easily shared and tracked between providers. This type of system offers a true continuum of care for patients served (Martin, 2018).

Different types of healthcare organizations envelope the various types of healthcare facilities; both have been discussed in this chapter. Managed care organizations comprising preferred provider organizations and health maintenance organizations have been devised to provide health care consumers with choices on the types and quality of products and services received based on cost of these products and services. One significant quality of a managed care organization is the assumption of risk associated with the provision of health care service.

This chapter provided fundamental knowledge—including an overview of payment and delivery of health care services, the various types of healthcare facilities and organizational structures—in hopes of propelling the reader to relish further learning elements that will continue throughout this book on healthcare organizations.

1.7 KEY POINTS

- Health is the function of several variables or determinants. Because of these determinants, the government must develop and maintain health policy to intervene in health-related issues. Health determinants refer to social, personal, economic, and environmental factors that affect individual and population-based health.

- Based on the premise that health care refers to services provided within a health care system to improve the health of an individual, a healthcare organization is an establishment that provides healthcare services.

- The World Health Organization (WHO) indicates that a well-functioning healthcare system operates according to the needs and expectations of the population (2010).

- Healthcare organizations rely on health policies, the healthcare market, organizational governing bodies, and the overall desire to improve patient satisfaction to dictate how work is structured and completed.

- Health policy plays a major role in health care organizations within the U.S. They are a collection of rules or laws that illustrate the distribution of resources, services, and political influences on the health of the population.

- The structure of an organization is outlined in reference to how specific activities are performed to ensure the mission and vision of the organization are achieved.

- There are many types of healthcare facilities, ranging from doctors' offices; to clinics; to urgent care centers; to large hospitals with cardiac, pediatric, and mental health wings; emergency rooms; and trauma centers.

1.8 KEY TERMS

Health, healthcare, health care, medical model, biomedical model, healthcare organizations, healthcare facilities, holistic medicine, holistic health.

1.9 QUESTIONS FOR REVIEW AND DISCUSSION

1. Explain the concept of hospice care and the types of services hospice provides.
2. Describe the significance of health policy to healthcare.
3. Compare and contrast the three types of organizational structures.
4. Explain the differences between primary care and specialty care. What are the differences between health, healthcare, and health care?
5. Explain the differences between holistic health and holistic medicine.

1.10 REFERENCES

Allcorn S. Using matrix organization to manage health care delivery organizations. Hosp Health Serv Adm. 1990;35(4):575–590.

Bach, O. (2018). Functional specialization in organization design is great until it isn't. Retrieved March 8, 2020 from https://www.managementkits.com/blog/2018/10/12-downsides-of-functional-specialization-in-unit-structures

Centers for Connected Health Policy: The National Telehealth Policy Resource Center. Retrieved December 12, 2019 from https://www.cchpca.org/about/about-telehealth

Delaune, J., & Everett, W.(2008). Waste and Inefficiency in the U.S. Health Care System. Clinical Care: A Comprehensive Analysis in Support of System-Wide Improvements. New England Health Institute (NEHI).. Retrieved from http://media.washingtonpost.com/wp-srv/nation/pdf/healthreport_092909.pdf

Elsaid, N.M., Okasha, A.E., & Abdelghaly, A.A. (2013). Defining and Solving the Organizational Structure Problems to Improve the Performance of Ministry of State for Environmental Affairs – Egypt. International Journal of Scientific and Research Publications, 3(10). Retrieved from http://www.ijsrp.org/research-paper-1013/ijsrp-p2244.pdf

Fine, K. (2016). A Look at Vertical Integration Between Payers and Providers. Retrieved March 7, 2020 from https://www.mdmag.com/physicians-money-digest/practice-management/a-look-at-vertical-integration-between-payers-and-providers

Flavin, B. (2018). 14 Types of Healthcare Facilities Where Medical Professionals Provide Care. Retrieved September 23, 2019 from, https://www.rasmussen.edu/degrees/health-sciences/blog/types-of-healthcare-facilities/

Fritscher, Lisa (2019). Medical Model use in Psychiatry. Accessed September 10, 2019, from https://www.verywellmind.com/medical-model-2671617

Gleeson, Patrick. "Advantages & Disadvantages of Matrix Organizational Structures in Business Organizations" last modified January 28, 2019. http://smallbusiness. chron.com/advantages-disadvantages-matrix-organizational-structures-business-organizations-26350.html

Health Maintenance Organization." 2019. Columbia Electronic Encyclopedia, 6th Edition, May, 1. http://search.ebscohost.com/login.aspx?direct=true&db=khh&AN=134519269&site=eds-live&scope=site.

Institute of Medicine (US) Committee on Assuring the Health of the Public in the 21st Century. The Future of the Public's Health in the 21st Century. Washington (DC): National Academies Press (US); 2002. 1, Assuring America's Health. Available from: https://www.ncbi.nlm.nih.gov/books/NBK221233/

Johnson, A., Roberts, L., & Elkins, G. (2019). Complementary and Alternative Medicine for Menopause. Journal of Evidence-Based Integrative Medicine Volume 24: 1-14. Retrieved from https://journals.sagepub.com/doi/pdf/10.1177/2515690X19829380

Kenton, W. (2020). Organizational Structure. Retrieved March 8, 2020 from https://www.investopedia.com/terms/o/organizational-structure.asp.

Kisacky, J. S. (2017). Rise of the Modern Hospital : An Architectural History of Health and Healing, 1870-1940. University of Pittsburgh Press.

Longest, B. B., & Association of University Programs in Health Administration. (2016). Health Policymaking in the United States, Sixth Edition: Vol. Sixth edition. Health Administration Press.

Martin, R. (2018). INTEGRATED DELIVERY NETWORKS What pharmaceutical companies need to know before engaging them. Retrieved March 10, 2020 from https://www.iqvia.com/-/media/iqvia/pdfs/us-location-site/market-access/integrated-delivery-networks.pdf

Merriam-Webster, s.v. (health), Accessed September 4, 2019, from https://www.merriam-webster.com/dictionary/health

Merriam-Webster, s.v. (health care), Accessed September 4, 2019, from https://www.merriam-webster.com/dictionary/health care

Mohan, C. What Is Holistic Medicine? WebMD. (June 12, 2017). Accessed September 13, 2019, from https://www.webmd.com/balance/guide/what-is-holistic-medicine#1-2

National Hospice and Palliative Care Organization, (2018). NHPCO Facts and Figures. Retrieved March 10, 2020 from https://www.nhpco.org/wp-content/uploads/2019/07/2018_NHPCO_Facts_Figures.pdf.

National Research Council. 1998. Biomedical Models and Resources: Current Needs and Future Opportunities. Washington, DC: The National Academies Press. https://doi.org/10.17226/6066. Retrieved September 16, 2019 from, https://www.nap.edu/catalog/6066/biomedical-models-and-resources-current-needs-and-future-opportunities

Niles, N.J. (2018). Basics of the U.S. Health Care System 3rd ed. Burlington, MA. Jones and Bartlett Learning.

Plugge, Emma, Nicola Douglas, and Ray Fitzpatrick. 2008. "Imprisoned Women's Concepts of Health and Illness: The Implications for Policy on Patient and Public Involvement in Healthcare." Journal of Public Health Policy 29 (4): 424–39. doi:10.1057/jphp.2008.32.

Rattan, S. I. S. (2013). Healthy ageing, but what is health? *Biogerontology, 14*(6), 673–677. https://doi.org/10.1007/s10522-013-9442-7

Ruhl, L. Healthcare vs. Health Care – What's the Difference? (February 2013)Retrieved September 13, 2019, from https://www.allphysicianjobs.com/blog/2018/02/13/healthcare-vs-health-care/

Segen's Medical Dictionary. s.v. "medical model of health." Retrieved September 10 2019 from https://medical-dictionary.thefreedictionary.com/medical+model+of+health

Selimen, Deniz, and Isil Isik Andsoy. "The Importance of a Holistic Approach during the Perioperative Period." AORN Journal 93, no. 4 (April 2011): 482–90. doi:10.1016/j.aorn.2010.09.029.AORN J. 2011 Apr; 93(4):482-7; quiz 488-90.

Shi, L. & Singh, D. (2015). Delivering Health Care in America: A systems Approach. 6th ed. Jones and Bartlett Learning.

Tomljenovic, A. (2014). Holistic Approach to Human Health and Disease:Life Circumstances and Inner Processing. Coll. Antropol. 38(2), 787-792

Walston, S. (2017). Organizational Behavior and Theory in Healthcare: Leadership Perspectives and Management. Health Administration Press.

World Health Organization (WHO), Constitution of the World Health Organization, s.v. (health) Assessed from https://www.who.int/about/who-we-are/constitution

World Health Organization. (2010). Health Service delivery. Retrieved March 8, 2020 from https://www.who.int/healthinfo/systems/WHO_MBHSS_2010_section1_web.pdf

World Health Organization (WHO). (2010). Key Components of a Well-Functioning Healthcare System. Assessed March 7, 2020 from https://www.who.int/healthsystems/EN_HSSkeycomponents.pdf?ua=1

Zamanzadeh, V., Jasemi, M., Valizadeh, L., Keogh, B., & Taleghani, F. (2015). Effective factors in providing holistic care: a qualitative study. *Indian journal of palliative care, 21*(2), 214–224. doi:10.4103/0973-1075.156506

2

OVERVIEW OF HEALTHCARE MANAGEMENT

2.1 LEARNING OBJECTIVES

- To introduce the role of managers in healthcare organizations
- To emphasize the various levels of management within a healthcare organization
- To highlight the role of managers in leadership development
- To convey an understanding of the use of strategy in healthcare organizations
- To discuss the manager's role in health policy

2.2 INTRODUCTION

Healthcare management plays an essential role in the success of healthcare organizations. The manager's role is multifaceted and diverse relative to their individual work environment. This role must be fluid to adapt to the ever-changing turbulent healthcare atmosphere. Health care management is the business of providing governance and guidance to organizations and their sub-units and departments that deliver healthcare services. Understanding basic concepts relative to managing healthcare organizations and organizational behavior can enhance the ability of an individual in becoming an effective leader. Grasping knowledge associated with how organizations behave is essential to organizational success. This chapter will introduce the functions, roles, and responsibilities inherent to managers within the healthcare setting. Several of this chapter's topics, including talent acquisition, managerial and leadership functions, inputs and outputs, the communication process and skills, motivation, market forces, and industry challenges, will receive additional discussion in later chapters. The later discussion will differently contextualize the information in this chapter. The goal is to expand on topics throughout the progression of the textbook to provide the reader with a better picture of its content.

2.3 MANAGERIAL ROLE IN HEALTHCARE ORGANIZATIONS

2.3.1 Leadership

Several studies, captured in response to a research study by Baker, Mathis, & Stites-Doe (2011), have been conducted on leadership in reference to theories, styles, behaviors, characteristics, use of power and influence, engaging effective teams, and organizational performance, among others. For example, Baker, Mathis, & Stites-Doe (2011) investigated leader and follower characteristics and found a significant correlation between the study's variables [embracing change ($r = 0.151$, $p < 0.05$), encouraging others to act ($r = 0.181$, $p < 0.01$), challenging the process ($r = 0.189$, $p < 0.01$), and the control variable of education. These results indicate respondents with higher levels of education performed better in relation to followership performance characteristics. Vast differences exist in how leadership and leader behaviors are defined. McConnell (2015) suggests that true leaders are defined by how well they are accepted by their followers, such that the followers willingly obey the position of the leader.

Further, many levels of leadership exist, including administrators, top executives, managers, and front-line workers such as housekeepers, nutrition staff, healthcare workers, social workers, nurses, laboratory technicians, x-ray technicians, etc. Healthcare administrators oversee functions, projects, divisions, regions or districts, or specific programs, such as emergency preparedness and response. They ensure that all tasks are performed and completed in a timely and efficient manner according to specified requirements (Marshall, 2017). Unsurprisingly, many types of leadership positions exist within organizations including healthcare organizations. These include the following: Chief Executive Officer, Chief Medical Officer (CMO), Chief Operating Officer, Chief Nursing Officer (CNO), Chief Financial Officer (CCO), Chief Human Resources Manager (CHRM), Chief Security Officer (CSO), Chief Analytics Officer (CAO), and Chief Data Officer (CDO). These positions are referred to as C-Level executives (or C-suite) because the word "chief" precedes each type of officer. The levels of such positions in healthcare organizations are based on the size, mission, and geographic location; thus, not every organization will comprise each position level. The table below explains the role of each position.

Table 2.1 Roles of Organizational Leaders	
Chief Executive Officer	Leads the organization and seeks input from other c-suite members of the organization in making decisions for the organization.
Chief Medical Officer	A physician who heads the medical services at the organization and leads the team of medical personnel including physicians, surgeons, psychiatrists, nurse practitioners, and physicians' assistants.

Chief Operating Officer	Ensures the organization's operating functions are in order, such as recruitment, training, payroll, legal, and administrative services. The COO is usually second in command to the CEO.
Chief Nursing Officer	Oversees leadership functions of governance and decision-making within organizations employing nurses.
Chief Financial Officer	Handles the finances of the organization, such as investments, accounting, and financial risk, and supervises a team of financial analysts and accountants.
Chief Compliance Officer	Ensures organizational compliance with internal policies, laws, regulations, and other governing bodies and that the organization meets legal requirements.
Chief Human Resources Manager	Oversees the human resource management policies, practices, and operations for an organization.
Chief Security Officer	Develops and oversees policies and programs that decrease the organization's risk related to compliance, operations, and finances.
Chief Analytics/Data Officer	Captures, processes, and analyzes data for the organization

Source: Original Work
Attribution: Dorothy Howell
License: CC BY-SA 4.0

2.3.2 Understanding Managerial Functions

Cunningham (1979) describes management as a process centered on a set of integrating principles or a process wherein managers perform functions specific to different departments or units. For example, a Nurse Manager would oversee the various levels of nurses within a specific nursing unit, such as oncology; whereas the Chief Nursing Officer would oversee nursing functions within the entire healthcare facility. Several principles are used in the management process, including planning, organizing, staffing, controlling, decision making, and directing. Planning represents what needs to be done, when it needs to be done, how it should be done, and who should do it. Organizing includes the identification, classification, and assignment of activities. Staffing includes ensuring the availability of appropriate, skilled, human resources through recruitment, selecting, training, and placement. Direction refers to ensuring the organization flourishes through effective leadership, communication and motivation. Coordinating refers to the development of teams to pursue common objectives. Controlling refers to establishing standards, measuring performance and taking corrective action as needed.

These management functions allow the manager to respond to day-to-day obstacles and ensure the acquisition, allocation, and use of resources. In other words, management requires "inputs of people, materials, resources, and equipment which systematically relate to certain processes and functions" (Cunningham, 1979, p. 658). Furthermore, managers need specific competencies or qualities to perform specified management functions that permit successful direction of their organizations. For example, key competencies or qualities required are the conceptual skills enabling critical analysis of difficult problems and the ability to develop solutions to identified problems. Another example of competency is the technical skills or proficiencies required to perform specific job responsibilities. Finally, interpersonal skills are important abilities that allow the manager to exhibit effective communication and the capacity to work with others (Buchbinder & Shank, 2017). The aforementioned competencies enable managerial proficiencies in understanding the ins and outs of the organization, the ability to lead and manage people and resources, and engage in effective communication. Communication is a message transmitted through a sign or signal to a recipient who is responsible for interpreting the message. Effective communication must be understood by the recipient.

Krajcovicova, et. al, (2012) believe these managerial proficiencies—of knowing the organization, leading and managing people, managing resources, and communicating effectively—are critical to the managerial role. Overall, management encompasses the ability to communicate, exhibit power, and operate the organization.

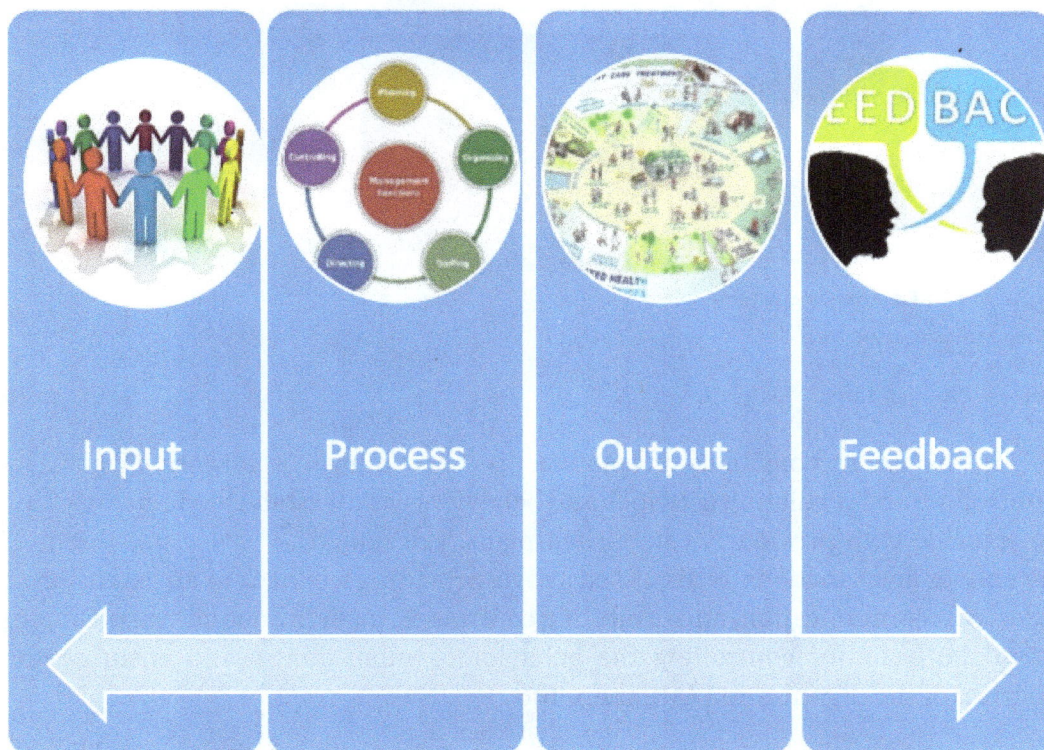

Figure 2.1: Input, Process, Output

Source: Original Work
Attribution: Dorothy Howell
License: CC BY-SA 4.0

As indicated above, managers are expected to exercise a certain degree of power or control. The exhibition of power represents the ability to act in a certain way and control others. Such power derives from two sources: (1) formal power consisting of authenticity, incentives, and sanctions and (2) informal power consisting of attraction and proficiency. The leveraging of power and control by managers and leaders to influence employees and reach organizational goals will be further explored in Chapter 9.

Managing organizational operations include the use of inputs and outputs to achieve set goals and objectives that will improve efficiency for the organization (Millman, 1962). Inputs are resources that are required to make the system function, such as humans, finances, materials, technology, and information. Processes are managerial functions that make the system work, such as planning, organizing, staffing, controlling, directing, and decision-making. Outputs are consistent with the performance of the organization and represent what is created from the inputs and processes, and they incorporate goals, products, services, efficiency, and effectiveness (Millman, 1962). Feedback is integral to organizational performance and performance improvement. Feedback informs the manager of how the output is responding to the input based on implemented processes. With this information, adjustments can be made to improve upon the process.

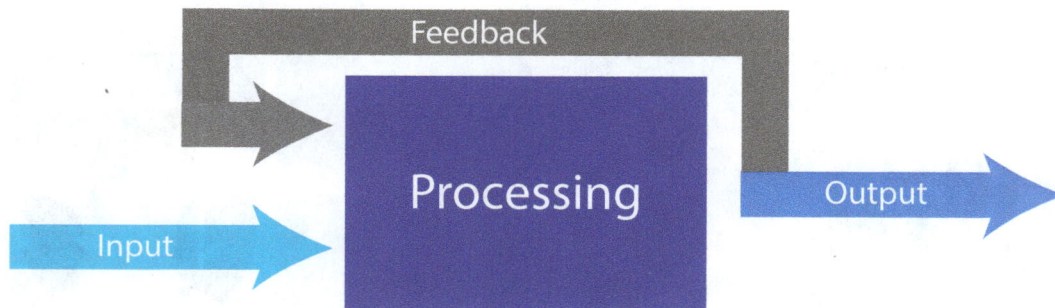

Figure 2.2: Feedback System

Source: Original Work
Attribution: Corey Parson
License: CC BY-SA 4.0

The overall responsibility of a manager is to accomplish organizational goals by controlling and regulating activities and behaviors within established relationships to coincide with previously established plans. Engaging the power subsystem of incentives and sanctions as discussed above, providing feedback as an extension of effective communication, and exhibiting controls through the operating subsystem form the basis for controlling the behavior of subordinates and ensuring the survival of the organization (Millman, 1962).

Stop and Apply

Review the case at the beginning of chapter 1. You have learned about the manager's role in healthcare organizations. Some members of the code team did not know how to get to the hospice center. As the manager of the hospice center, how might you remedy this?

2.3.3 Need for Managers in Healthcare Organizations

In many cases, healthcare delivery has witnessed a transition from professional to managerial authority. Physicians are no longer the decision makers in healthcare organizations, as managers have been given the responsibility of ensuring efficiency and cost effectiveness due to internal and external economic stressors (Embertson, 2006). The reduction in physicians' control over healthcare delivery is partly due to the rise in managed care and consolidation by hospital centered institutions. However, physicians are now becoming owners of specialty care centers, which has enabled them to regain control of healthcare delivery (Shi & Singh, 2015).

Healthcare managers possess a substantial role in ensuring that the scope, complexity, and dynamics of individual task performance are carried out appropriately in health care organizations (Buchbinder & Shanks, 2017). Providing a patient experience wherein the patient feels that their needs have been met through the provision of quality services is paramount to the organization's sustainability. The patient, providers, payers—such as private and public insurance—regulators— such as the Food and Drug Administration (FDA) and the Centers for Disease Control and Prevention (CDC)—pharmacies, clinical support, and vendors of medical devices and supplies all expect high-quality healthcare services, the delivery of which enriches the patient experience and patient satisfaction (Schultz, 2004). The manager achieves this patient satisfaction by establishing a mission and vision for the organization that focuses on patient centered care. The tasks required to produce healthcare services demand the management of highly specialized disciplines that work together as a cohesive unit in providing this care (Buchbinder & Shanks, 2017). Therefore, another significant requirement of a successful healthcare organization is the acquisition of professional talent (a management function) that lends itself to achieving the mission and vision of the organization. Professionalism encompasses a knowledge base and skill set that represents competence in a specific field. Healthcare professionals additionally adhere to high standards of honesty, integrity, unselfishness, accountability, and respect (Peters, et. al, 2014).

Managers shape the organization and make decisions that affect organizational performance. These decisions, again, include enlisting skilled personnel as well as acquiring and allocating the resources required to sustain the organization. Healthcare managers make decisions that safeguard high-quality patient care services and allow the organization to achieve desired performance objectives that will propel the group above its counterparts (Buchbinder & Shanks, 2017).

Previously, senior managers were held responsible for organizational performance. This task now falls to middle and first line managers and the employees of the organization. First line managers comprise people who oversee the employees who perform hands-on tasks. An example of a first line manager would be a housekeeping supervisor. Middle managers reside between the first line and senior managers, such as the CEO or COO. This current practice facilitates interchange of authority and information in an organization (Embertson, 2006). Regardless of their managerial level within the organizational structure, managers must be able to engage in and accomplish specific functions to ensure the organization is performing in the desired manner. These functions are discussed below.

2.3.4 Talent Acquisition and Management

One of the managerial functions discussed above is staffing, which requires the manager to employ various strategies to acquire and retain skilled talent. Ensuring that various management functions are accomplished necessitates an essential number of qualified, talented, and motivated employees. Successful organizational performance therefore involves recruiting, developing or training, and retaining highly skilled employees. Talent management involves obtaining candidates based on their knowledge, competencies, and abilities to achieve the mission, vision, goals, and objectives of the organization (Buchbinder & Shanks, 2017). The objective is to find the right person who fits the organization while also ensuring that the organization fits the person. Organizational fit is commensurate with organizational values or with the demands and offerings of the job (Levesque, 2005).

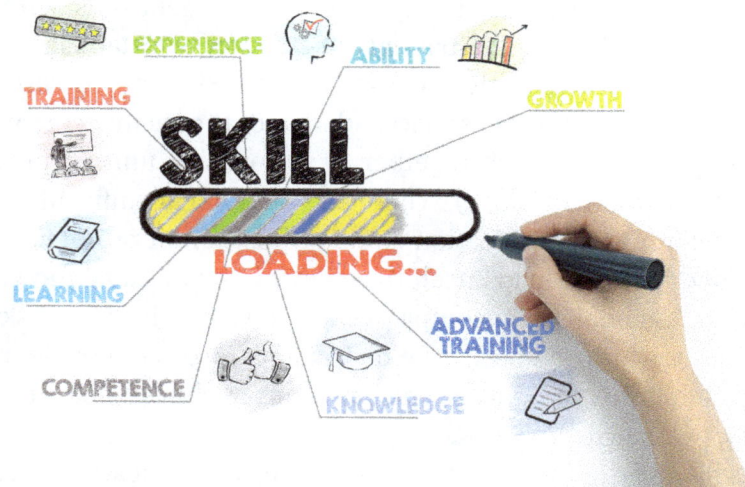

Figure 2.3: Talent Management

Source: 123rf.com
Attribution: 123rf.com
License: © 123rf.com. Used with permission.

Lack of talented staff and healthcare professionals affects the quality of care provided to patients. Expectations of health systems and patients are that patients receive safe, effective, efficient, and patient centered care by sufficient numbers of motivated, well trained healthcare professionals. This expectation is difficult to achieve in rural areas due to shortages of physicians, nurses, allied professionals, support workers and administrators. For example, one fifth of the population in the U.S. lives outside of metropolitan or urban areas, while only 12% of physicians practice in rural areas. In reference to overall shortages in both the urban and rural sectors, it is projected that the shortage of registered nurses in the United States (U.S.) could reach as high as 500,000 by 2025, with a projected deficit of 200,000 physicians by 2020 (Dubois & Singh, 2009). As a result, many individuals seeking healthcare must travel to urban areas to receive care and treatment. The problem behind this situation is that obtaining talented healthcare professionals can be challenging in rural areas. This difficulty may be caused by a perceived increase in workload and lower pay associated with working in rural areas due to the percentage of patients requiring services, existing comorbidities, and fewer opportunities for healthcare professionals to obtain continuing education (McQueen, et. al, 2018). Solving this problem requires policy makers to provide incentives to physicians and other healthcare professionals, such as decreased tuition or education loan forgiveness if they agree to work in a rural area. Rural healthcare organizations can also offer pay increases or develop resources for continuing education.

Claus (2019) denotes a reinvention of talent management that focuses on "agility, customized solutions, letting go of control, and finding the sustainability sweet spot." Organizational complexity, potential changes, and problems associated with the day-to-day operations within the organization should be the emphasis of talent acquisition. The goal is that employees will be able to adapt to the changing internal and external environments of the organization. The use of necessary strategic thinking compels the organization to be creative in developing solutions to organizational challenges and generate meaningful experiences for their employees. New talent management forfeits command and control in lieu of researching and testing contemporary solutions based on stakeholders' needs and organizational expectations (Claus, 2019).

Several trends are unfolding regarding talent management. For example, the use of social media and the internet have proven successful in the acquisition of skilled employees. Social networks are also useful in forming communities and talent searches (Fajčíková, 2018). The following methods of using social media in talent management are suggested by Szwarcbart (2013): (1) organizations develop and open Facebook pages highlighting the greatness of the employees' journey through employment with them; (2) organizations develop enterprise websites to display real employees speaking about how satisfying it is to work there; (3) organizations establish Twitter accounts and encourage followers to discover how great it is to work for them; and (4) organizations use LinkedIn accounts to approach candidates through discussion groups and to evaluate potential candidates based on their view of specific topics. Another trend in attracting the best candidate is the use of organizational branding or strengthening the employer's image (Fajčíková, 2018).

Other best practices to ensure that newly hired talent are ready to engage within their new work environment include the institution of welcoming programs, such as transporting the candidate from the airport and providing meals during the interview process, ensuring the availability of supplies once the candidate has been hired, and meeting with upper management to acknowledge and support candidates' choice of the organization for employment (Szwarcbart, 2013). Organizations may also consider having a feedback system in place to gain the perspective of employee attitudes regarding organizational culture, work environment, compensation, training, supervision, and communication. Gathering this information facilitates employee engagement in the workplace and improves work performance (Chhabra & Aparna, 2008). Incorporating other methods of engagement, such as periodic employee appraisals, performing rounds, and managing employee relations are additional useful tools to keep employees engaged (Buchbinder & Shanks, 2017).

Another reason to acquire, retain, and engage skilled talent is to improve the performance of the organization through strategic management and planning, which is initiated by the Board of Directors or the CEO of the organization. The board is responsible for either initiating the planning process or supporting and approving the directives of the CEO regarding the strategic plan. The CEO initiates, coordinates, implements, evaluates and monitors the strategic plan. The strategic plan focuses on building and allocating resources to meet current and future needs of the organization through the development and implementation of a strategic plan. The plan outlines the mission, vision, goals, objectives, strategies and actions to be taken (Walston, 2017). The mission, vision, values, and goals cannot be achieved without human resources. Consequently, strategic management entails overseeing and directing organizational activities to ensure the mission and vision are attained and that the staff buy-in and participate for success. Providing quality services are critical to successful organizational performance and growth which requires resources (including people) and finances. The following section provides more in-depth discussion on performance improvement.

2.3.5 Performance Improvement

A major managerial objective is to increase the operational and service performance within the organization. Understanding how an organization performs directly relates to meeting the strategic goals and objectives set by the organization that ultimately aid in achieving the organization's mission and vision. The mission mandates what the organization is attempting to achieve. The vision stipulates the direction the organization would like to go in. Both are engrained by organizational top and middle managers in the needs and expectations of the organization.

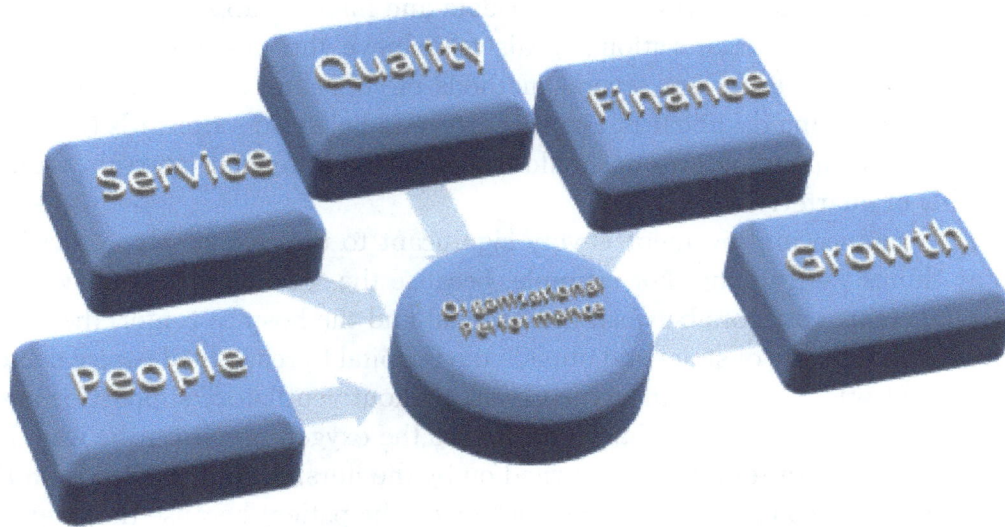

Figure 2.4: Organizational Performance

Source: Original Work
Attribution: Dorothy Howell
License: CC BY-SA 4.0

Organizations are developing codes of conduct or behavior that employees must follow to aid the organization in meeting its goal and objectives. The manager's role is to set employee expectations and monitor employee behavior while modeling appropriate behavior themselves. This was not the case in the following scenario. Dr. Paul Griner, Professor Emeritus of Medicine at the University of Rochester, discusses a scenario in which the chief medical officer was reviewed as a poor leader with substandard work performance causing potential risk to patient care and safety. Physicians under his leadership began documenting work related and behavioral issues, such as poor patient care, absenteeism, and professional incompetence, and made a report to hospital leadership. Several months later, the CMO in question was moved to another facility.

Organization performance requires support from what Buchbinder and Shank describe as people, quality, service, finance, and growth. People include doctors, nurses, patients, employees, etc. who provide and receive services. Services are goods, medicine, and medical or surgical treatment—including mental health, laboratory care, diagnostic, preventive care, substance abuse treatment, dentistry, nutritional support, physical, occupational or speech therapy, or optometric— required as a result of illness, sickness, disability or injury (ORS, 2017). Quality is the degree to which services lead to desired outcomes based on professional knowledge. In its simplest terms, finance implies funds required to operate an organization. Organizational growth, then, represents survival, power, efficiency, prestige, and the ability to withstand market fluctuations.

Performance management requires monitoring to determine what and if progress is being made. Adjustments can be made based on the findings from the monitoring activities. Monitoring is achieved using the right metrics (called key performance indicators, KPIs) to gather data and institute appropriate processes based on strategic organizational goals to achieve the mission and vision of the organization. There are several methods of collecting data and monitoring progress, including dashboards, Gantt charts, and balanced scorecards (Walston, 2017). Monitoring of indicators should be completed at regular intervals, weekly, monthly or quarterly.

Performance improvement is very significant to the case of Mr. Rodriquez. Many things went wrong. For example, because the code team was unaware of the connecting corridors between the hospital and the hospice center, they went down several flights of stairs and outside the hospital to reach the hospice center; the patient was placed on an oxygen mask without ventilatory support or chest compressions; the mask had been attached to the oxygen nozzle on the wall, but the oxygen had not initially been turned on by the nursing staff; the leads on the monitor were incompatible with the stickers on the patient because they were 10 years old; and the patient had requested not to be resuscitated, yet his chart did not indicate this information. The manager of the hospice center, the CEO of the hospital, the chief nursing officer, chief medical officer, chief data analyst and the staff involved in the incident will need to come together to identify the problems and develop solutions and policies to prevent similar incidents in the future. As mentioned above, performance improvement activities, such as identifying and monitoring how an organization is performing, can be achieved using dashboards and scorecards.

2.3.6 Dashboards

Dashboards, scorecards, and balanced scorecards are color coded (red, yellow, and green) so that managers can readily see how the organization is performing. A red status color indicates below-target performance or underlying critical risks. Yellow indicates a narrowly missed target or poorly trending performance that may impact end-of-year targets. The color green implies on-target performance.

A **dashboard** is a visual representation that houses all organizational data and KPI metrics in a single, easy-to-access location analogous to the dashboard or instrument panel of an automobile wherein the driver can review such key performance metrics as speed, oil and fuel levels, tire pressure, etc. Just as the dashboard of an automobile can assist the driver to track the process of driving a car in real-time, so also does the dashboard perform the same service for the healthcare manager (Joshi, et. al, 2014). Leaders within the hospice center and hospital can use a dashboard in the case with Mr. Rodriquez, for instance, to monitor and improve the time it takes to begin a code blue or resuscitation event and the time it takes to initiate each step in the resuscitation process.

Vital to measuring healthcare quality is the frequently used indicator of patient satisfaction. Patient satisfaction influences the timely, efficient, and patient-centered delivery of quality health care, which in turn influences clinical outcomes, patient retention, and medical malpractice claims. It is a critical factor in ensuring that healthcare practitioners and the healthcare facility is successful in attaining its goals. Therefore, senior and direct line leadership should use these metrics to assist in monitoring the performance of the organization (Prakash, 2010). The dashboard allows managers a clear view of how each metric is performing. Patients are asked to agree or disagree with two statements regarding patient satisfaction. The target goal for patient satisfaction is 80%. In this instance, 71% of the patients agreed that the staff explained procedures to them. Sixty four percent of the patients agreed with the statement that staff answered their questions. As you can see, the organization has not met their target goal. Review the targets for lab turn around by reviewing the image at this link: https://www.datapine.com/dashboard-examples-and-templates/healthcare. Can you tell if Saint Martin's met their goal? Saint Martin's has set a patient fall rate of less than 4.99%. Have they met this target? Review wait times for the patient to get a bed, see the doctor, and get treatment. How well are they performing?

2.3.7 Scorecards and Balanced Scorecards

Dashboards and scorecards differ in that a dashboard, like the dashboard of a car, indicates the status at a specific point in time; a scorecard, on the other hand, displays progress over time. **Scorecards** reflect outcome measures that assist the unit manager and other organizational leaders to record and report on past or previous performance of the organization rather than real-time process measures. An example of this is a final grade received by a student for completing a college course. Although there is a break between the time the student enrolled in and completed the course and the time they received the final grade, the final grade can be used to assist the student in determining future outcomes, such as enrolling in further courses until graduation requirements are met (Joshi, 2014). Review the scorecard from Government and Public Works (https://csipbl.com/resources/scorecard-examples/), which measures customer service, people, and operations. Targets have been set for the items to be measured. The person assigned to monitor performance of these goals has been determined. Monitoring will occur on a monthly basis. This scorecard reveals data from January-March of 2013 and contains a column informing the reviewer/manager of the organization's performance year to date. Sometimes a manager might set different monthly targets from the annual target. In this instance, the organization may be performing well on a monthly basis, but not enough time has elapsed to meet the annual or year to date target.

2.3.8 Balanced Scorecards

Balanced scorecards are reporting tools that portray both financial and nonfinancial performance measures, such as patient satisfaction and organizational processes that provide a comprehensive picture of organizational performance. Finances, customers and stakeholders, internal operations, and learning and growth are significant measures of the balanced scorecard and are substantial factors in organizational performance and growth. These measures center on the mission and vision of the organization. Financial metrics allow the organization to respond to how stakeholders or those providing funding to the organization. This metric includes profits, revenue growth, return on investment, and expense reductions. The production costs and volumes related to labor, materials, supplies, and overhead are components of the internal business processes of the organization that measure the successful operations required for the organization to attract and retain customers and key stakeholders. Customers and stakeholders' metrics provide the organization with information on how the customers and stakeholders view the products and services provided by the organization. This metric measures customer satisfaction, acquisition, and retention. Learning and growth measures include any new services required, examine what the organization should be doing to get better, and employee satisfaction and retention. Healthcare organizations also measure healthcare quality, outcomes, access, etc. (Walston, 2017). These quality improvement measures include safety, efficiency and timeliness, care that is patient centered and equitable, decreasing waste due to ineffective processes, etc. You might ask why are quality, outcomes, and access important to a healthcare organization?

The purpose of a healthcare organization is to serve its patients through the services provided by the healthcare professionals employed at the organization. For an organization to operate effectively, it must have a set of practices enabling it to optimize how it functions. In other words, how quickly and successfully does it achieve what is intended, especially in comparison to competitors? Many times, patients are dissatisfied with the quality of healthcare services they receive, which reflects negatively upon the organization. This negative response can over time adversely affect the financial viability of the organizations in general. As you can see from this discussion, it is important for an organization to establish a monitoring system to review its performance of strategic objectives.

2.3.9 Gantt Charts

As a healthcare manager, you might be tasked with developing a project for your department. Once you and your team devise the goals, objectives, and steps to complete the project, you will need a way to keep the project on schedule and determine the resources required to complete it. One way of doing this is by using a Gantt chart. Gantt charts are bar charts or graphs that display timetables for a single project or multiple projects. The graph includes start and end dates and percentages of completion along the continuum. The purpose of the chart is to see how long the project will take, determine the type and number of resources needed, and direct the completion of tasks. It serves to keep the project on schedule. Please review the video on Gant Charts in the Appendix Section of this book.

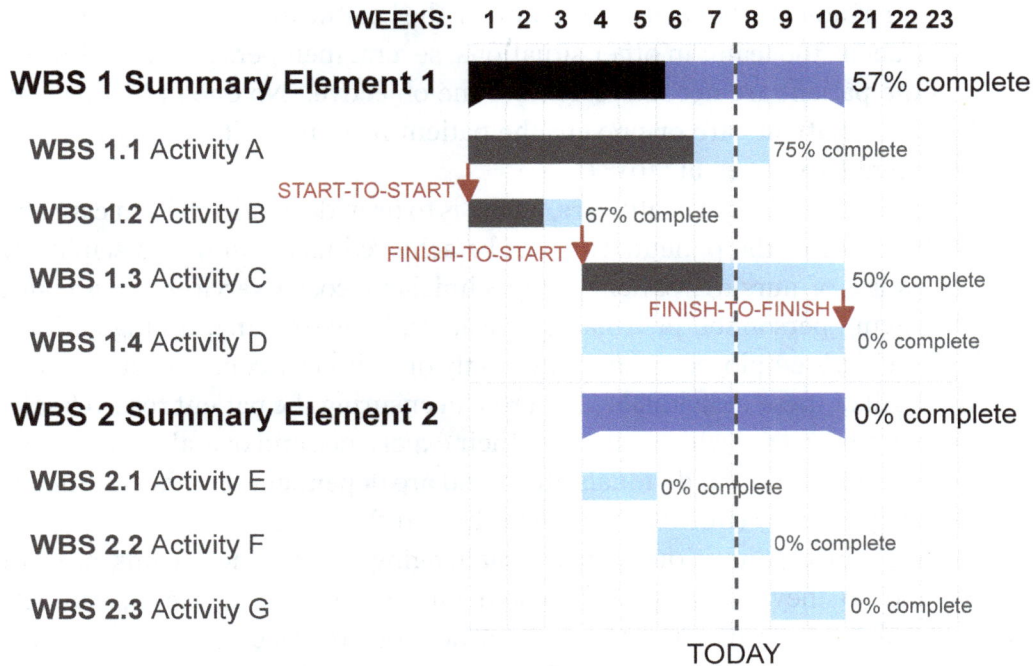

Figure 2.5: Gantt Chart

Source: Wikimedia Commons
Attribution: Unknown
License: Public Domain

2.3.10 Team Building

Many times, teamwork is required to complete tasks and projects for the organization or resolve issues within the organization that will lead to improving its performance, as outlined in the section above. Teams are required in almost every situation. From early childhood, as we play with others, we begin working in groups or teams. Families work as teams to complete chores or projects. We join such teams within the church or the community as choir, girl scouts, or eagle scouts. A team is a group of people who come together to accomplish a common goal. For example, a student may be required to join a team to complete a project on organizational leadership or assist the American Red Cross with a blood drive. Health care organizations are no different in that teams are required to carry out day-to-day operations. For example, Casimiro, Hall, Kuziemsky, O'Connor, & Varpio (2015) conducted a study that included 140 participants in a Canadian hospital to review the types and characteristics of teamwork that enabled patient-participatory care and how various situations affect team behaviors. The following patterns were noted: (1) **uniprofessional**—a healthcare professional collaborates one-on-one with the patient to address a situation; (2) **multiprofessional**—more than one healthcare professional from various disciplines collaborates with the patient and/or their family to address the patient's concerns or goals; and (3) **interprofessional**—an interdisciplinary team of professionals combine their expertise and include the patient and their family in the decision making process.

These patterns indicate that in some situations, the healthcare professional and the patient can act as the team; in other situations, several members of the healthcare team and the patient are needed to achieve the objective. No one individual can provide quality patient care or prevent the patient from receiving injury or harm from treatment (Rosen, et. al, 2018).

One important aspect of healthcare, again, is to provide quality patient care and support the needs of the patient. This can be achieved using an interdisciplinary team consisting of nursing, patient care technicians, social services, physicians, lab and imaging personnel, pharmacy, educators, housekeeping, dining staff, or any of the facility's employees who may directly or indirectly come in contact with the patient. All of these individuals play a role in ensuring the patient receives safe, effective, and timely care which enhances their experience and overall satisfaction. The tasks of each of these individuals affect and are dependent on others, which is called interdependency (Buchbinder & Shanks, 2017).

Teamwork in organizations can be challenging. Sometimes teams are not effective and so they need to be dissolved due to contrasting views, conflicts among members, or when team members do not embrace teamwork. Teams must be able to work together in an effective manner and overcome issues, such as role clarification, team unity, communication, decision making and leadership. The process of teamwork cannot be initiated unless individuals understand that they cannot operate in siloes but must instead learn to work together. Without this understanding, problems cannot be solved, decisions cannot be made, and outcomes cannot be achieved (Gafà, et. al, 2005). Although developing and facilitating team activities are management functions, managers are not trained during their formal education on team building, retention, and task completion, but must acquire this skill on the job (Buchbinder & shanks, 2017).

Successful organizations increase their competitive advantage by fostering teamwork. Delivering outstanding coordinated care through teamwork promotes patient satisfaction, quality services, and a more engaged workforce, all of which are strategic imperatives that lead to increased financial performance for healthcare organizations (Lee, 2016). Building a team is contingent on finding the best fit between the project and members, based on how potential members think and behave. Meetings should not end in major disagreements or fighting among team members. Good leaders and followers are needed to ensure the project is completed in a timely manner and successfully. Buchbinder and Shanks relay the following characteristics in figure 2.6 as attributable to successful and unsuccessful teams.

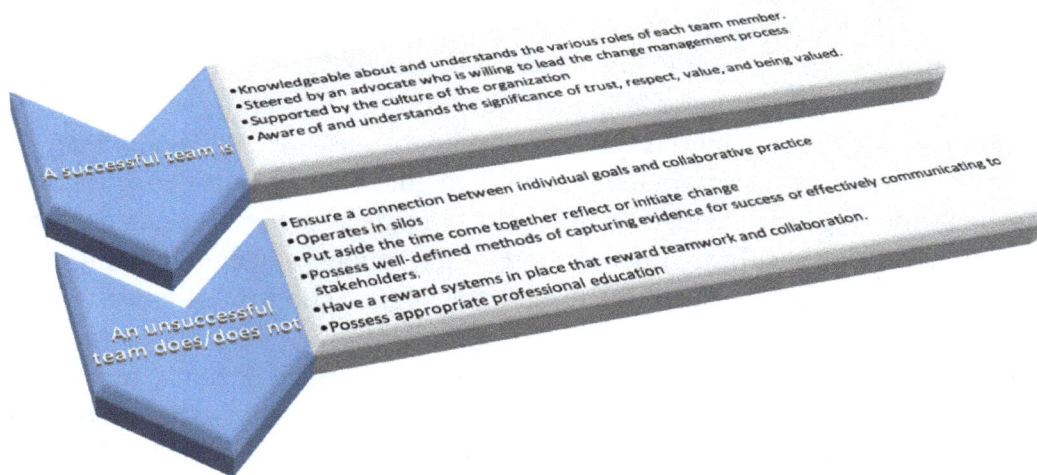

Figure 2.6: Successful and Unsuccessful Teams

Source: Original Work

Attribution: Dorothy Howell

License: CC BY-SA 4.0

Stop and Apply

As the manager of the code team, make a list of what went wrong with Mr. Rodriquez's code. What can you do to reduce the likelihood of these process issues in the future? Do you need to pull the code team together to answer this question?

2.3.11 Developing Leaders

One of a leader's many tasks is building and working with teams. Their work is essential to the success of the mission and vision of the organization. How can you (as the leader) keep the team motivated, or how can you keep employees, in general, engaged and motivated? How will you find, train, encourage, educate, and support employees within the organization to take over if you desire to leave for a new position or retirement? Managers are responsible for not only ensuring the organization is performing but also developing successors within the organization who will support and follow the vision.

Motivation

Motivation is important for many reasons. It provides the employees with a sense of personal investment within the organization. They appear happier, work harder and stay with the organization for longer periods of time than do employees who are not motivated. Managers therefore must understand the job-related needs of the employees and ensure these needs are met. In addition, managers must acknowledge their role in maintaining the culture and diversity of the organization by employing a variety of individuals, such as women, minorities, baby boomers, and millennials, and incorporating them into different areas within their departments. Employees who are engaged and motivated can increase work and organizational performance, which can propel the organization into a dominant position in the healthcare market (Buchbinder & Shanks, 2017).

Motivating staff is achieved through various means; for instance, money is generally viewed as a positive motivator, but it might not be the most effective one. Knowing which type of incentives to include during the hiring process can improve the bottom line for healthcare organizations and go a long way in motivating staff to increase performance and remain with the organization. McKinnies (2016) reports the top four incentives for attracting and retaining staff are as follows: professional development, tuition reimbursement, retirement benefits, and health care insurance. Although important to motivation, neither starting salaries nor sign on bonuses were the most significant issues related to retention efforts. The goal is to put incentives in place that fit employee needs. However, it is important that organizations monitor their incentive packages on a continuous basis to increase the organizations' appeal to potential employees and retain them after hiring.

Employees play a substantial role in ensuring the vision and mission of the organization is achieved. Organizational leaders must obtain employee buy-in or a sense of connection in reference to achieving the vision. It should be tied to team and achievable goals, since such ties serve to increase their motivation in achieving the vision. Motivation occurs based on psychological factors that encourage an employee to complete work activities and can be intrinsic or extrinsic as noted in Figure 2.7. Motivation can be intrinsic because the employee finds it satisfying and stimulating or extrinsic because of an incentive such as money or status. Intrinsic motivation leads to better work performance, goal attainment, and job satisfaction and is increased by a supportive work environment. Individuals who place too much emphasis on extrinsic motivation may experience job burn out, health problems, low performance, and job turnover (Kotera, et.al, 2017). The following figure depicts the characteristics of intrinsic and extrinsic rewards (Buchbinder and Shanks, 2017).

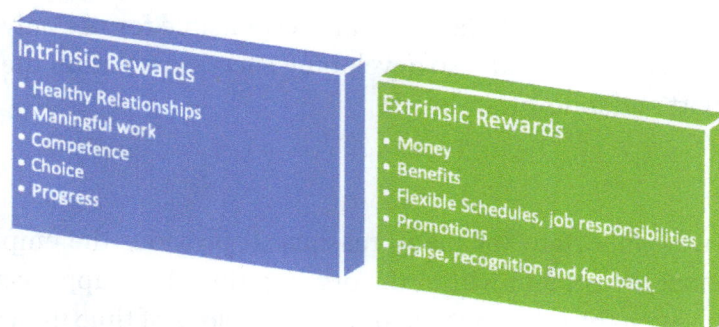

Figure 2.7: Intrinsic and Extrinsic Rewards

Source: Original Work
Attribution: Dorothy Howell
License: CC BY-SA 4.0

Managers can use the following strategies to motivate their employees. One strategy is to make employees aware of work expectations. They need goals, training, coaching, counseling, and feedback to increase their productivity. Another strategy is to incorporate methods for employees' improving their professional skills. Providing employees responsibility in the decision-making process and showing them that they can be trusted to do their jobs is another strategy. Other strategies include the following: (1) attempting to recruit and hire motivated employees, (2) improving job titles and responsibilities to deserving employees, (3) knowing employees and their behaviors, (4) being fair, consistent, supportive, and respectful, and (5) leading by example (McConnell, 2018).

Shaping Successors

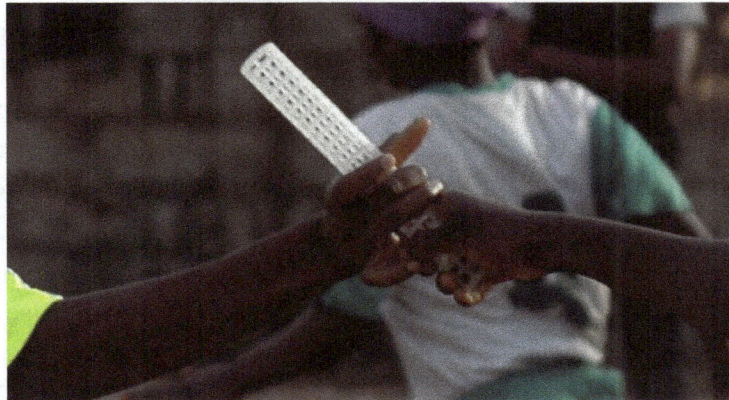

Figure 2.8: Successors

Source: Wikimedia Commons
Attribution: Fowosire Damilola
License: CC BY-SA 4.0

Although motivation is an important factor for healthcare leaders in supporting the mission and vision of the organization, also important is the leader's shaping a successor to take their place if they decide to leave. To whom will you pass the baton to, and how will you do it? Succession planning is the process of putting steps into place to allow employees the opportunity to move into management positions within the organization following the vacation of a current management position due to retirement or transitioning to another position (Buchbinder & Shanks, 2017). Walston (2017) discusses the following key succession plan practices that will improve the function and competence of an organization:

- Top Leadership Support. Executive leadership supports and funds programs that prepare subordinate staff to assume leadership roles.

- Link to Strategic Plan. Succession planning should be engrained within the strategic plan of the organization as a method of ensuring the mission and vision of the organization are achieved.

- Locate employees within the organization with leadership capabilities. High-performing employees should be rewarded by including them in programs that will improve their knowledge base and skills in preparation for management positions.

- Assign developmental activities and formal training. Providing employees with assignments across the organization allows them to participate in new roles and activities that will reinforce their skills and competencies and provide new ones.

- Address human capital challenges. Organizational challenges associated with employees are diversity, leadership, capacity, and retention. Organizations must be able to respond to shifts and changes within the internal and external environment through succession planning efforts.

- Enable change. Changes may be required for an organization to achieve its mission and vision. Organizations must make changes in their products, services, and processes to maintain its control or share in the market. For this purpose, it is crucial for the organization to be able to select appropriate candidates who will foster change.

Coaching and/or mentoring are integral to leadership development and aid in transferring acquired and learned competencies and expertise within the organization. In a healthcare organization, coaching/mentoring is a mutually agreed upon one-on-one relationship between the manager and the employee with the goal of improving the skills of the employee. A successful coaching relationship begins with the establishment of mutual trust and respect between the manager and the employee. The next step involves establishing needs, developing a plan, and setting goals and objectives that will meet the needs. The manager should begin the coaching process and monitor progress and provide feedback to the mentee along the way (Al Shamsi, et. al, 2015).

Training up appropriate successors is key to successful healthcare organizations. Doing so provides potential managers the opportunity to improve on their management skills. Training can be achieved through leadership development programs that provide education on various leadership topics through structured learning and competency-based assessments and didactic courses on leadership and management, offered via face-to-face, hybrid, or online formats (Buchbinder & Shanks, 2017). Training potential managers can be achieved in several steps. Employees can participate on cross-functional committees and be provided with activities outside of their current skillset. Managers can assist employees to build a reputation within the organization so that they can be noticed by top executives and/or other significant stakeholders. Managers can also provide employees with feedback on assigned tasks and suggestions on how to improve themselves for leadership positions (Grupe, et. al, 2003).

2.4 STRATEGY IN HEALTHCARE ORGANIZATIONS

Throughout this chapter, we have discussed the role of leaders and managers in performing various functions within the healthcare organization. These roles have included planning, organizing, staffing, controlling, making decisions, directing, communicating, and improving performance using various monitoring tools. Other roles of leaders include building and working with teams and developing successors. Organizational leaders, again, must be able to fulfill their roles if they expect to be successful in forwarding the mission and vision of the organization. Also again, the mission and vision are accomplished by developing strategy or strategic goals and objectives that set the organization apart from its competitors. The next section of this chapter discusses why strategy is needed and how to develop, implement, and evaluate it. This section on strategy also discusses the importance of establishing strategic alliances that will be beneficial to all organizations involved in the alliance.

2.4.1 The Purpose of Strategy

For students to understand the purpose of strategy, they must know its meaning. Strategy is a thoroughly devised plan to ensure a specific set of goals and objectives are achieved. Knowledge of strengths and weaknesses are essential elements of strategy. Organizations must be able to use their strengths to their advantage and reduce or eliminate weaknesses that will prevent them from attaining their mission and vision. Strategy consists of mechanisms that will enable the organization to provide for the needs of their customers (patients), position themselves above their competition, and make appropriate changes based on positive and negative circumstances within the internal and external environments. Strategic management represents the decisions and activities required to develop strategy to assist the organization in achieving its goals. It focuses on producing new markets, technology, and products. Strategic management determines required actions, people responsible for performing the actions, and the means by and times at which the actions will be performed. It is vital to the survival and growth of the organization.

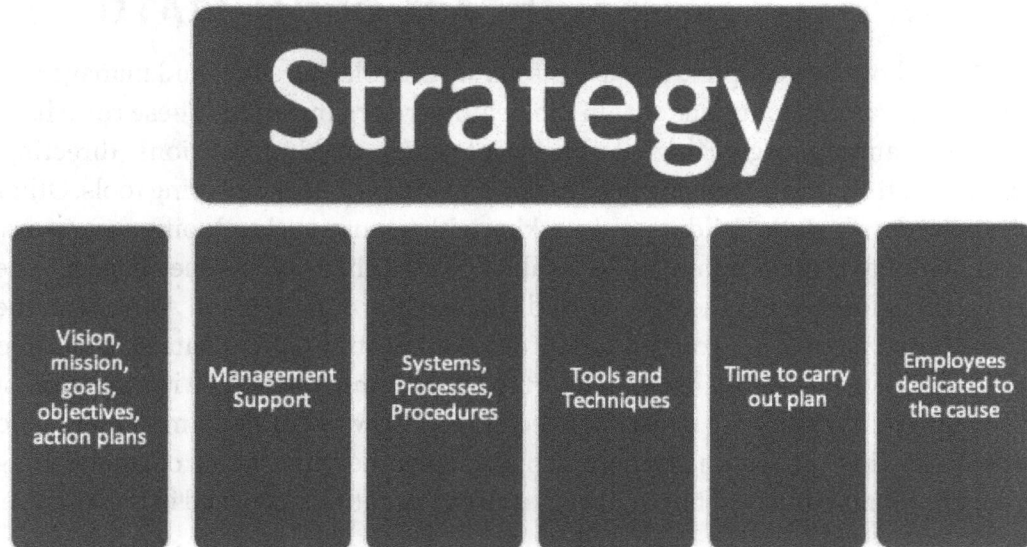

Figure 2.9: Strategy

Source: Original Work
Attribution: Dorothy Howell
License: CC BY-SA 4.0

Strategic planning focuses on the future of the organization. In other words, it helps leaders to determine what the organization wants and needs to be doing in the next five, ten, or more years. Executive level managers use it to set organizational priorities and identify actions required to ensure the priorities materialize. The following solutions are integral to improving organizational strategy. The mission and vision of the organization are the driving forces that indicate the purpose (the who, what, and how) and the future state of the organization. Goals, objectives, and action plans are developed to assist the organization in meeting the mission and vision. The manager's role is to provide support in the form of employee trust and the allocation of resources required to accomplish the action plan. Systems, processes, and procedures are guides that outline and standardize how things should be done.

Tools and techniques represent essential resources needed to implement, monitor, and evaluate the success of the strategic plan. Time required to complete the strategic plan is contingent upon the size and complexity of the organization and the specific elements of the strategic plan. The strategy cannot be completed without the commitment of dedicated employees who have a stake in the mission and vision of the organization (McConnell, 2018).

An example of using strategy in a healthcare organization would be the Hospice Center where Mr. Rodriquez resided. A part of the center's mission and vision would be providing quality care to their patients. As a reminder of the case, the leads attached to Mr. Rodriquez were outdated by 10 years and did not fit the monitor from the hospital. The hospice care center leaders would need to formulate a strategy to ensure the hospice center maintains the latest supplies, products, and technology for their patients. They could begin by inventorying their supplies, products, and supporting technology and updating those that are outdated with the most current ones. This task might be a massive undertaking that would require large capital to support it (especially if expensive equipment is required). The timing of obtaining up-to-date products, supplies, and technology would be contingent upon those that were most critical to save the lives of the patient.

2.4.2 Planning Strategy

Now that you know why strategy is needed in healthcare organizations, you need to know the steps in planning strategy. Good strategic plans begin with a team that includes board members, senior and middle managers, employees from the technical support, and other stakeholders as needed coming together to obtain the following information: (1) what is the current position of the organization as compared to where it wants to go, (2) how can the mission and vision be achieved, (3) what goals and objectives are needed, (4) what actions are required, (5) how can the goals and objectives be put into action, and (6) what evaluation and monitoring tools are needed to determine if objectives have been achieved. This information gathering is called an environmental analysis because it leads to any gaps between what is desired and what is needed. The gap is the basis for development of strategic options, goals and objectives, action plans, marketing plans, implementation and evaluation.

However, your having completed the environmental analysis does not mean you will be successful in carrying out the plan. Both controllable and uncontrollable market forces exist that can prevent the organization from becoming a success. **Market forces** are economic considerations that influence pricing, as well as demand for and availability of health care services and products. Porter's Five Forces Model provides a framework that influences competition in an industry. These forces include the possibility of new entrants, threat of substitute products, degree of buyers' power, and rivalry among competing sellers (Walston, 2018). In addition, all industries are influenced by driving forces, such as changes in technology, demographics, politics, culture, and economics. The following forces are common in the healthcare sector: (1) changes in consumer demand wherein consumers are included in the decision making regarding healthcare they receive; (2) technological changes affecting how individuals interact, share information, and generate activities useful in the planning process; (3) workforce availability, which refers to shortages of skilled personnel and services; and (4) political change, which refers to laws that affect access to healthcare and reimbursement (Walston, 2018). Strategic planning assists the organization in identifying and determining the effect of market forces on the success of the organization and in devising a plan to eliminate or counteract the forces or use them to their advantage. The strategic plan also serves to keep the organization focused on attaining its vision (Buchbinder & Shanks, 2017).

In most cases, strategic planning is based on data driven decisions. However, in the absence of quantifiable data, front-line to executive managerial decisions can be derived from informed judgements. In effect, strategic planning requires a step-by-step process, brainstorming sessions, data or information, organizational focus, data driven decisions, external environmental scans allowing consensus on organizational fit, and documentation of results (Ginter, Ducan, & Swayne, 2015) It is also influenced by the internal environment, which indicates what the organization can do based on its resources, ability, and expertise.

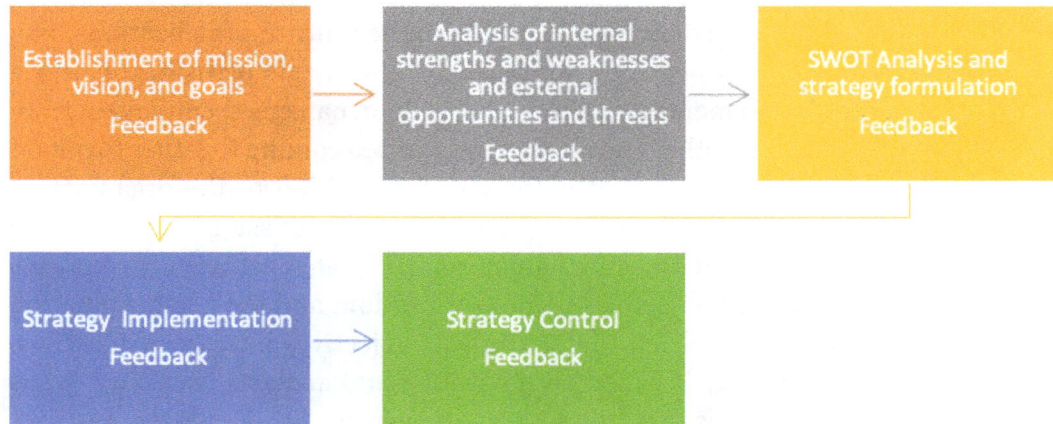

Figure 2.10: Steps in Strategic Planning Process

Source: Original Work
Attribution: Dorothy Howell
License: CC BY-SA 4.0

The planning process begins with an analysis to identify both positive and negative attributes of the organization. Among these are a political, economic, social, technological analysis (PEST analysis), force field analysis, scenario analysis, strengths, weaknesses, opportunities, threats (SWOT) or TOWS analysis, and portfolio analysis. The **PEST Analysis** is an analytical method reviewing driving forces for the organization. This analysis involves reviewing laws, regulations, and governmental polices supporting or perhaps impeding the plans of the organization. The economic factors comprise a review of purchasing power, distribution of wealth, availability of the workforce, and ability of the organization to increase its financial status. Social factors refer to population demographics and their attitudes. Technology focuses on research and innovation and the rate at which the technology is adopted. **Force field analysis** is an extension of the PEST analysis. It is used to determine if environmental forces encourage (through long-term finances, executive level support, etc.) or hinder (through layoffs, short-term expenses, population attitudes, etc.) the organization's strategic planning efforts.

The **scenario analysis** proposes alternative solutions in response to changes in the environment. It assists the leaders of the organization to plan for the future. **SWOT Analysis** refers to strengths, weaknesses, opportunities, and threats affecting the organization. This allows the organization to view what is happening within their external and internal environments. Adaptations are then made based on findings through the identification and selection of prioritized strategies to prevent the organization from becoming overwhelmed with too many new policies. The **TOWS analysis** is an expansion of the SWOT analysis. It enhances the decision-making abilities of organizational leaders as they compare external opportunities and threats to internal strengths and weaknesses to make decisions regarding what strengths can be leveraged and what threats or weaknesses can be minimized.

The **portfolio analysis** represents the products and services offered by the organization. Its purpose is to evaluate whether the products and services offered will sustain the future of the organization based on organizational performance, cash flow, and allocation of resources (Walston, 2018). As a manager, you will need to have knowledge concerning various types of problem-solving strategies and how to select the best one(s) for your organization. Once the appropriate strategies are selected and a plan is devised and implemented, monitoring and control occur. Feedback occurs along each step of the process (Buchbinder & Shanks, 2017).

2.4.3 Implementing

Once the type has been selected and formulated, the manager must realize that the strategy can fail at the implementation phase, which requires buy-in and support from all members of the organization. Only 45-to-50% of all hospital strategies that are formulated get implemented (Walston, 2017). Implementation involves putting the organization's strategy into practice. In other words, implementation begins as the organization's step by step process in accomplishing the strategic plan's goals and objectives (Lindsay, Jack, & Ambrosini, 2018).

Successful implementation is initiated through planning, budgeting, implementing, controlling, and monitoring, which warrants communicating the strategy to all levels of the organization. Stakeholders, such as governing boards, payers, suppliers, organizational leaders, and employees, must view the plan as an impetus for change in order to improve the organization, which also provides them with the motivation to be critically engaged in the process. An internal champion for the change must lead the process and ensure that all the plan's activities are achieved by completing a feasibility study, completing environmental assessments, developing timetables, and formulating evaluation guidelines. The strategic planning and implementation process incorporates the governing board that manages and directs the organization; the strategic planning committee who is responsible for organizing and leading the process; medical staff that serves on both the governing board of community leaders from the business units and strategic planning committee, and consultants who develop the strategic plan (Walston, 2018). All of these entities must provide support for successful implementation.

Besides stakeholders, specific tools, such as resources and organizational competencies, are also required for strategy implementation. Capital, such as physical space, tools, equipment, human resources, and control and reporting systems are all linked to strategy implementation. Capital resources are finances or money needed for the organization to implement the plan. Human resources are the skilled, capable, motivated, engaged, and willing employees who have bought-in to the process and desire to see positive outcomes. The organization must possess the appropriate amount of physical space and necessary equipment to carry out the plan's activities. The system includes policy, procedures, employees, electronic processing and communication equipment, such as accounting and budgeting systems, management information, compensation and rewards, and planning systems. Figure 2.11 depicts the processes required to implement strategy (Moseley, 2018).

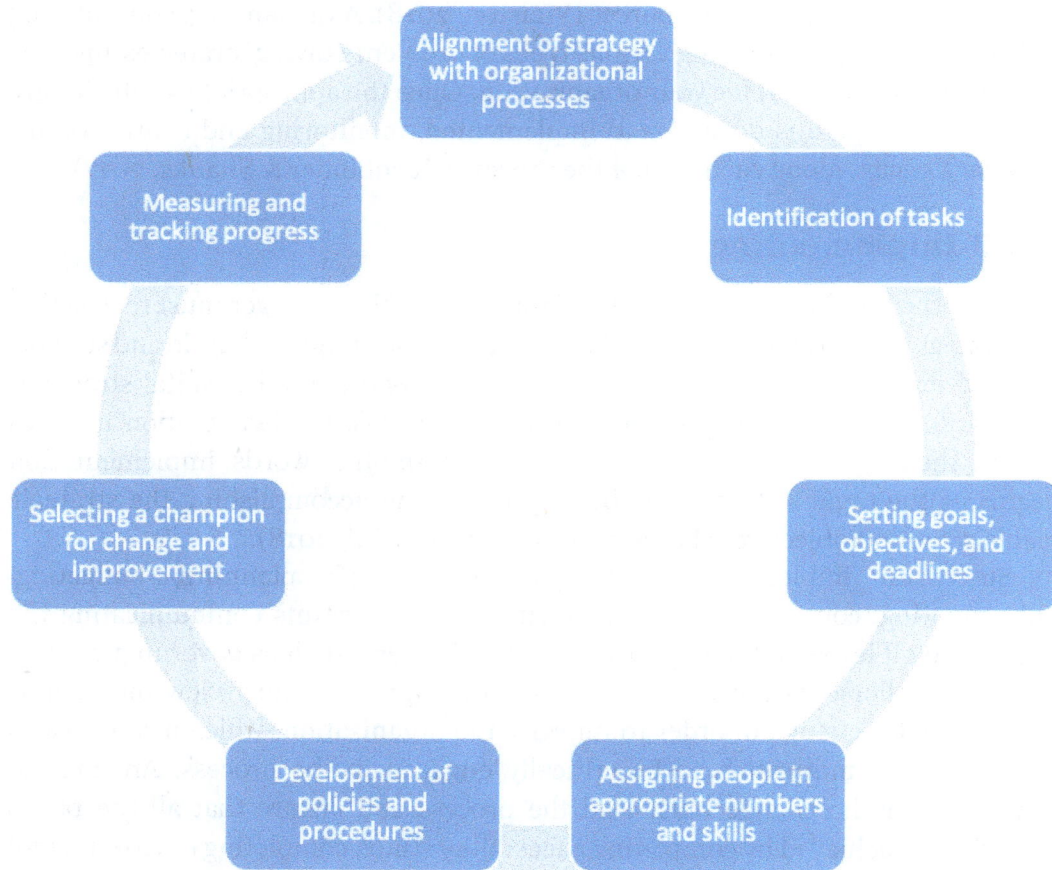

Figure 2.11: Process for Implementing Strategy

Source: Original Work
Attribution: Dorothy Howell
License: CC BY-SA 4.0

2.4.4 Evaluation

In relation to the strategic planning process, evaluation occurs after the strategic plan has been implemented. It is a method of assessing and monitoring the progress of the implemented activities in the plan. Evaluating is essential to its success. Monitoring should occur either weekly, monthly, or quarterly. Monitoring involves developing and assigning measurable key performance indicators to each strategic objective. Monitoring and evaluation are achieved by tracking organizational trends and comparing organizational data to data from other organizations (Walston, 2018).

Monitoring strategic plan outcomes is achieved using tools such as dashboards, Gantt charts, and balanced scorecards. **Dashboards** monitor the organization's performance related to strategic, operational, and financial outcomes over time based on the needs of the organization (Buchbinder & Shanks, 2018). **Gantt charts** depict schedules, steps, and timeframes of a project. **Balanced scorecards** evaluate metrics and collect feedback on the strategic plan's progress.

The purpose of monitoring is to be apprised of changes in the external and internal environments related to the organization's strategic performance or preferences so that the strategy can be adjusted as needed. Once the strategic plan is implemented, current organizational performance is mapped back to the original strategic goals to establish any gaps between the two. Reducing and eliminating the potential loss in market share organizational failure is contingent on closing the gaps identified through the evaluation process (Moseley, 2018).

The Southern California Injury Prevention Research Center (SCIPRC, 2018) suggests the following reasons for strategy evaluation: to see if the strategy is accomplishing the goals and objectives it was intended to achieve, determine if costs outweigh the benefits, monitor progress post implementation so needed changes can be made, and keep stakeholders apprised of successes and challenges during implementation.

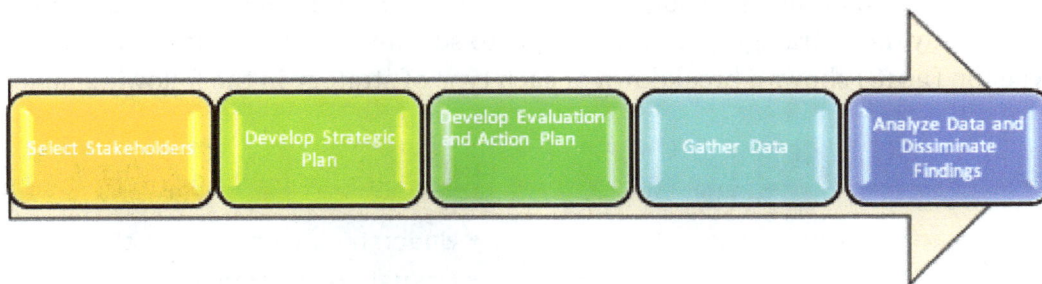

Figure 2.12: Monitoring Strategy

Source: Original Work
Attribution: Dorothy Howell
License: CC BY-SA 4.0

Process and outcomes are two types of evaluations used in strategy implementation. **Process evaluation** allows the organization to establish if the strategy was implemented as planned and if it reached the intended stakeholders. **Outcome evaluation** helps the organization to visualize if the strategy was effective (SCIPRC, 2018).

Monitoring allows the organization to draw conclusions from the data or make changes to the strategic plan. For example, the strategy can be cancelled if it no longer meets the needs of the organization or the customers, if it no longer fits within the market segment, or if the competitors have added similar strategies. A strategy can by adjusted or new strategies added based on findings from the data. Resources may require reallocation or the addition of new resources to ensure the strategic plan is accomplished. Strategic objectives may also require changes if they are not accomplishing the mission (Moseley, 2018). Another type of strategy involves developing a relationship between your organization and other organizations to allow financial leverage, as this arrangement is mutually beneficial to all organizations involved. This type of relationship is called a strategic alliance.

2.4.5 Types and Selections of Strategies for Healthcare Management

Strategy can be prospective or emergent. **Prospective strategy** is forward in that it plans for the organization's future. Prospective strategy provides the opportunity for the organization to place its footprint of its competition using purposeful and strategic designing, planning, and positioning. This strategy takes into consideration the organization's behavior and aligns it with the organization's mission and vision. Managers use prospective strategy to attain planned outcomes and forecast human and capital resource needs.

Emergent strategy is retrospective in that it pulls from the past experiences of the organization's market behavior to establish correlations that can be modified to advance its market position among the competitors. With this strategy, organizations can review the actions of its competitors and use them to their advantage. It also allows the organization to learn from its successes and failures and modify their strategic plan accordingly to sustain the organization's presence. Walston (2018) shows a breakdown of each type of strategy in the following table.

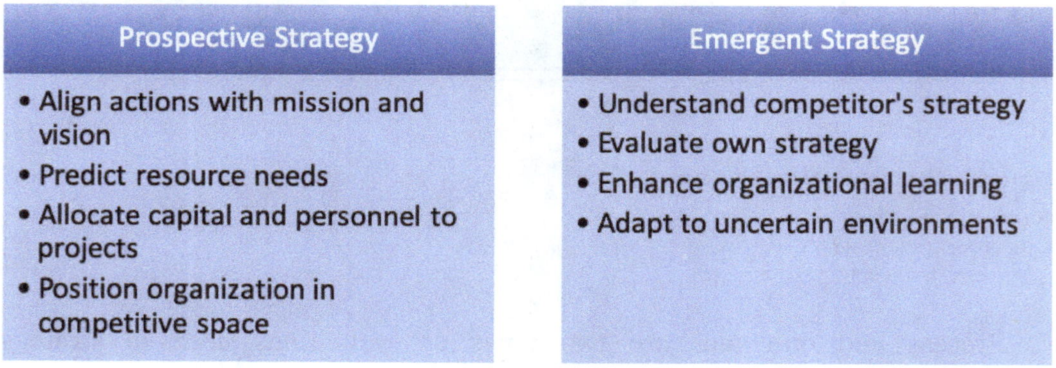

Prospective Strategy	Emergent Strategy
• Align actions with mission and vision • Predict resource needs • Allocate capital and personnel to projects • Position organization in competitive space	• Understand competitor's strategy • Evaluate own strategy • Enhance organizational learning • Adapt to uncertain environments

Figure 2.13: Prospective and Emergent Strategy

Source: Walston
Attribution: Walston
License: © Walston. Fair use.

Along with types of strategies are three levels of strategies: corporate, business unit, and functional as seen in Figure 2.14. Top executives, corporate staff, and board of directors reside at the highest level and make business decisions for the organization. Managers at the **corporate level** establish strategy significant to the sustainability of the organization. These top executives understand the organization and what is needed to contribute to its competitive advantage. The organization's mission, vision, values, focus areas, strategic goals, and key performance indicators provide the foundation for developing strategy at this level. Allocation of resources and determining what, when, and how to enter and exit existing industries or whether to develop new industries occurs at the corporate level. For example, an organization may enter or exit existing industries based on the possibility of new entrants, substitute products or services, power of buyers, or rivalry among competitors. Corporate strategies are broad and cover a 3–5 year period.

Business and functional level strategies are extracted from the corporate level strategies. **Business level strategies** represent specific strategic business units and relate to a distinct product-market area, such as the Hospital Corporation of America (HCA). **Business units** refer to departments or a functional group within an organization that handles the issues and affairs for specific activities. Examples of business units include marketing, finance, operations, accounting, sales, human resources, and research and development divisions. It involves defining the competitive position of a strategic business unit. The purpose of business strategy is to achieve the goals of a business within the corporation. The business level is directed by division managers and staff.

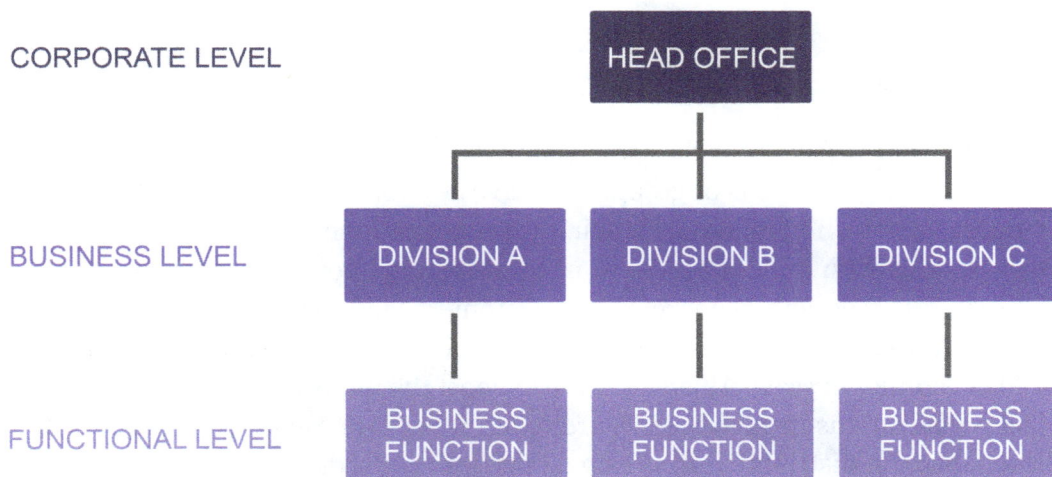

CORPORATE LEVEL		HEAD OFFICE	
BUSINESS LEVEL	DIVISION A	DIVISION B	DIVISION C
FUNCTIONAL LEVEL	BUSINESS FUNCTION	BUSINESS FUNCTION	BUSINESS FUNCTION

Figure 2.14: Levels of Strategy

Source: Original Work
Attribution: Corey Parson
License: CC BY-SA 4.0

The emphasis of **functional level strategy** is on how a division or department operates and is grounded in products and services. Functional level strategy focuses on how the various functions of an organization contribute to the business and corporate strategy levels. Functional level strategies include marketing, finance, manufacturing, human resources, etc. These strategies support the day-to-day operations of a healthcare organization (Ordenes, 2018). An example of each level of strategy in use can be seen with Hospital Corporation of America or HCA, which is in 20 U.S. states and the United Kingdom.

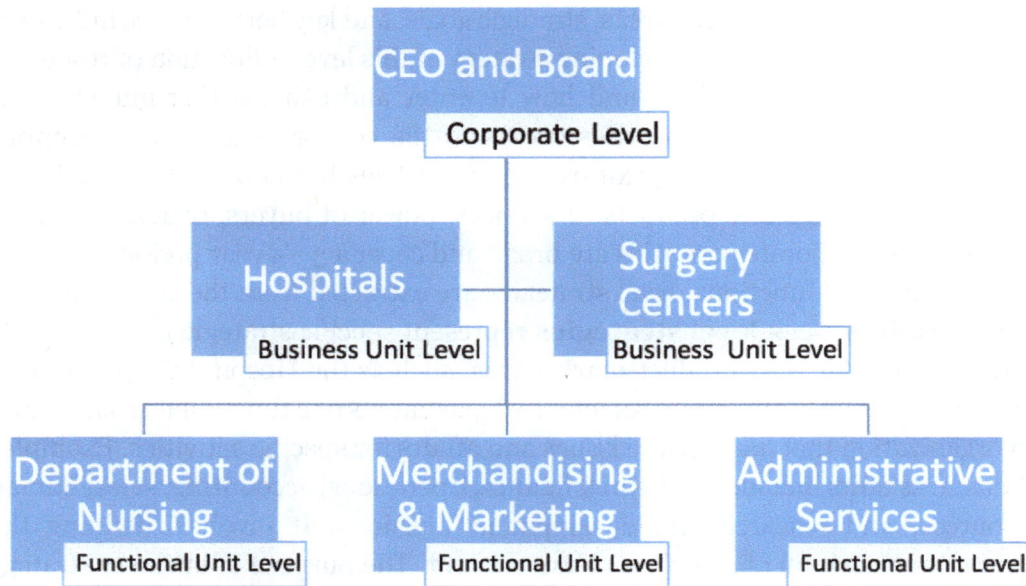

Figure 2.15: Corporate, Business, and Functional Strategy

Source: Original Work
Attribution: Dorothy Howell
License: CC BY-SA 4.0

2.4.6 Strategic Alliances

A **strategic alliance** is the establishment of a long-term relationship between two or more organizations or groups that have developed mutually beneficial goals or needs but do not relinquish their independent functions. Alliances provide organizations with greater access to new technology, new industries, new goods and services, geographic markets, new customers, and new talent. They provide opportunities to share resources, research, and development investments, as well as build economies of scale. Alliances serve to boost the innovativeness and branding of all organizations involved. Risks are reduced because each organization within the alliance can distribute risk among all parties involved.

Alliances are usually formed based on uncertainties within the environment. Along with these uncertainties comes increased risks. However, if the alliance is to be successful, the organizations' missions and cultures must be aligned. Failure of the alliance will occur without collaboration, cooperation, and coordination of goals and objectives. Successful alliances permit organizations within the alliance to provide patient-centered care because of the alliance's benefits.

Organizations need to understand the steps required to form an alliance. The first step is deciding whether to enter one. If the organization believes that the alliance would aid in the accomplishment of strategic objectives, it will have to develop a plan outlining the project especially regarding required resources.

The next step involves securing a comparable partner by analyzing strengths, weaknesses, management styles, mission, vision, and available resources of the potential partner in order to determine compatibility. The next step involves both partners outlining the terms of the alliance through a written contract defining contributions, duties and obligations, incentives, policies and procedures governing the alliance, determining how to manage conflicts, devising a system for monitoring and evaluating outcomes, as well as determining when the contract can be terminated. The next step involves starting the alliance and determining how it will function. The final step outlines when, how, reasons why, and if the alliance will be terminated (Moseley, 2018).

Alliances can be vertical or horizontal. A **horizontal alliance** is a partnership between organizations that are similar in that they provide the same products and services and compete. This type of alliance is formed to boost market position and power as compared to other competitors in the marketplace. A **vertical alliance** is a partnership of an organization and its suppliers, wherein the organization and the supplier(s) operate in different industries.

There are several ways of entering strategic alliances based on how the members have designated the degree of control and equity between the members. For example, learning alliances and purchasing alliances have a low degree of control and equity, while a franchise and joint venture alliance have a high degree of control and equity. Learning and purchasing alliances require a fee to participate and have little to no control over the direction of the alliance. A **joint venture alliance** is one wherein the parties combine resources and share ownership and a large percentage of control. This type of alliance produces value for each of the members. An example is a medical service organization created by a hospital and physicians. **Pooled alliances** develop from many members who come together to share resources that will bring value to the organization's. An example is group purchasing organizations who save money for their members by negotiating prices. A **network outsource alliance** outsources or contracts out portions of its operations (Walston, 2018).

2.5 HEALTHCARE POLICY

Regardless of leadership functions, practices, or strategies, the organization cannot be successful without internal and external rules and regulations that govern its performance. Managers must not only be aware of and engaged in external policy development by governmental agencies (e.g., accreditation, regulation, etc.) but also engaged in policy development within the organization. The following section discusses the manager's role in health policy development.

2.5.1 Management's Role in Health Policy

Organizational policies are rules or laws that are constructed from the mission and vision of the organization to provide structure to health behavior and provide governance and accountability. The potential for litigation increases the need for and significance of health policy within healthcare organizations. They also decrease confusion among the employees and thereby lead to better performance and outcomes. Poorly worded policies or the absence of policies increase time wasted by managers in revisiting and revamping previously made decisions and re-answering questions. Managers should assure policies that contain such specific information as (1) salary and benefits, (2) staffing and scheduling practices, (3) smoking and drug use, (4) Right to Know laws, (5) caring for AIDS patients, (6) sexual harassment, (7) Health Insurance Portability and Accountability Act (HIPAA), (8) cultural diversity, (9) discrimination, (10) Persons with Disabilities, and (11) Accreditation and Regulatory bodies (McConnell, 2018).

Employees within the organization must have a clear picture of the policies and procedures governing their behaviors and receive disciplinary action if they disregard policies. Managers must thoroughly comprehend policies and enforce them without favoritism even when policies are difficult to enforce. They must also understand when and how to modify polices and develop new policies as need arises. There are times when a manager may take a risk and bend policies based on specific circumstances. For example, a nurse manager may make rounds and find that one of the nurses has left the building outside of the break time. Her first decision was to call the nurse in for a verbal warning against such activity as it is against unit and hospital policy. Upon further reexamination, the nurse manager finds out that the nurse had left her sick child at home and had gone home (5 minutes away from the hospital) to give the child some medication. The manager in this case can elect to overlook this policy under the circumstances.

Understanding the healthcare environment requires realizing challenges that invoke a need for new policies. Having a grasp on this knowledge and using it proactively to inform strategic formulation and decisions rather than reacting to established policies can increase the organization's competitive advantage (Longest, 2012).

2.6 EXPANSION AND COMPLEXITY OF HEALTH LAW AND REGULATION

Healthcare is governed by local, state, and federal guidelines (and laws and policies). Many of these policies are developed as measures to reduce or prevent diseases or discourage the spread of diseases. Specifically, health policies are geared toward enhancing healthcare quality (e.g., reducing medical errors), reducing healthcare costs, or improving healthcare access. The purpose of health policy is to develop a system to enhance public health. The Centers for Medicare and Medicaid, Centers for Disease Control and Prevention, Veterans Administration, Health Resources and Service Administration, Indian Health Services, The Food and Drug Administration, and the Occupational Health and Safety Administration develop and enforce policies at the federal level. Other entities that develop and enforce health and safety standards include state health departments, insurance agencies, and environmental agencies (Ginter, Duncan, & Swayne, 2015).

The current health care regulatory structure is fragmented. Health care is regulated by the federal, local, and state governments as well as private organizations, thus making coordination difficult. One of the problems with health law involves tension over control between federal, state, and local governments. Although day-to-day governance of activities is usually done at the state level, the federal government has sovereign control. The state licenses and manages healthcare players, such as physicians, hospitals, and insurance companies, with the federal government again having supreme authority. Other entities under state and local control include public health programs, such as sanitation, restaurant inspections, and investigations of epidemics, while the federal government controls organizations such as the CDC and HRSA. Today healthcare professions among others are governed by their own authority. For example, the American Medical Association governs physicians, and the American Nursing Association governs and licenses the profession of nursing. Control at all levels of government serve as a system of checks and balances preventing any one level from gaining too much power. In addition, this type of control makes provision for collaboration between the regulatory agencies (Field, 2008).

Stop and Apply

Earlier in this chapter, you made a list of things that went wrong with Mr. Rodriquez's code. You were asked to devise a plan to reduce the likelihood of these issues from happening in the future. Think about this---as a manager, you have just engaged in strategy formulation. Give yourself a pat on the back. Now think in terms of implementation and evaluation and whether or not you need to put a policy into place at the hospice center to improve performance.

2.7 CONCLUSION

Healthcare managers inform decisions at all levels of the organization. These managers must possess specific skills and knowledge to perform management functions of planning, organizing, staffing, directing, and making decisions. The manager's ability to direct teams to formulate, implement, and evaluate strategic plans for the organization is critical to its success. They should be forward thinking in planning what needs to be done to give the organization greater market share and a competitive advantage among their competitors. Another important management function is acquiring and retaining talent for the organization and building leaders within it. Understanding the internal and external environments of an organization helps managers make informed decisions while also implementing and evaluating strategic plans. It is crucial that managers absorb knowledge about the external environment and understand the role that this information plays in health policies. These policies are instituted by local, state, and federal regulatory bodies that have a direct relationship with the delivery of healthcare by healthcare organizations. Leading an organization requires an awareness and comprehension of the correlation between health policy and reduction of risk and how policy can be used to improve the quality of care provided by the organization, which increases customer satisfaction.

2.8 KEY POINTS

- Many levels of leadership exist, including administrators, top executives, managers, and such front-line workers as housekeepers, nutrition staff, healthcare workers, social workers, nurses, laboratory technicians, and x-ray technicians.

- Several principles are used in the management process, such as planning, organizing, staffing, controlling, decision making, and directing.

- Healthcare managers possess a substantial role in ensuring the scope, complexity, and dynamics of individual performances of tasks so that they are carried out appropriately in health care organizations.

- Talent management focuses on "agility, customized solutions, letting go of control, and finding the sustainability sweet spot."

- Acquiring, retaining, and engaging skilled talent improves the performance of the organization through strategic management and planning, which is initiated by the Board of Directors or the CEO of the organization.

- Understanding how an organization performs directly relates to meeting the strategic goals and objectives set by the organization that lead to the attainment of the organization's mission and vision.

- Performance management requires monitoring through dashboards and scorecards to determine what and if progress is being made.

- Teamwork is required to complete tasks and projects for the organization and/or resolve issues that will lead to an improvement in the organization's performance.

- Strategy is a thoroughly devised plan to ensure a specific set of goals and objectives are achieved.

- Implementation of the strategic plan involves putting the organization's strategy into practice. In other words, implementation begins as a means for the organization to engage in a step by step process that accomplishes the goals and objectives within the strategic plan.

- Monitoring keeps managers and supervisors up to date with changes in the external and internal environments related to the organization's strategic performance or preferences so that the working strategy can be adjusted as needed.

- A strategic alliance is the establishment of a long-term relationship between two or more organizations or groups that have developed mutually beneficial goals or needs but do not relinquish their independent functions.

- Alliances are usually formed based on uncertainties within the environment.

- Organizational policies are rules or laws that are constructed from the organization's mission and vision to provide structure to health behavior, governance, and accountability.

- In order to develop effective new policies within the healthcare environment, managers and employees must thoroughly understand the industry's specific challenges while using critical thinking to solve problems.

- Healthcare is governed by local, state, and federal guidelines (and laws and policies). Many of these policies are developed as measures to reduce, prevent, and discourage the spread of diseases.

2.9 KEY TERMS

Healthcare management, strategic management, talent acquisition, health policy, management functions, shaping successors, intrinsic and extrinsic rewards, team building, teamwork

2.10 QUESTIONS FOR REVIEW AND DISCUSSION

1. Distinguish the difference between healthcare management and health care managers.
2. Describe the functions carried out by health care managers.
3. What is the healthcare manager's role in ensuring high performance within an organization?
4. Why is it important for employees to be motivated?
5. Explain extrinsic and intrinsic rewards. Which is more important?
6. Why is it important to have complete and current organizational policies?

2.11 REFERENCES

Al Shamsi, Saeed Ali Obaid, Christopher Dixon, Chowdhury Golam Hossan, and Marina Papanastassiou. 2015. "Coaching Constructs and Leadership Development at an Oil and Gas Company in the United Arab Emirates." Journal of Competitiveness Studies 23 (1/2): 13. https://ezproxy.mga.edu/login?url=http://search.ebscohost.com/login.aspx?direct=true&db=aqh&AN=112289254&site=eds-live&scope=site.

Buchbinder, S. & Shanks, N. (2017). *Introduction to Healthcare Management*, 3rd ed., Burlington, MA: Jones & Bartlett

Chhabra, N.L., and Aparna, M. 2008. "Talent Management and Employer Branding: Retention Battle Strategies." ICFAI Journal of Management Research 7 (11): 50–61. https://ezproxy.mga.edu/login?url=http://search.ebscohost.com/login.aspx?direct=true&db=bth&AN=35765718&site=eds-live&scope=site.

Claus, Lisbeth. 2019. "HR Disruption—Time Already to Reinvent Talent Management." BRQ Business Research Quarterly 22 (3): 207–15. doi:10.1016/j.brq.2019.04.002.

Cunningham, J. Barton. 1979. "The Management System: Its Functions and Processes." Management Science 25 (7): 657–70. doi:10.1287/mnsc.25.7.657.

Dubois, C., Singh, D. "From staff-mix to skill-mix and beyond: towards a systemic approach to health workforce management." Human Resource Health 7, 87 (2009). https://doi.org/10.1186/1478-4491-7-87

Embertson, Marl K. 2006. "The Importance of Middle Managers in Healthcare Organizations." Journal of Healthcare Management 51 (4): 223. doi:10.1097/00115514-200607000-00005.

Southern California Injury Prevention Research Center (SCIPRC), (2018). *A Guidebook to Strategy Evaluation: Evaluating Your City's Approach to Community Safety and Youth Violence Prevention*. Retrieved October 3, 2019, from http://www.ph.ucla.edu/sciprc/pdf/Evaluation_Guidebook_July08.pdf

Fajčíková, Adéla, Hana Urbancová, and Martina Fejfarová. 2018. "New Trends in the Recruitment of Employees in Czech Ict Organizations." Scientific Papers of the University of Pardubice. Series D, Faculty of Economics & Administration 25 (43): 39–49. https://ezproxy.mga.edu/login?url=http://search.ebscohost.com/login.aspx?direct=true&db=a9h&AN=132031637&site=eds-live&scope=site.

Field, R. (2008). "Why Is Health Care Regulation So Complex?" Pharmacy & Therapeutics. 33(10). Retrieved from https://www.ptcommunity.com/system/files/pdf/ptj3310607.pdf

Gafà, M., A. Fenech, C. Scerri, and D. Price. 2005. "Teamwork in Healthcare Organizations." Pharmacy Education 5 (2): 113–19. doi:10.1080/15602210500174474.

Griner, P. (n.d.) Mutiny. Retrieved from http://www.ihi.org/education/IHIOpenSchool/resources/Pages/Activities/Mutiny.aspx

Grupe, Fritz H., Simon Jooste, and Nilesh Patel. 2003. "Passing the Baton: Helping Your

Successor to Succeed." Information Systems Management 20 (2): 19. doi:10.1201/107 8/43204.20.2.20030301/41466.4.

Kotera, Yasuhiro1, Y.Kotera@derby.ac.uk, Prateek1 Adhikari, and William1 Van Gordon. 2018. "Motivation Types and Mental Health of UK Hospitality Workers." International Journal of Mental Health & Addiction 16 (3): 751–63. doi:10.1007/ s11469-018-9874-z.

Krajcovicova, K.; Caganova, D.; & Cambal, M., (2012). "Key Managerial Competencies and Competency Models in Industrial Enterprises." Annals of DAAAM for 2012 & Proceedings of the 23rd International DAAAM Symposium, 23(1). Retrieved September 26, 2019, from https://pdfs.semanticscholar.org/2388/ ac2160d872a1ede8b9d700dea2c63b3b01b4.pdf

Lee, Thomas H. 2016. "Teamwork: The Competitive Differentiator for the New Marketplace." Hfm (Healthcare Financial Management) 70 (12): 1–4. https:// ezproxy.mga.edu/login?url=http://search.ebscohost.com/login.aspx?direct=true&db =fth&AN=120651240&site=eds-live&scope=site.

Levesque, Laurie L. 2005. "Opportunistic Hiring and Employee Fit." Human Resource Management 44 (3): 301–17. doi:10.1002/hrm.20072.

Lindsay, S., Jack, G., and Ambrosini, V.. 2018. "A Critical Diversity Framework to Better Educate Students About Strategy Implementation." Academy of Management Learning & Education 17 (3): 241–58. doi:10.5465/amle.2017.0150.

Longest, B. B. Jr. 2012. "Management Challenges at the Intersection of Public Policy Environments and Strategic Decision Making in Public Hospitals." Journal of Health and Human Services Administration 35 (2): 207. https://ezproxy.mga.edu/ login?url=http://search.ebscohost.com/login.aspx?direct=true&db=edsjsr&AN=edsj sr.41709983&site=eds-live&scope=site.

Marshall, D. (2107). "Differences between and administrator and executive job title." Retrieved March 11, 2020 from https://careertrend.com/difference-between- executive-director-administrator-job-title-35384.html

McConnell, C.R. (2018). *Management Skills for the New Health Care Supervisor*. 7th ed. Burlington, MA: Jones and Bartlett Learning.

Mckinnies, Richard, Sandra Collins, Sandra Watts, and Cristian Lieneck. 2016. "Employee Incentives in Healthcare: An Eight Year Comparison." Radiology Management 38 (5): 43–48. https://ezproxy.mga.edu/login?url=http://search. ebscohost.com/login.aspx?direct=true&db=mnh&AN=30726598&site=eds- live&scope=site.

MacQueen, I. T., Maggard-Gibbons, M., Capra, G., Raaen, L., Ulloa, J. G., Shekelle, P. G., Miake-Lye, I., Beroes, J. M., & Hempel, S. (2018). "Recruiting Rural Healthcare Providers Today: a Systematic Review of Training Program Success and Determinants of Geographic Choices." Journal of general internal medicine, 33(2), 191–199. https://doi.org/10.1007/s11606-017-4210-z

Millman, R.W. 1962. "A General Systems Approach to the Analysis of Managerial

Functions." Academy of Management Proceedings (00650668), December, 133–38. doi:10.5465/AMBPP.1962.5068287.

Moseley, G.B. (2018). *Managing Health Care Business Strategy*. 2nd ed. Burlington, MA: Jones and Bartlett Learning.

Odom, Curtis L., Curtis.odom@prescientstrategists.com. 2013. "Hiring the Best Candidate Not the Best Resume." Financial Executive 29 (2): 61–63. https://ezproxy. mga.edu/login?url=http://search.ebscohost.com/login.aspx?direct=true&db=bft&A N=85919994&site=eds-live&scope=site.

Ordenes, P. (2018). "Strategy Levels and How To Apply Them In Your Business." Retrieved October 2, 2019, from https://www.executestrategy.net/blog/strategy-levels

ORS, (2017). Health care Services. Oregon Legislature. Retrieved September 27, 2019 from, https://www.oregonlaws.org/glossary/definition/health_care_services

Peters, Dawn E., Susan A. Casale, Michele Y. Halyard, Keith A. Frey, Brian E. Bunkers, and Suzanne L. Caubet. 2014. "The Evolution of Leadership: A Perspective from Mayo Clinic." Physician Executive 40 (3): 24–32.

Prakash B. (2010). "Patient satisfaction." Journal of cutaneous and aesthetic surgery, 3(3), 151–155. https://doi.org/10.4103/0974-2077.74491

Schultz, Frank C., and Shoma Pal. 2004. "Who Should Lead a Healthcare Organization: MDs or MBAs?" Journal of Healthcare Management 49 (2): 103. doi:10.1097/00115514-200403000-00007.

Susan D. Baker, Christopher J. Mathis, and Susan Stites-Doe. 2011. "An Exploratory Study Investigating Leader and Follower Characteristics at U.S. Healthcare Organizations." Journal of Managerial Issues 23 (3): 341. https://search.ebscohost. com/login.aspx?direct=true&AuthType=ip,shib&db=edsjsr&AN=edsjsr.23209120&si te=eds-live&scope=site.

Szwarcbart, Bernardo. 2013. "Talent Attraction and the Technology Challenge." Workforce Solutions Review 4 (4): 36–37. https://ezproxy.mga.edu/ login?url=http://search.ebscohost.com/login.aspx?direct=true&db=bth&AN=915972 65&site=eds-live&scope=site.

3 HEALTHCARE TECHNOLOGY AND INFORMATION STRATEGIES

3.1 LEARNING OBJECTIVES

- To examine the meaning and role of information technology in healthcare organizations
- To investigate factors influencing the establishment, distribution, and utilization of technology
- To discuss information systems unique to healthcare organizations
- To describe various types of information technology relative to patient information
- To analyze the future directions of information technology in healthcare

3.2 INTRODUCTION

Technology is transforming the healthcare environment. Healthcare consumers and healthcare professionals rely on technology in healthcare for reference, diagnosis, treatment, surgery, enhancing patient care coordination, using the electronic health record, etc., all of which has led to increased demand and usage. Technology integration has changed how medical services are organized and delivered. One of the major improvements is the institution of the electronic medical or health record in all healthcare organizations including private physician's practices. Although technology is useful, it has raised some social and ethical concerns. This chapter explores various categories encompassing the diffusion of information technology in healthcare.

3.3 INFORMATION SYSTEMS

3.3.1 Information Systems in Healthcare Organizations

In Chapter 1, we learned about health and healthcare. We defined health as a state of well-being wherein a person uses social, spiritual, mental, and physical ability to function in various situations. Health care was defined as the deeds or acts between the healthcare provider and the patient to maintain or improve the patient's health status. Many health care organizations abide by joint commission standards that focus on processes within the organization that are essential to delivering safe, high quality patient care. This criteria can be met by ensuring that patients receive quality healthcare services through the institution of such measures as ensuring patient safety, ensuring that care is patient centered, coordinating care amongst caregivers, promoting effective prevention and treatment measures, using best practices, maintaining efficiency, and increasing access to healthcare (Joshi, Ransom, Nash, & Ransom, 2014). The joint commission has developed a set of national patient safety goals specific to various health care organizations, such as ambulatory care, behavioral health, hospitals, home care, office-based surgery, and nursing center care. These objectives include but are not limited to correctly identifying patients, safely using medications, preventing infections, preventing mistakes in surgery, etc. (The Joint Commission, 2020). What happens when something goes wrong in the provision of health care? Health care mistakes and medical errors lead to poor health care outcomes, which increases length of stay and even deaths. They also contribute to rising healthcare costs in the U.S. (Fichman, Kohli, & Krishnan, 2011). The Institute of Medicine (IOM) defines medical errors as incomplete actions or using the wrong plan to achieve a goal. Due to how serious healthcare mistakes and medical errors are, the IOM issued a series of reports. Two of these reports, issued in 1999, are called, *To Err is Human* and *Crossing the Quality Chasm*. According to the first piece, between 44,000 and 98,000 medical errors occur each year, costing between $17 billion and $29 billion. The following medical errors can occur in the healthcare setting: adverse drug events and improper transfusions, surgical injuries and wrong-site surgery, suicides, restraint-related injuries or death, falls, burns, pressure ulcers, and mistaken patient identities. These errors occur as a result of faulty systems, processes, and conditions that lead people to make mistakes or fail to prevent them (IOM, 1999). *Crossing the Quality Chasm* focuses on redesigning the health care system in this country so that all Americans can receive state-of-the art quality health care. One of the steps identified in effecting change in healthcare delivery is instituting information technology through patient-specific clinical information systems (IOM, 2001).

Stop and Apply

Have you or anyone you know been affected by a medical error? How did this situation make you or your loved one feel? How could you or your loved one have been treated differently?

Information systems are integrated sets of components for collecting, storing, and processing data. These systems also provide information, knowledge, and digital products to users. Hardware, software, data, people, and processes make up the components of the overarching system. The system's hardware refers to any part that can be touched, such as computers, keyboards, disk drives, iPads, and flash drives. **Software** tells the hardware what to do. **Data** is a directory of facts that have been organized and grouped into a database for a specific purpose. **People** in information systems include help desk workers, systems analysts, programmers and chief information officers. **Process** refers to the series of steps taken to achieve a goal (Bourgeois & Bourgeois, 2019). Before we delve into information systems, we need to have a clear understanding of clinical, health, and medical informatics, which are closely related. The purpose of clinical informatics is to manage and organize information better. Health informatics include using information technology to make delivering healthcare services more consistent, efficient, and accurate. Medical informatics is using information technology in healthcare. The schema below (Figure 3.2) depicts clinical, health, and medical informatics as they coexist and work together. The key is to integrate healthcare and information technology. Clinical, health, and medical informatics center on managing and organizing information and technology to improve health care services and outcomes.

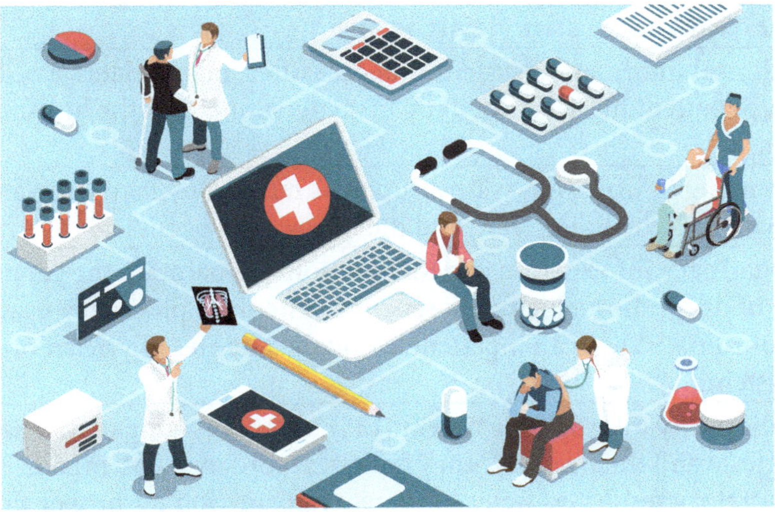

Figure 3.1: Information System

Source: 123rf.com
Attribution: User "aurielaki"
License: aurielaki © 123rf.com. Used with permission.

Computers in healthcare assist healthcare professionals achieve the following purposes: diagnosing, monitoring and treating patients; informing, supporting, and enhancing education, research, and pharmacy; and complete administrative tasks such as office managing, scheduling, and accounting. Health information systems is an umbrella term that encompasses how computers are used to improve managing and organizing patients' data and their information related to finance, pharmacy, laboratory results, and radiology outcomes (Burke & Weill, 2019). This chapter discusses the various systems that are used in healthcare. Many of them overlap in relation to the services they can provide to healthcare professionals.

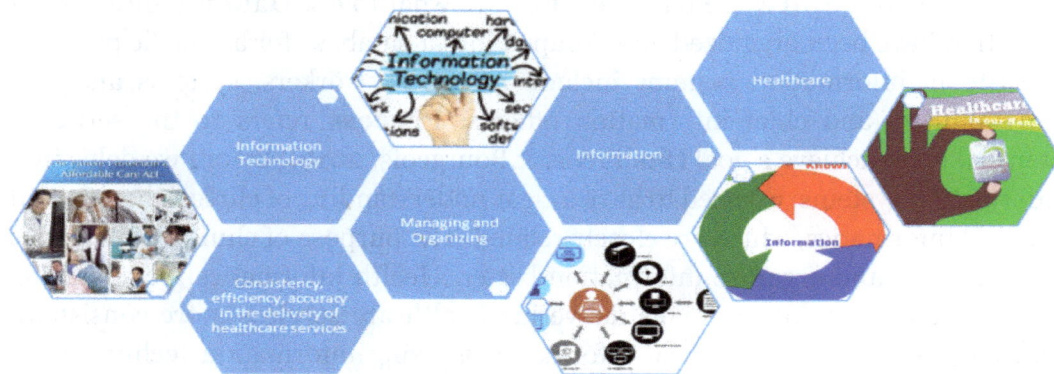

Figure 3.2: Schema of Clinical, Health, and Medical Informatics

Source: Original Work
Attribution: Dorothy Howell
License: CC BY-SA 4.0

Table 3.1 Computers in Healthcare
CIS: The clinical information system collects, stores, manipulates, and ensures availability of patient information to medical personnel and the healthcare delivery process
NIS: The nursing information system supports nursing by managing and improving charting, scheduling staff, and the integration of clinical information.
PIS: The pharmacy information system functions to maintain the supply and organization of drugs through either a separate system for pharmacy usage only, or it can be coordinated with an inpatient hospital computer physician order entry (CPOE) system.
LIS: The laboratory information system (LIS) uses computers to manage patients' laboratory tests and their results. They collect, record, present, organize, and archive laboratory results, as well as generate information for proper financial management of the laboratory.

PACS: The picture archiving and communication system (PACS) manages digital images and allows for immediate visualization to the computer monitor and their transport to shared networks regardless of their location.
FIS: The financial information system (FIS) in conjunction with the decision support system is used at the administrative level to enhance financial planning and decision-making and improve outcomes for the organization.

Source: Original Work
Attribution: Dorothy Howell
License: CC BY-SA 4.0

3.3.2 Clinical Information Systems (CIS)

The clinical information system requires using computers to manage clinical information, such as the patient's history (Burke & Weill, 2019). The clinical information system (CIS) collects, stores, manipulates, and ensures patient information so that it is available to medical personnel and the healthcare delivery process in its most updated form. It stores patients' illness histories, interactions with care providers, and healthcare outcomes. The system can also network with the computers in other departments, such as pathology and radiology, and pulls all patient related information into an electronic patient record, which clinicians can see at the patient's bedside. Furthermore, it improves patient care outcomes as it aids in the communication between healthcare professionals caring for the patient, signals other departments, such as radiology or the lab, that the patient needs x-rays or bloodwork, among completing other tasks. CIS allows healthcare professionals to make better decisions regarding the patient's care, encourages quality improvement, and makes it easier to conduct clinical research. Without a CIS, healthcare professionals are left to collect patient information using a paper chart. Therefore, it saves time, decreases and contains costs, and reduces errors (Or, Dolton, & Tan, 2014). The electronic medical record is an example of a clinical information system.

3.3.3 Nursing Information Systems (NIS)

The nursing information system (NIS) is similar in function to the clinical information system. The nursing information system supports nursing by managing and improving charting, scheduling staff, and integrating clinical information. This system's goal is to minimize paperwork and improve care given to patients (Burke & Weill, 2019). The nursing information system (NIS) can be mobile so that nurses can use it for documentation purposes in a patient's room. NIS reduces redundancy or duplication in documentation and automatic data processing, such as automatic visualized vital signs, nursing diagnosis accompanied by disease diagnosis, and ultimately patient care outcomes (Lee, Sun, Kou, & Yeh, 2017). Although these systems are beneficial, they also have a few drawbacks that nurses consistently voice concerns about. Among these complaints include the fact that nurses must stand to enter information in the system, often in the hallway or in the patient's room, which can violate HIPAA recommendations to keep patient information safe. Nurses are not able to use the system when handing over the patient to the on-coming nurse. Instead, the nurse must use a paper reporting system. In addition, it is difficult for the NIS to summarize patient information if the patient is being admitted or discharged. Nurses also report that the NIS does not support their duties or workflow (Cheng, Chan, Chen, & Guo, 2019).

3.3.4 Pharmacy Information Systems (PIS)

The pharmacy information system (PIS) can be used within the hospital setting (inpatient) or in community-based settings (outpatient). A pharmacy information system (PIS) functions by maintaining drug supply and organization through either a separate system for pharmacy use only or coordination with an inpatient hospital computer physician order entry (CPOE) system. A PIS paired with a CPOE allows for an easier transfer of information. This system monitors a patient's drug allergies and interactions. In addition, the PIS determines if the appropriate dosage has been given based on the patient's age, weight and other physiological factors. It can also detect when a patient's prescription needs to be refilled and make labels based on the prescriptions to inform the patient when and how to take the medication. The PIS is also helpful when functioning within the pharmacy due to the system's ability to track inventory and create drug profiles for each patient. It also warns pharmacists against medication errors by sending alert messages and warnings. In addition, the PIS will reject filling a medication if it detects that the drug may be a potential error for the patient (El. Mahalli, El-Khafif, & Yamani, 2016). The PIS generates reports related to medication usage patterns, drug costs, purchases, and dispensations. This system can interact with the CIS for access to patient information and the financial information system (FIS) for billing purposes (Burke & Weill, 2019).

3.3.5 Laboratory Information System (LIS)

The laboratory information system (LIS) uses computers to manage patients' laboratory tests and results. They collect, record, present, organize, and archive laboratory results, as well as generate information for the laboratory's proper financial management (Sepulveda & Young, 2013). The following functions are included in a laboratory information system:

1. Patient management, including admission date, admitting physician, ordering department, specimen type, etc.
2. Patient data tracking
3. Decision support, including lab order comparisons with their respective ICD-9 codes
4. Standard test ordering and specimen tracking

5. Test ordering for point-of-care, molecular, and genetic testing
6. Quality assurance
7. Workload and management reporting
8. Analytical reporting
9. Workflow management
10. Billing
11. Third-party software integration

The LIS has supported public health institutions (like hospitals and clinics) by managing and reporting critical data concerning "the status of infections, immunology, and care and treatment status of patients." Some laboratory information systems interface with a patient's electronic health record to send results automatically. At other times, results are mailed or faxed to the physician for entry into the patient's record (Burke & Weill, 2019).

3.3.6 Radiology Information Systems (RIS)

The radiology information system (RIS) manages a patient's visit to the radiology department. It can be used to register, schedule appointments, and report test results. Radiology information systems allow healthcare professionals to integrate multiple functions into one comprehensive system. It reduces redundancy and provides access to crucial patient data to make decisions regarding patient care easier. It is efficient and thereby saves time and money. The system allows better patient care coordination between all the patient's caregivers. However, to send this information electronically, the system must interface with the patient's electronic health record (Burke & Weill, 2019).

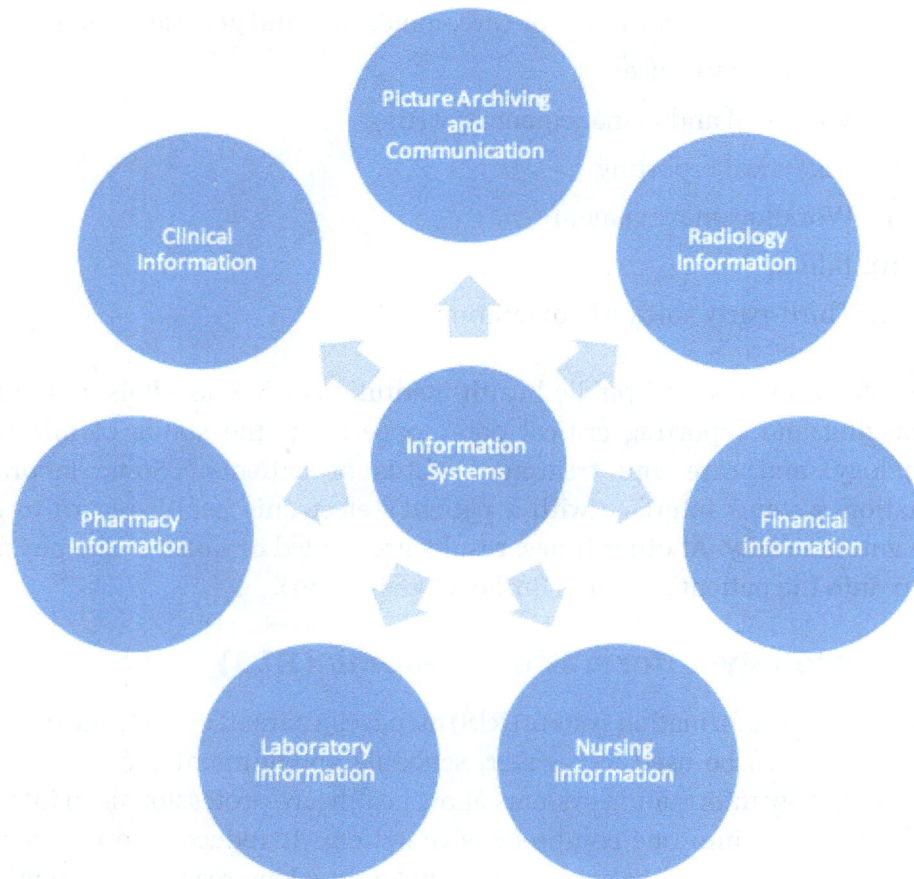

Figure 3.3: Information Systems

Source: Original Work
Attribution: Dorothy Howell
License: CC BY-SA 4.0

3.3.7 Picture Archiving and Communication System (PACS)

The picture archiving and communication system (PACS) manages digital images, allows for immediate visualization to the computer monitor, and provides imaging transportation to shared networks regardless of their location. These systems are used in radiology, nuclear medicine, cardiology, pathology, oncology, dermatology, etc. Images from this system allow for analysis, diagnosis, and patient treatment. This system replaces hard copy films, thereby allowing physicians to obtain remote access of digital images. The system interfaces with RIS and the electronic health record (EHR) (Burke & Weill, 2019).

3.3.8 Financial Information Systems (FIS)

Thus far we have discussed information systems used in providing patient care. The financial information system (FIS), in conjunction with the decision support system, is used at the administrative level to enhance financial planning and decision-making and improve outcomes for the organization. This type of system is associated with payroll; accounting, such as patient charges; accounts payable; accounts receivable; general ledger and assets; claims; and contract management (Burke & Weill, 2019). It produces data related to operating and capital, budgets and reports, accounting reports, and estimating cash flow. If you have received healthcare services, you may receive a bill after the insurance company has submitted their share of the payment for services rendered on your behalf.

3.3.9 Information Technology in Healthcare Organizations

Now that you have a picture of how information systems are used in healthcare, let's review how information systems differ from information technology (IT). Information systems and information technology differ in that information systems integrate people, technology, and processes related to information. Information technology is the design and implementation of information, or data, within the information system. Information technology refers to improving computer literacy and using computers and communication networks in healthcare by transforming data into useful information (Fichman, Kohli, & Krishnan, 2011). Data requirements, such as what is needed, how to get it, and how to report it to end users, are information technology components. End users can be any of the following: health care professionals, managers, payers, patients, researchers, or governmental agencies. Most healthcare organizations have an IT department.

Health care IT includes many of the systems described in the previous section. Information technology is applied to health care organizations in three ways: clinical information systems, administrative information systems, and decision support systems. As per our previous discussion, clinical information systems include methods of processing, storing, and retrieving information related to delivering healthcare. Examples of these functions include the electronic health record, which allows healthcare providers to deliver quality patient care, and computerized physician order entry, which gives healthcare providers the ability to transmit orders from the patient's bedside. Administrative information systems support financial and administrative activities, such as payroll, billing, and budgeting. Decision support systems provide information and analytical tools to aid managers and clinicians in making better decisions pertinent to patient care (Shi & Singh, 2015). Computerized healthcare information systems that interface with other information systems will continue to improve medical care and public health, lower costs, increase efficiency, reduce errors and improve patient satisfaction, while also optimizing reimbursement for ambulatory and inpatient healthcare providers. The following discussion indicates the specific types of information technology used in healthcare.

3.3.10 eHealth and mHealth

Electronic health (eHealth) is a type of information technology that encompasses all forms of electronic health care delivered over the internet (Shi & Singh, 2015).

Gunther Eysenbach, editor of the *Journal of Medical Internet Research*, describes eHealth as health services and information delivered or enhanced through the internet and related technologies. Examples of such devices include computers, mobile phones, and satellite communications. Mobile health (mHealth) uses such wireless communication devices as smart phones or portable devices in healthcare. Both eHealth and mHealth embody various healthcare services, including electronic prescribing, medical records, and text messages reminding patients about medications (Moss, Süle, & Kohl, 2019).

3.3.11 Telemedicine and Telehealth

Telemedicine refers to a health care professional's use of telecommunications technology to diagnose patient conditions and provide patient care from a distance. Telemedicine requires no face-to-face visits. This type of medicine is very important for individuals who live in rural areas and require healthcare access; about 19% of the total United States population falls into this category (CDC 2019). Patients living in these areas usually have access to small hospitals. However, the facility may be 15-20 miles away from them. For this reason, it is paramount for the hospitals to use telemedicine that allows patients in rural areas to receive quality care. In addition, those who use telehealth resources experience lower health care costs due to fewer readmissions and emergency room visits. Furthermore, these patients can be monitored from their homes, which reduces the number of visits to health care practitioners (CDC, 2019).

Telemedicine and telehealth are accomplished using the internet and videoconferencing, wherein the patient and physician talk to each other through a computer or other audio-visual link. They store-and-forward imaging, allowing the patient's recorded health history to be sent electronically to a health care specialist or practitioner. Telemedicine and telehealth are also accomplished through streaming media as well as terrestrial and wireless communications. The patient's health and medical data can be monitored from any location by their health care provider (Shi & Singh, 2015). For example, a health care provider can view the patient's data from their residence while the patient is in the hospital. The patient can also receive text messages and email notifications regarding their health care or disease outbreaks, such as the Coronavirus. Additionally, patients can access their health information from their home by filling out account information on the healthcare facility's website. Several types of specialized medical services can be provided using telemedicine, such as teleradiology (transmitting x-rays and scans), telepathology (using video microscopes to view tissue), telesurgery (using robots to perform surgery from a distance), and providing consultations by healthcare specialists. Telemedicine can occur in real time through interactive videoconferencing, or it can allow information to be viewed later due to store-and-forward features. Telehealth goes beyond telemedicine in that it encompasses education, research, administrative, and clinical applications using various types of healthcare professionals (Shi & Singh, 2015).

3.3.12 E-prescribing

Porterfield et. al (2014) describes electronic prescribing (e-prescribing or e-Rx) as electronically sending a patient's prescription to their pharmacy via their healthcare provider. The e-prescribing system is accessed through the patient's electronic health record. It replaces the patient's paper based or faxed copied prescription. The computer is used to generate, transmit, and fill the prescription. The system allows the provider access to patient allergies and medication history. This knowledge reduces medication prescription errors and helps the healthcare provider make better clinical decisions. Here is an example of how this system works. Ann was seen by her primary care physician with complaints of frequent urination, pain, and burning with urination. She was diagnosed with a urinary tract infection and prescribed antibiotics. The physician implemented electronic prescribing and forwarded Ann's prescription to her preferred pharmacy. Ann was directed to go to the pharmacy to pick up her medication. Electronic prescriptions are accurate and can be sent with minimal errors, thereby being easily understood by the pharmacist. The system also reduces issues with substance abuse and misusing controlled substance prescriptions by limiting drug and doctor shopping, as well as cracking down on physicians who prescribe drugs for non-medical purposes. Drug diversion is a medical and legal concept involving the transfer of any legally prescribed controlled substance from the individual for whom it was prescribed to another person for any illicit use. An example would include a healthcare provider's stealing prescription medicines or such controlled substances as opioids for their own use (CDC, 2019). Sansone & Sansone (2012) describe doctor shopping as seeing multiple treatment providers, either during a single illness episode or to procure prescription medications unlawfully. In addition, prescriptions can be easily renewed or alternate medications ordered if the current one is ineffective. With this system, patients can electronically access their prescriptions at the pharmacy and request refills. In the case that a prescription has no more refills, the pharmacy can send an alert to the patient's healthcare provider to renew the patient's prescription.

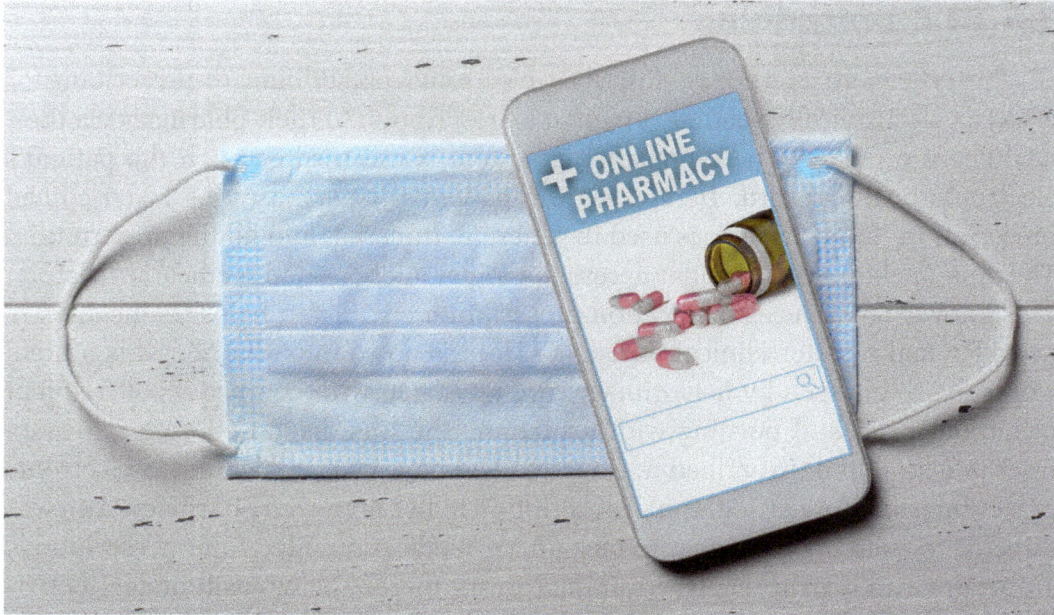

Figure 3.4: Electronic Prescriptions

Source: 123rf.com
Attribution: Andrey Mitrofanov
License: Andrey Mitrofanov © 123rf.com. Used with permission.

3.3.13 Analytics

Analytics are needed in healthcare organizations is due to healthcare's growth and complexity, rising healthcare costs, inefficiencient policies, and poor-quality services. Healthcare organizations are investing in and implementing various types of information technology systems to assist with these issues. The information technology systems generate vast sums of patient and other data that needs to be translated into meaningful use. Meaningful use refers to how healthcare providers use information technology through the EHR to improve patient care. There are 15 core objectives of meaningful use, such as maintaining the patient's active medication and allergy list, recording and charting vital signs, exchanging key clinical information between health care providers, and protecting the patient's information (Hamilton, 2013). Meaningful use is an important factor in adopting electronic health records for health care organizations and health information exchange. This task is where healthcare analytics can help. Healthcare analytics tools can capture, share, and aggregate patient data to be used by the organization to improve quality and lower care costs. Analytics can extract this data from information systems and assist managers in making decisions for the organization (Islam, Hasan, Wang, Germack, & Noor-E-Alam, 2018). Descriptive, operational, predictive, and prescriptive are the four types of analytics that will be explored in this chapter.

Descriptive analytics refer to how policies or programs that have already been implemented are reviewed to see if they are performing as planned, which is based on historical data. For example, how many patients were admitted to the hospital last week? This data can be obtained using simple statistical measures, such as counts or averages. Collecting a patient's personal data can help the health care practitioner determine how the patient's history will influence the patient's current treatment plan. Collecting historical data can also provide information to the organization on how well it is performing (Hagan, Kassivajjala, & Scalzi, 2019).

Diagnostic analytics (also based on historical data) are an extension of descriptive analytics as they provide information on why an event occurred. They also allow for further analysis of a situation. For example, what led to the patient's admission to the hospital (Usvyat & Long, 2019)?

Operational analytics answers the question, "where are we now?" In other words, what is our current admission rate? Healthcare managers can create dashboards using this data and provide feedback to subordinate staff (Hagan, Kassivajjala, & Scalzi, 2019). If the organization is not where it should be in reference to the provision of quality patient care, measures can be put into place to ensure the objectives are carried out.

Predictive analytics refer to the future of the organization and provide information to managers on what can be expected in the future. For example, which patients will have the highest risk of hospitalization next week? Historical and operational data can be used as inputs into the system to predict the future of an organization (Hagan, Kassivajjala, & Scalzi, 2019). From these predictions, the organizational managers can calculate risk scores for each patient and identify which patients may need additional attention (Usvyat & Long, 2019).

Prescriptive analytics pull from predictive analytics outputs to allow organizations the ability to create, test, and implement new or revised policies and procedures, and see their performance in real time (Hagan, Kassivajjala, & Scalzi, 2019). In other words, they provide information on what needs to be done in order to avoid negative predictions. For example, having a leukemia patient avoid contact with infected, or viral, individuals can reduce the patient's readmission to the hospital. Using prescriptive analytics can lead to better healthcare outcomes.

3.3.14 Patient Information

We have discussed how information systems and information technology are used in healthcare. The electronic medical record (EMR), EHR, mhealth, ehealth, telehealth, and telemedicine, as discussed throughout this chapter, require using patient information. The Agency for Healthcare, Research, and Quality, which supports research to help improve health care quality, describes patient information as demographic or other information about the patient, such as medical and surgical history, mental health history, or family history. Patient information, which is found in the patient's medical record, includes self-reported information from the patient along with physician's notes about the patient's presenting problems, diagnoses, and treatments. From the patient's medical record, health care providers can view the patient's health status over time. In addition, the medical record can enhance continuity and quality of care provided to the patient. Therefore, data entered into the patient's record must be accurate and complete.

Adopting the electronic health record has aided in providing accurate, complete information for healthcare organizations. The information technology systems and software applications imbedded within the EHR must be capable of communicating, exchanging data, and using the information that has been exchanged across the organization. For example, the laboratory, nursing, or pharmacy information systems must be able to communicate with the clinical information system so that pertinent patient information is shared when and where needed. The medical record can be a paper or electronic chart depending on the healthcare provider and its available resources (Abiy, Gashu, Asemaw, Mitiku, Fekadie, Abebaw ... & Tilahun, 2018).

3.3.15 The Paper Medical Record

Prior to implementing electronic medical records, health care practitioners recorded and stored self-reported patient information and clinical diagnostic notes on paper-based charts. Even today, some healthcare professionals continue to use these paper charts. According to Bendix (2018), 14% of physicians continue using paper charts because of implementation costs for electronic records, personal preference, impediments within the patient-physician relationship, and because they are not required for healthcare providers to complete their work effectively.

Paper chart advantages include ease of use without additional training, low maintenance, and low cost. Another advantage of paper medical records is that the form is customizable to each hospital or doctor's requirements with no technology required. These charts are available when the system goes down or when electricity is absent. This chart contains all files and data pertinent to the patient, such as blood pressure readings, labs, x-rays, medications, family history, etc.

Disadvantages for paper charts include the need for storage space and there being no way to replace charts if they are destroyed in fires or floods. They are time consuming, given the time required to document and find previous related entries. The data is prone to errors because it is handwritten. Inconsistent layout from one chart to another or from one practitioner to another is another issue. Paper records don't provide a method for audits or histories in reference to who made changes and when they were made (True North ITG, 2019)

3.3.16 The Personal Health Record

The Personal Health Record (PHR) is an electronic portal for patient information that can be accessed and maintained by the patient. An example of a device used for this purpose is one developed by Apple, as shown in in figure 3.6. Other companies, such as Deloitte's and the American Society of Health System Pharmacists, use this technology through the PDAs, iPads, iPhones or iPods. The PHR is connected through the internet to a secure medical practice website. With the PHR, patients can become interactive with their medical information and share it with others. Patients can schedule appointments, receive reminders, request medication refills, access lab and radiology results and ask questions concerning their health (Hamilton, 2013, p. 8). The PHR was introduced through the Meaningful Use (MU) Mandate supported by the HITECH Act. The PHR contains the patient's diagnoses, medications, immunizations, family medical histories, and provider contact information and can be maintained in any secure environment of the patient's choice. PHRs can include information from a variety of sources, including clinicians, home monitoring devices, and patients themselves (Healthit. gov, 2019). This type of system serves to enhance the patient's engagement with their care. Patients who have accessed their medical records have reported a broader knowledge base of their own health concerns, the ability to communicate more effectively with their physicians, initiating additional efforts to improve their health, and decreased utilization of healthcare services. PHRs can help make patients aware of their health conditions, which could initiate changes in their healthcare plan.

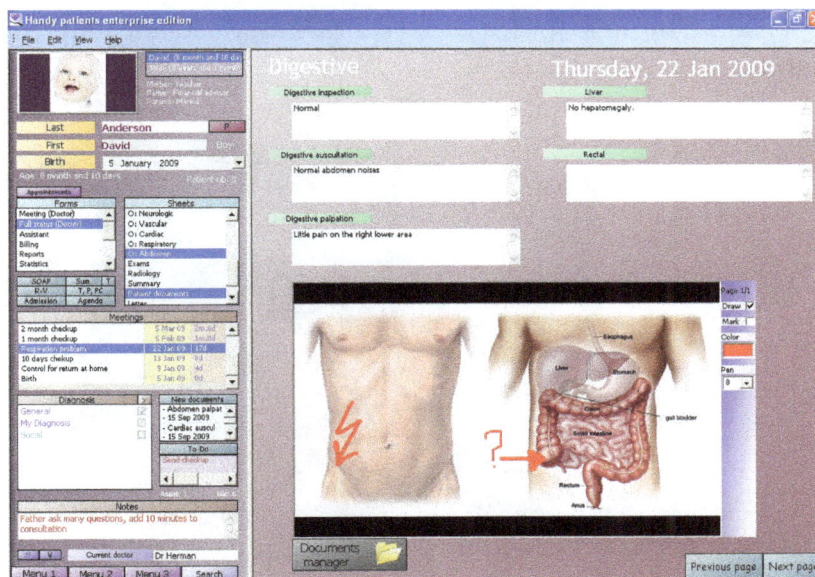

Figure 3.5: The Personal Health Record

Source: Wikimedia Commons
Attribution: User "DaCarpenther"
License: GNU General Public License

3.3.17 The Electronic Medical Record (EMR)

Electronic Medical Records (EMR) are real-time digital versions of the paper charts. Each facility can have an EMR for a patient. Health care practitioners and medical professionals and staff use the EMRs to document notes and information about the patient's condition, diagnosis and treatment. Patient data contained in the EMR allows health care providers to track data over time, practice preventive medicine, monitor patients, and improve health care quality (Healthit.gov,

2019). The EMR is maintained in the practitioner's office and must be printed and hand delivered, faxed, or emailed for it to be reviewed by another healthcare provider or member of the healthcare team. Because of this inconvenience, they are like paper records (Garrett & Seidman, 2011). In this respect, it is different from the EHR, in that the EHR can be accessed across facilities by any member of the healthcare team.

Adoption of the EMR has been slow because of the capital required to implement this type of system. Implementation is an ongoing process to maintain the system's effectiveness. The Health Information Technology for Economic and Clinical Health (HITECH) Act of 2009 directed grants and financial incentives to encourage hospitals and physicians into adopting the EMR (Shi & Singh, 2015). Healthcare practitioners were required to meet specific criteria beginning in 2011 to receive a bonus or incentive payment from the Centers for Medicare and Medicaid Services (CDC). These incentives ranged from $18,000-$44,000 over a five-year period or more than $63,000 over a six-year period (Hamilton, 2013). Physicians practicing in areas where there was a shortage of healthcare professionals would receive an additional 10% bonus. Physicians who had not adopted the EHR by 2015 were penalized by up to 3% for each year that they had not adopted the EMR (Worzala, 2009).

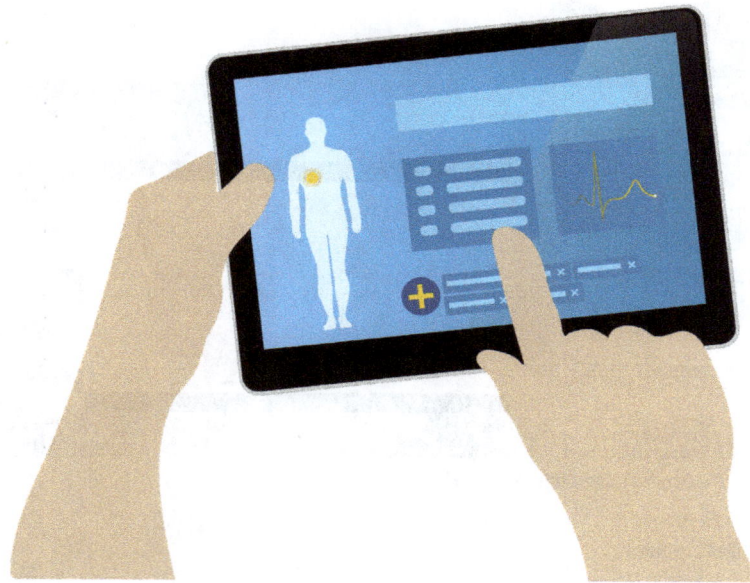

Figure 3.6: EMR

Source: Pixabay
Attribution: User "mcmurryjulie"
License: Pixabay License

3.3.18 The Electronic Health Record

The Electronic Health Record (EHR) is different from the EMR in that the EHR contains patient information from all health care clinicians who have provided care to the patient, whereas the EMR contains the patient's information from one facility. In other words, the EHR provides a look at the total health of the patient. The EHR can share information with other health care providers because of its ability to follow the patient electronically from one facility to another. Any clinicians taking care of the patient can access the patient's data because of its digital format (Healthit.gov, 2019). The EHR provides the following benefits. The patient's data can be seen by any clinician with a right to the information, even if the patient is unconscious. The patient can review their own information, such as lab results of blood pressure readings from a computer or mobile device as long as they have established an account with the facility. Finally, discharge instructions, prescriptions, follow-up care, lab, and other test results can be automatically transmitted to the patient's EHR to follow the patient as needed. The table below depicts the differences between the PHR, EHR, and EMR (PHR, 2008).

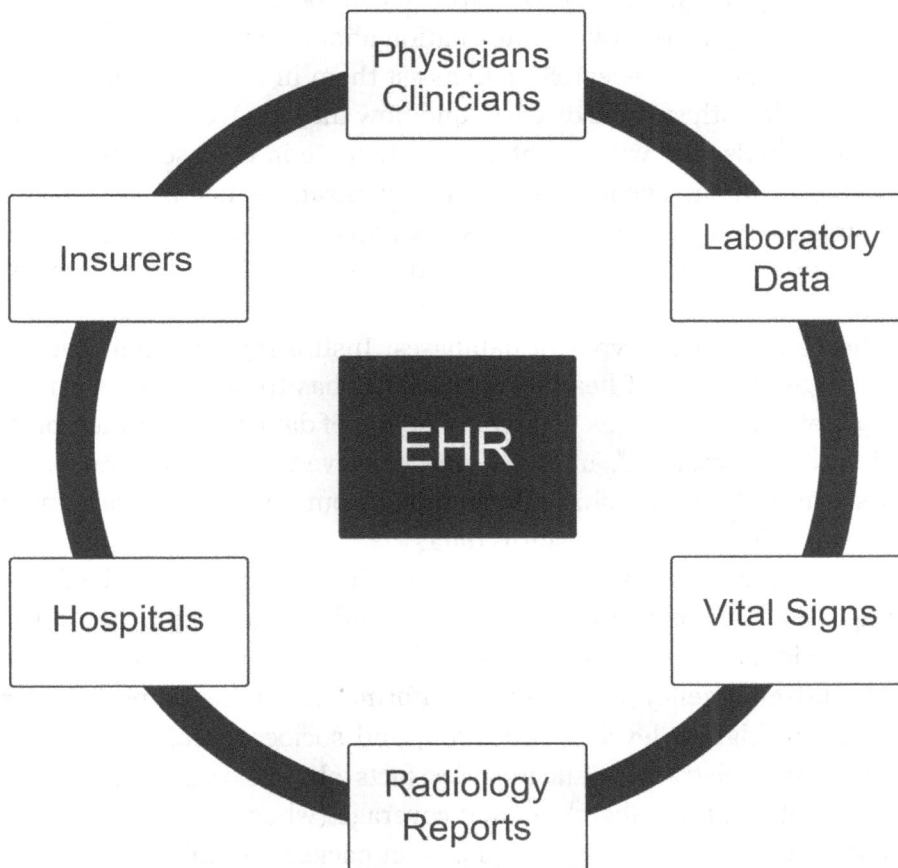

Figure 3.7: Electronic Health Record

Source: Original Work
Attribution: Corey Parson
License: CC BY-SA 4.0

Table 3.2 PHR, EMR, EHR		
PHR	EMR	EHR
The PHR includes electronic copies of information that patients have received from their providers and may include data they enter themselves.	The EMR contains the results of encounters between a health care professional and a patient which occur during episodes of patient care	The EHR integrates a person's multiple, physician-generated EMRs and their patient- generated and maintained PHR

Source: Original Work
Attribution: Dorothy Howell
License: CC BY-SA 4.0

3.3.19 Registries and Databases

According to the National Institute of Health (2019), information about specific diseases, diagnoses, or conditions can be found in a registry. The purpose of a registry is to provide information about certain health conditions to healthcare providers and researchers to assist them in tracking trends about the number of people with specific diseases and how they are treated. Registries also seek out individuals who will voluntarily participate in disease specific research studies. A government agency, nonprofit organization, health care facility, or private company can sponsor registries. Examples of registries include cancer, Alzheimer's prevention, congenital heart disease, cystic fibrosis, rare disease, death, etc.

Healthcare uses many types of databases. Instituting electronic records has generated large amounts of healthcare data that has to be stored. A database is defined by Merriam Webster as "a large collection of data in a computer, organized so that it can be expanded, updated, and retrieved rapidly for various uses." Databases contain demographic information about the patient, administrative data and health risks and health status data.

Demographic data consist of facts regarding the patient's personal information, such as age (or date of birth), gender, race and ethnic origin, marital status, address of residence, names of and other information about immediate family members, and emergency information. Information about employment status (and employer), highest level of education, and socioeconomic status may also be included. Administrative data includes facts about health insurance status, such as eligibility and membership, dual coverage (when relevant), and required copayments and deductibles for a given benefit package. Administrative data also includes the amount charged and paid for services provided.

Healthcare providers are identified using a unique system, perhaps with letters and numbers indicating the type of provider, practice, institution, and location. Health risk information indicates the behavior and lifestyle of a patient, such as tobacco and alcohol usage and facts about family history and genetic factors, such as cancer history. Health status (or health-related quality of life) is self-reported and reflects the level of physical, mental, emotional, cognitive, and social functioning. It also includes the patient's perception of their health status. Health status and quality-of-life measures are deemed as healthcare outcomes. Researchers and evaluators also use this information to analyze disease severity, patient demographics and other pertinent information (IOM, 1994).

3.3.20 Protecting Health Information

The U.S. Department of Health and Human Services provided an example of improperly disclosing patient information wherein a nurse and patient care assistant discussed a patient's AIDS/HIV diagnosis in the presence of other patients. The hospital administration discovered the incident and initiated disciplinary action against the employees; they were placed on leave. The patient care assistant resigned; the nurse received a written reprimand, probation, peer review proceedings, and HIPAA privacy training. The patient's family was awarded a monetary settlement (HHS.gov, n.d.)

As seen from the above incident, patient information in healthcare organizations is not exempt from security breaches, data spill, and data hacking. One of the concerns associated with the EMR is ensuring patient information is kept confidential and secure. Protecting patient information requires that healthcare managers ensure they have installed the latest security updates for their specific systems and that the patient health information is encrypted. Employees must be taught about HIPAA violations and measures put in place to prevent the patient's information from being compromised (Buchbinder & Shanks, (2107).

The U.S. Department of Health and Human Services established the privacy rule standards to address how organizations subject to the privacy rule should appropriately use and disclose individuals' health information. The department also created new criteria regarding individuals' privacy rights so that healthcare organizations and providers could understand and control how their health information was used (HHS.gov). The Health Insurance Portability and Accountability Act (HIPAA) of 1996 stipulates that only those individuals with a right to know can have access to a patient's personal or health information. This process was clearly breached in the incident above. Individuals with the right to know must be providing direct health care, operations, or reimbursement to the patient without disclosing personal information to unauthorized individuals (Shi & Singh, 2015).

A healthcare organization, also known as a "covered entity," may use patient information to treat, diagnose, or receive payment for services rendered. In addition, an organization can use patient information to support the following operating activities: quality assessment and improvement activities, competency related to credentialing and accreditation; planning for medical reviews or legal services, insurance functions, and business management or administrative activities, such as creating data sets or fundraising. Administrative concerns with this system revolve around patient literacy that may cause inaccurate information. Another concern is the potential for the patient to delete information concerning their condition. Providers are also apprehensive regarding whether the patient would be able to interpret and understand their treatment regimen without additional medical knowledge (Lester, et. al, 2016).

3.3.21 Innovation, Diffusion, and Utilization of Information Technology

In 1962, E.M. Rogers developed the Diffusion of Innovation Theory (DOI) to explain the adoption of information technology and how it is spread from one consumer, community, population, or social system to the next. The theory explains innovation as a different, unfamiliar, or new idea, process, product, technique, technology, or service that appeals to others, including healthcare consumers (Zhang, Yu, Yan, Ton, & Spil, 2015). Those who adopt innovative objects or policies possess specific characteristics as described here (Lamorte, 2019).

- Innovators - These people are risk takers who want to be the first to try or develop a new object or concept.

- Early Adopters - These are leaders who easily embrace opportunities for change and do not need information to convince them to change.

- Early Majority - These people are rarely leaders, but they do adopt new ideas based on evidence that the innovation is effective.

- Late Majority - These people do not like change and will only adopt an innovation after it has been tried by the majority.

- Laggards - These people are bound by tradition and quite conservative, therefore such individuals find it very difficult to adopt change.

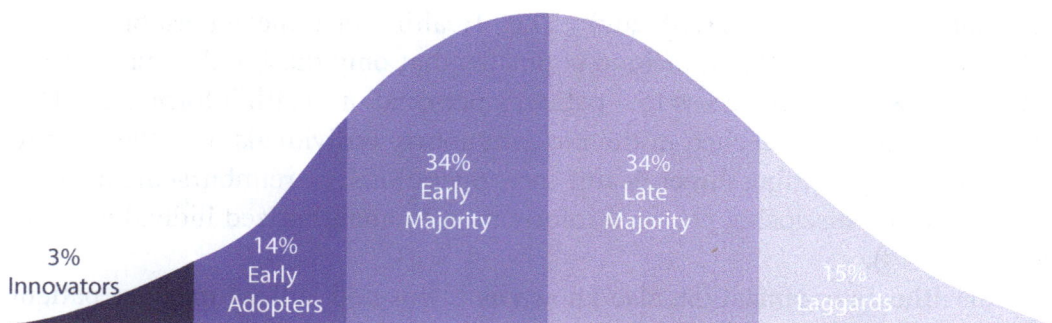

Figure 3.8: Adoption of Innovation

Source: Original Work
Attribution: Corey Parson
License: CC BY-SA 4.0

The following list displays five factors that affect the adoption of an innovation (Zhang, et. al, 2015).

- Relative Advantage - The degree to which an innovation is seen as better than the idea, program, or product it replaces.

- Compatibility - How consistent the innovation is with the potential adopter's values, experiences, and needs.

- Complexity - How difficult the innovation is to understand and/or use.

- Trialability - The extent to which the innovation can be tested or experimented with before a commitment to adopt is made.

- Observability - The extent to which the innovation provides tangible results.

Technology diffusion occurs when these products, techniques, and services spread throughout society. The innovative service's coverage by the third-party payment system, the degree to which the innovation is perceived as beneficial to consumers, and compatibility with the adopter's values and needs increase the technology's likelihood of being adopted or utilized. This is referred to as rapid diffusion. The following factors have influenced information technology usage in the U.S. (Shi & Singh, 2015).

Anthro-Cultural Beliefs and Values

Anthropology is a method of viewing humans and their cultural, social, biological, and environmental aspects of life in the past and the present. American beliefs and values influence the nature of health care delivery and, as such, Americans have high expectations regarding how technology can be used towards disease prevention or improving health status. They want the best medications, procedures, and equipment, which illustrates that anthro-cultural values relate to beliefs, practices, the human population's cognitive and social organization, and how individuals share their beliefs and practices with others. This knowledge sharing will enhance technology usage in healthcare indefinitely (Shi & Singh, 2015).

Medical Specialization

Technology is used in many healthcare facilities today, and consumer needs and desires continue to drive increased innovation. Therefore, physicians need exposure to technology early in their residency training programs. Their usage in training increases their usage in acute care hospitals that specialize in high intensity care.

Financing and Payment

Because of the costs associated with using a new technology, consumers are concerned with how a new technology that can be used in their care will be paid for. This decision is relocated to the insurance companies' discretion.

Technology-Driven Competition

Patients seek quality healthcare services, especially if they are insured. This can lead to competition between health care providers as one adopts new technology, techniques, or services while another provider does not. An example of this situation is a physician practice with its own laboratory and imaging services or same day surgery services versus a physician practice without this technology. Competition between the providers drives up costs for the healthcare consumer. Healthcare facilities provide the perception of higher quality services based on implementing state-of-the-art technology. These facilities advertise the new technology in hopes of attracting new patients. The patient then pays more for services because of the new technology (Shi & Singh, 2015).

Expenditures on Research and Development

Research and development (R&D) refer to the activities companies take on to innovate and introduce new products and services. The U.S. spends more than any other country on R&D.

Government Policy

Although government policy plays a major role in determining which types of technology are made available to the public, the government has not been successful in maintaining direct control over innovation, diffusion, and utilization of technology.

Stop and Apply

This chapter has provided you with information on using information systems in healthcare. Recall the story of Mr. Rodriquez. He went into cardiac arrest and CPR was performed. Do you think that information systems were used in Mr. Rodriquez's case? If so, which one(s) from this discussion would have been most helpful and why? What could have been done to prevent the initiation of CPR on Mr. Rodriquez since he was a do not resuscitate (DNR)?

3.3.22 Future Directions

Because of how information technology is influencing healthcare, it will continue to affect the management and delivery of healthcare in this country. Organizations not willing to embrace the advancement of information technology will not be able to maintain a competitive edge in the healthcare market and will experience increased pressure as a result. Proactive providers will understand the need to increase their organization's footprint on the healthcare market by continuing to invest in digital systems if they wish to remain ahead of the curve. Although healthcare organizations have invested millions in implementing EHR, they will need to continue making investments in innovative technology to meet consumers' demand. Authors Fitz & Shaikh (2018) suggest four strategies that proactive managers will need to implement to maintain viable organizational success in the future.

The first strategy is that organizations will need to commit to an integrated planning process that includes continuing to apply and integrate information technology into the organization's day-to-day operations while also allocating capital to sustain technology initiatives. Making an investment in technology requires the organization to analyze and understand its current position in the healthcare market and determine how to gain a competitive advantage, which is the second strategy in the process. Organizations that are ready for the future of information technology will ensure measures are in place to support nursing, laboratory, radiology, pharmacy, financial, and clinical information systems as well as picture archiving and communication systems. Meeting technologically perceptive consumers' needs will be the key focus of organizations in the future. After understanding the current state, the next step, or strategy, is to understand where the organization wishes to go and the technology that will be required to get there. The final step in the process is developing and implementing an action plan outlining how the organization will get to the next level. The action plan should consider sequencing objectives and priorities, timing towards implementation, tracking performance and risks, and ensuring that resources are properly allocated to maintain the organization's position.

3.4 CONCLUSION

Information technology in the healthcare setting has had, and will continue to have, a great impact on managers and the healthcare industry. Computers are used by healthcare providers to aid in the diagnosis, monitoring, and treatment of patients. Additionally, they assist management by informing, supporting, and enhancing education and research. Computers also aid in administrative functions, such as office managing, scheduling, and accounting. Virtual dashboards and scoreboards have increased healthcare organization's ability to monitor the status of their strategic objectives and organizational performance overall.

Technology in healthcare has improved the quality of services provided to healthcare consumers and their quality of life, especially with the adoption and implementation of the Electronic Medical and Health Records. The patient's information can follow them to any healthcare facility. However, managers will have to ensure they maintain cybersecurity measures to ensure patient data is kept confidential and secure. Technology has also increased life expectancy and decreased mortality rates worldwide. Penn Wharton's Budget Model (2016) cites several reasons for this occurrence, which are "advances in the understanding of infectious diseases and investments in sanitation, water purification, and other public health improvements eliminated infectious disease as a major cause of death. Scientific innovations of new drugs, treatments, and medical devices together with improved health behaviors related to smoking, nutrition, and obesity further reduced mortality from cancer and cardiac diseases." The use of eHealth, mHealth, telemedicine, and telehealth will continue to expand. While the increasing use of innovation and diffusion of information technology in the healthcare sector may increase health care costs that are passed on to consumers, we must not forget the benefits of this technology. They include enhanced accessibility to clinical information, improved patient safety, enhanced quality of care, and the overall efficiency and savings of using technology (Hamilton, 2013).

This chapter has provided basic information on health information systems useful to the healthcare manager. Clinical information is available to clinicians to provide and maintain continuity of patient care. Policies instituted by the federal government and other governing bodies have made it easier for information technology to be desired by healthcare consumers and adopted by healthcare institutions. As a result, managers will need to acquire the skill sets necessary to handle the demand.

3.5 KEY POINTS

- The joint commission has developed a set of national patient safety goals specific to various health care organizations, such as ambulatory care, behavioral health, hospitals, home care, office-based surgery, and nursing center care. These include but are not limited to correctly identifying patients, safely using medications, preventing infections, preventing mistakes in surgery, etc.

- Software tells the hardware what to do. Data is a directory of facts that have been organized and grouped into a database for a specific purpose.

- Computers assist healthcare providers in the following ways: diagnosing, monitoring, and treating patients; informing, supporting, and enhancing education, research, and pharmacy; and for administrative purposes, such as office managing, scheduling, and accounting.

- Information systems and information technology differ in that information systems integrate people, technology, and processes related to information. Information technology is the design and implementation of information, or data, within the information system.

- Innovation refers to developing new products, techniques, and services to appeal to healthcare consumers. Technology diffusion occurs when these products, techniques, and services spread throughout society.

3.6 KEY TERMS

Information systems, patient information, mHealth, eHealth, telehealth, clinical information systems, nursing information system, pharmacy information systems, laboratory information systems, radiology information systems, electronic health record, electronic medical record, personal health record

3.7 QUESTIONS FOR REVIEW AND DISCUSSION

1. What are medical errors?
2. What role do computers play in healthcare?
3. Explain the various types of health information systems.
4. Perform some research to answer the following question. A large physician podiatry practice will be adopting the EHR. You are the manager for this practice and are responsible for overseeing this process. What key features should you be looking for and how will you integrate them into the practice? Be mindful that physicians might object to implementing the EHR and usually show resistance during the monthly practice meeting. Develop a proposal of your idea to present to the managing partners for the system you think would work best for the practice. Assuming the partners approve the system, how would you implement the system? Provide timelines, deliverables, responsible persons, and a plan to train the staff.
5. Provide a brief overview of how technology influences the quality of medical care.

3.8 REFERENCES

Abiy, R., Gashu, K., Asemaw, T., Mitiku, M., Fekadie, B., Abebaw, Z., ... Tilahun, B. (2018). "A Comparison of Electronic Medical Record Data to Paper Records in Antiretroviral Therapy Clinic in Ethiopia: What is affecting the Quality of the Data?." Online journal of public health informatics, 10(2), e212. doi:10.5210/ojphi. v10i2.8309

Agency for Healthcare Research and Quality. Patient Information Form. Retrieved from, https://ushik.ahrq.gov/ViewItemDetails?system=ps&itemKey=88337000

BENDIX, J. (2018). "The paper chart holdouts: Why some physicians have resisted electronic health records systems and still rely on paper." Medical Economics, 95(20), 27–31.

Bourgeois, D. & Bourgeois, D. (2019). *Information Systems for Business and Beyond.* Retrieved from, https://opentextbook.site/informationsystems2019/

Centers for Disease Control (CDC) National Center for Chronic Disease Prevention and Health Promotion (2019). "Telehealth in Rural Communities." Retrieved March 17, 2020 from https://www.cdc.gov/chronicdisease/pdf/factsheets/Rural-Health-Telehealth-H.pdf

Cheng, C.-C., Chan, C.-L., Chen, L., & Guo, S. H.-M. (2019). "Evaluation of the Implementation of a Mobile Nursing Information System." Online Journal of Nursing Informatics, 23(3), 1.Database."

Dulac, Jennie D., Scott R. Engel, Therese A. Fitzpatrick, and Jay Spence. "Return on Analytics: Addressing the 'Signals' in the 'Noise.'" Hfm (Healthcare Financial Management), March 2019, 1–8. https://search.ebscohost.com/login.aspx?direct=true&AuthType=ip,shib&db=fth&AN=135146014&site=eds-live&scope=site

El. Mahalli, A., El-Khafif, S. H., & Yamani, W. (2016). "Assessment of Pharmacy Information System Performance in Three Hospitals in Eastern Province, Saudi Arabia." *Perspectives in Health Information Management*, 1–25.

Eysenbach G. (2001). "What is e-health?." Journal of medical Internet research, 3(2), E20. doi:10.2196/jmir.3.2.e20

Fichman, R.G., Kohli, R., Krishnan, R. (2011). "The Role of Information Systems in Healthcare: Current Research and Future Trends." Information Systems Research, *22*(3). http://dx.doi.org/10.1287/isre.1110.0382

Fitz, T., & Shaikh, M. (2018). "4 Tactics of Effective Strategic Technology Planning for the Digital Future." Hfm (Healthcare Financial Management), 1–10. Retrieved from https://search.ebscohost.com/login.aspx?direct=true&AuthType=ip,shib&db=hxh&AN=132859159&site=eds-live&scope=site

Garrett, P., & Seidman, J. (2011). "EMR vs EHR – What is the Difference?" Retrieved from https://www.healthit.gov/buzz-blog/electronic-health-and-medical-records/emr-vs-ehr-difference

Hagan, J. J.1, Vamsi Chandra2 Kassivajjala, and Guy3 Scalzi. "Data Analytics: A Powerful Tool for Corrections Professionals." *Corrections Today*, January 2019, 62–71. https://search.ebscohost.com/login.aspx?direct=true&AuthType=ip,shib&db=ssf&AN=134873068&site=eds-live&scope=site.

Healthit.gov (2019). "What are the differences between electronic medical records, electronic health records, and personal health records?" Retrieved from https://www.healthit.gov/faq/what-are-differences-between-electronic-medical-records-electronic-health-records-and-personal

HHS.gov. Health Information Privacy. "Summary of the HIPAA Privacy Rule." Retrieved March 18, 2020 from https://www.hhs.gov/hipaa/for-professionals/privacy/laws-regulations/index.html

Institute of Medicine (US) Committee on Regional Health Data Networks; Donaldson MS, Lohr KN, editors. Health Data in the Information Age: Use, Disclosure, and Privacy. Washington (DC): National Academies Press (US); 1994. 2, Health Databases and Health Database Organizations: Uses, Benefits, and Concerns. Available from: https://www.ncbi.nlm.nih.gov/books/NBK236556/

Institute of Medicine. (1999). *To Err is Human: Building a safer health system.* Retrieved from: http://www.nationalacademies.org/hmd/~/media/Files/Report%20 Files/1999/To-Err-is-Human/To%20Err%20is%20Human%201999%20%20 report%20brief.pdf

Institute of Medicine. (2001). *Crossing the Quality Chasm: A New Health System For The 21st Century.* Retrieved from: http://www.nationalacademies.org/hmd/~/ media/Files/Report%20Files/2001/Crossing-the-Quality-Chasm/Quality%20 Chasm%202001%20%20report%20brief.pdf

Islam, M. S., Hasan, M. M., Wang, X., Germack, H. D., & Noor-E-Alam, M. (2018). "A Systematic Review on Healthcare Analytics: Application and Theoretical Perspective of Data Mining." Healthcare (Basel, Switzerland), 6(2), 54. doi:10.3390/ healthcare6020054

Joshi, M.S., Ransom, E. R., Nash, D. B., & Ransom, S. B. (2014). *The Healthcare Quality Book: Vision, Strategy and Tools*, (3rd ed.) Foundation of the American College of Healthcare Executives.

LaMorte, W. W. (2019). "Diffusion of Innovation Theory." Boston University School of Public Health. Retrieved from, http://sphweb.bumc.bu.edu/otlt/MPH-Modules/SB/ BehavioralChangeTheories/BehavioralChangeTheories4.html

Lee, T.Y., Sun, G.T., Kou, L.T., & Yeh, M.L. (2017). "The use of information technology to enhance patient safety and nursing efficiency." Technology and Health Care, 25(5), 917-928. doi:10.3233/THC-170848

Lester, M., Boateng, S; Studeny J. & Coustasse, A. (2016). "Personal Health Records: Beneficial or Burdensome for Patients and Healthcare Providers?" Retrieved March 18, 2020 from, https://perspectives.ahima.org/personal-health-records-beneficial- or-burdensome-for-patients-and-healthcare-providers/

Merriam-Webster.com Dictionary, Merriam-Webster, https://www.merriam-webster. com/dictionary/database. Accessed 19 Mar. 2020.

Moss RJ, Süle A, Kohl S. eHealth and mHealthEuropean Journal of Hospital Pharmacy 2019;26:57-58. Retrieved from, https://ejhp.bmj.com/content/26/1/57

National Institute of Health. (2019). "Clinical research Trials and You. List of Registries." Retrieved March 18, 2020 from https://www.nih.gov/health-information/nih- clinical-research-trials-you/list-registries

Or, C., Dohan, M., & Tan, J. (2014). "Understanding Critical Barriers to Implementing a Clinical Information System in a Nursing Home Through the Lens of a Socio- Technical Perspective." Journal of Medical Systems, 38(9), 1–10. https://doi. org/10.1007/s10916-014-0099-9

Penn Wharton University: "Budget Model." (2016). Mortality in the United States: Past, Present, and Future. Retrieved March 19, 2020 from https://budgetmodel.wharton.upenn.edu/issues/2016/1/25/mortality-in-the-united-states-past-present-and-future

"Personal health records: an emerging trend." (2008). Journal of oncology practice, 4(4), 200–202. https://doi.org/10.1200/JOP.0842508

Sansone, R. A., & Sansone, L. A. (2012). "Doctor shopping: a phenomenon of many themes." Innovations in clinical neuroscience, 9(11-12), 42–46.

Sepulveda, J. L., & Young, D. S. (2013). "The Ideal Laboratory Information System." Archives of Pathology & Laboratory Medicine, 137(8), 1129–1140. https://doi.org/10.5858/arpa.2012-0362-RA

The Joint Commission. (2020) "Ambulatory Health Care and National Patient Safety Goals." Retrieved March 17, 2020 from, https://www.jointcommission.org/-/media/tjc/documents/standards/national-patient-safety-goals/2020-ahc-npsg-goals-final.pdf

True North ITG, Inc., (2019). "Advantages and Disadvantages of Paper Medical Records." Retrieved October 22, 2019, from https://www.truenorthitg.com/pros-cons-paper-medical-records

U.S department of Health and Human Services. "State Hospital Sanctions Employees for Disclosing Patient's PHI." Retrieved from https://www.hhs.gov/hipaa/for-professionals/compliance-enforcement/examples/all-cases/index.html

Usvyat, L. & Long, A. (2019). "4 Types of Healthcare Analytics to Use in Your Practice." Retrieved from, https://fmcna.com/insights/education/types-of-healthcare-analytics/

Webster's New World Dictionary, 2002.

Worzala C. (2009). "Policy Update: Federal Incentives for the Adoption of Electronic Health Records." Journal of oncology practice, 5(5), 262–263. https://doi.org/10.1200/JOP.091034

Zhang, X., Yu, P., Yan, J., & Ton A M Spil, I. (2015). "Using diffusion of innovation theory to understand the factors impacting patient acceptance and use of consumer e-health innovations: a case study in a primary care clinic." BMC health services research, 15, 71. https://doi.org/10.1186/s12913-015-0726-2

4 EMERGING TRENDS IN HEALTHCARE ORGANIZATIONS AND THEIR MANAGERIAL IMPLICATIONS

4.1 LEARNING OBJECTIVES

- To identify trends impacting the healthcare industry
- To examine trends influencing information technology in healthcare organizations
- To review trends affecting nursing homes
- To evaluate trends within accountable care organizations

4.2 INTRODUCTION

Healthcare is shifting at an accelerated momentum, requiring managers to be forward thinkers in improving their healthcare organizations' current, and future, status and quality along with the care they provide. If it swings too far in one direction, healthcare costs will continue to rise without an equal rise in healthcare quality and outcomes. As a result, managers are leading healthcare organizations to monitor, pursue, and adapt to the emerging trends that will continue to propel the future survival and success of healthcare. For example, current and future trends include cost containment, person-centered or personalization of healthcare services, launching uber health to provide increased patient access, the shift to value-based care, ensuring that individuals have access to healthcare insurance, etc. (Brown & Grossbart, 2019). This chapter focuses on evolving developments influencing the healthcare industry.

4.3 OVERVIEW OF TRENDS

A healthcare organization's purpose is to take care of patients, which may explain why healthcare is such a big industry in the U.S. Public and private practices, clinics, pharmacies, insurance companies, and hospitals are engaging in mergers, acquisitions, and consolidations as a continued trend in efforts to improve healthcare's quality and efficiency at lower costs, increase survival and longevity, increase service coverage, and increase service availability. For example, community-based hospitals are collaborating with large regional players; larger regional, statewide, and multistate health systems are combining in mega-mergers; and nonprofit healthcare systems are buying for-profit hospitals (Elisco, 2019). Several trends will affect healthcare, such as an increase in patients becoming informed healthcare consumers, expansion of well-defined quality measures, innovative provider payment models, rise in cost of care, healthcare reform and advances in information technology.

4.4 IMPROVEMENT IN HEALTHCARE QUALITY

Improving quality is an important factor in delivering healthcare services. For example, in 2004, a large, U.S. based, urban, acute-care academic hospital reviewed patient experience ratings collected through the National Research Corporation's Picker Hospital Survey (PHS) and the Consumer Assessment of Healthcare Providers and Systems (CAHPS) Survey in response to complaints concerning inpatient care that indicated nurses were slack in providing emotional support to the hospital's patients. The hospital developed an ongoing quality improvement plan to remedy this issue. The plan included collecting information to substantiate the claims, developing measures and setting goals for improvement, writing an action plan, implementing the plan, evaluating the plan's success or areas of failure and revising the plan as needed, and monitoring improvements to ensure they are maintained. By 2006, the hospital noted sustained improvement in the quality improvement plan to improve emotional support provided to their patients (Quigley, Wiseman, & Farley, 2010). So, what is healthcare quality?

The Institute of Medicine (IOM) describes quality of care as "the degree to which health services for individuals and populations increase the likelihood of desired health outcomes based on current professional knowledge." Lacking effective quality care emphasizes the need for change, as noted in such reports by the Institute of Medicine as *To Err is Human: Building a Safer Health System* and *Crossing the Quality Chasm: A New Health system for the 21ˢᵗ Century*. The IOM suggests that healthcare should be safe, effective, efficient, timely, patient centered, and equitable (Joshi, Ransom, Nash, & Ransom, 2014).

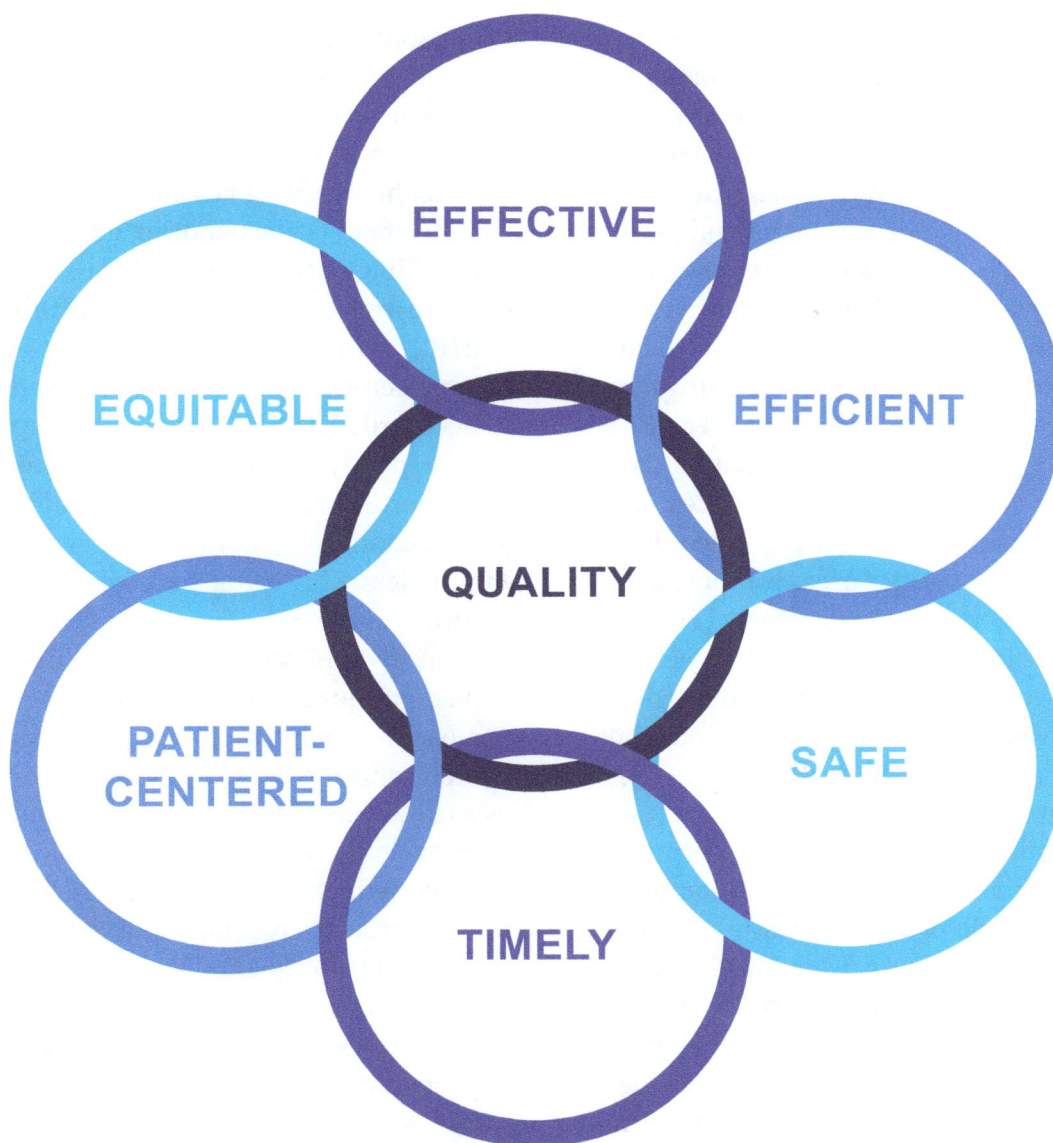

Figure 4.1: Quality of Care

Source: Original Work
Attribution: Corey Parson
License: CC BY-SA 4.0

Improving healthcare quality is a major concern for healthcare providers and one of the various initiatives for many national programs, such as the joint commission, Centers for Medicare and Medicaid Services (CMS), National Committee for Quality Assurance (NCQA), American Medical Association (AMA), Utilization Review Accreditation Committee (URAC), US Department of Health and Human Services (HHS), The Institute of Medicine (IOM), Agency for Healthcare Research and Quality (AHRQ), the Centers for Disease Control (CDC), and the National Quality Forum (NQF). Balachandran (2016) supports the premise that the joint commission has been involved in performance measurement since the 1980s and began monitoring hospital quality a few years later. This organization established a set of core measures that guide hospital operations and contribute to improving healthcare quality. The CMS mandates that healthcare providers, organizations, and institutions that manufacture or provide healthcare products or services report quality measures. The NQF focuses on fostering agreements between healthcare institutions regarding national healthcare goals and priorities for quality measurement and performance improvement (Balachandran, 2016).

The AMA emphasizes the importance of providing patient-centered care and developed quality measure sets to assist health care organizations in providing this care. Patient centered care is defined by the AHRQ as the provision of care that is respectful of and responsive to individual patient preferences, needs, and values and ensuring that patient values guide all clinical decisions. The AHRQ is a repository for collecting and distributing data pertaining to quality measures, coordinating evidence-based best practices, and annually reporting national clinical quality measures. The URAC is a healthcare quality accreditation organization for health plans, provider organizations, and physician practices with various accreditation and certification programs (Balachandran, 2016).

Improving healthcare quality can be achieved by implementing standardized performance measures through the principles of quality improvement that evaluate structure, process, outcomes, and the patient's perception of care (Joshi, Ransom, Nash, & Ransom, 2014). Structure refers to the setting where care is provided and characteristics of the providers such as certification, education, and training. The thought process is that, if care is provided by well-qualified providers in a high quality setting, then the patient will receive high quality healthcare. An example of structure is the percentage of board-certified physicians that use the EMR. However, we know that structure does not equate to quality. We also must take into consideration the role that processes and outcomes play in healthcare quality. Process refers to the steps that allow us to get from one event to the next. In healthcare, it refers to the sequence of actions that take place during the provision of healthcare to the consumer. These actions must be appropriate based on presenting circumstances, executed with skill and proficiency, and completed in a timely manner. An example of process is the percentage of people receiving such preventive services as mammograms, colonoscopies, or prostate exams. Outcomes refer to whether the goals were achieved. In other words, did the patient get better, and was the patient satisfied with the care they received (Joshi, Ransom, Nash, & Ransom, 2014)? Examples of outcomes are the rate of decubitus ulcers, falls, or hospital acquired infections. Organizational leaders should ensure that safe, effective, patient-centered systems are in place that will assist the organization in improving the quality of care provided to the patient. Several issues will need to be addressed in ensuring quality care, such as access to care, hospitals, practitioners; decreasing wait times for services and test results; ensuring patients receive information and instruction about medications, procedures, and all other services they may encounter; and administrative procedures (e.g. admissions and discharge). In addition, quality care is enhanced by trained, skilled, and proficient personnel, properly working high tech equipment and instruments, and the latest technology and medications (Rao, 2002). Leaders should also be mindful that because baby boomers (born between 1946-1964) will be replaced by millennials (born 1981-1996), therefore new healthcare needs and costs will emerge, along with growth in the use of telehealth and online resources (Volgenberg & Santilli 2018).

Stop and Apply

Review the case of Mr. Rodriquez. We have discussed quality in healthcare. Assume you are in the role of the hospice manager. Determine if Mr. Rodriquez received safe, effective, patient-centered care. Perform some research to determine how Mr. Rodriquez's care could have been improved.

4.5 INCREASE IN COSTS

Healthcare is one of the largest industries in the U.S., as it boasts the most advanced healthcare and technology of any other country in the world. The size of the healthcare industry is superseded by finance and insurance, state and local government, and real estate (Sawe, 2017). The continued advances in technology include the introduction of new medical equipment, treatments, procedures, and medications, which serve to intensify the care received by consumers. Increasing the intensity of care is directly related to disease detection and regulatory compliance. For example, the need to maintain HIPAA regulations will continue to raise healthcare costs. Although these technological advances increase the intensity of care provided to consumers, they also increase the cost of healthcare, insurance premiums, and claims (Parmenter, 2004).

The cost of healthcare can have various meanings. One meaning refers to the price of healthcare, such as with bills, procedures, or medications; or it can refer to how much is spent on healthcare, in general, worldwide or by a country. It can also refer to the cost of producing healthcare services. Healthcare policy has tried to contain healthcare costs over the past few years. However, consumers have seen little relief (Shi & Singh, 2015). These costs are associated with higher deductibles and out of pocket charges associated with doctors' visits, tests, treatment, hospital stays, etc., and expenses associated with treating chronic diseases. For example, the cost of treating leukemia can be more than $700,000 of out of pocket costs for the patient depending on insurance coverage.

In addition to the previously mentioned reasons for the rise in healthcare costs, Shi & Singh (2015) suggest these reasons as well: third party payment through the government or private insurance companies, which reduces out of pocket costs and makes patients insensitive to healthcare costs. The U.S. health care utilization and delivery system operates under an imperfect market. Imperfect market refers to an economic market that does not meet the high standards of a competitive market. In this market, utilization of services is unchecked. Patients are charged more for healthcare services than the cost for producing the service, which leads to higher healthcare costs. The continued technology growth continues to drive up healthcare costs in this country due to the costs incurred in the research and development of new technology. Additional reasons are the medical model of healthcare delivery which focuses on treating symptoms rather than on prevention and lifestyle behavioral changes; treating health related problems which are more costly than putting measures in place, such as diet and exercise or smoking cessation programs, to prevent medical conditions from occurring; and the use of defensive medicine by healthcare providers to avoid litigation. For example, an obstetrician may perform an unnecessary caesarean section to allow an easier defense of a potential birth injury case. This practice involves instances when the physician goes beyond what is usually necessary for diagnosing and treating the patient so they can ensure that they are not missing any unlikely, but possible, conditions.

Other costs increases are related to multipayer systems, and administrative costs are another reason for increasing healthcare costs. Multipayer systems include private insurance plans, Medicaid, Medicare, and employer financed health plans, wherein plan benefits and reimbursements are not standardized. In other words, these plans do not offer the same coverage or reimbursement rates for services rendered by a physician. Some physicians do not accept Medicaid as their reimbursement rates for service may be lower than an employer health plan. These systems deny payment to the provider, requiring rebilling for services rendered along with explanations for the service. Utilization reviews and authorization for care further increase healthcare costs. Administrative costs are related to how organizations manage financing, insurance, delivery, and payment functions. Fraud and abuse, which occur when billing claims and cost reports are intentionally falsified, provision of unnecessary services, or billing for services that were not provided also increase healthcare costs. Healthcare professionals also engage in practice variations wherein patients with similar conditions are treated differently. Decreasing healthcare costs can be achieved by rectifying the above cited issues, reducing the number of written prescriptions, and reducing pharmaceutical prices and the costs of prescription drugs (Syed, 2019).

Another reason for the increase in health care costs is the longer life span of Americans resulting from increased consumer knowledge about the importance of diet and exercise. Fifty percent of men and 60% of women will reach age 90. Nearly half of the American population will live to be age 100. The prospect that Americans are living longer will add to their inability to afford healthcare as they age (Porkorsi & Berg, 2017). Although Americans are living longer, many of them have chronic diseases, such as diabetes or heart disease. Amadeo (2020) contends that chronic diseases (experienced by half of the American population) are responsible for 85% of health care costs, with the sickest 5% consuming 50% of the total costs.

The increase in insurance coverage through private insurance, Medicare, and Medicaid has increased the demand and usage of healthcare services. Along with the increase in demand for services now comes increase in the costs of services.

Additionally, consideration should be provided to the uninsured. These individuals rely on emergency services to meet their medical and health needs, which further drives up the cost of healthcare. The Patient Protection and Affordable Care Act (ACA) or Obamacare was signed into law in early 2010 to remedy this problem. The ACA was developed as a measure to ensure that individuals in this country had access to essential healthcare, as its purpose was to expand insurance coverage even if the individual had a preexisting condition, such as diabetes, renal disease, or cancer. The ACA also increased consumer protections, emphasized prevention and wellness, improved quality and system performance, and curbed rising health care costs. Other provisions of this plan were covering dependents through age 25, granting income-based subsidies for enrollees, etc. (Kaiser Family Foundation, 2020)

Morrisey (2005) asserts that many individuals in the U.S. have some form of health insurance through employers, ACA, or other government plans, such as Medicare, Medicaid, or CHIP. Health insurance provides a buffer between the healthcare consumer and a provided service's total costs as the consumer only pays the minimum cost out of the total, usually in the form of a co-pay. Because consumers do not pay the full cost for services, they tend to overuse high-cost technologies and services. In addition, employer-based insurance plans through tax laws lower the price of benefits as we pay for them using pre-tax dollars. Because of the insensitivity to the cost of medical care and premiums, healthcare costs will continue to rise.

Price sensitivity is generally defined in terms of elasticity. Price elasticity is a measure of how consumers react to the prices of products and services. Generally, demand tends to decline as prices go up. However, depending on the product or service and the market, consumers' reaction to price changes can vary. Morrisey provides ways to decrease the insensitivity to increased use of services. Examples include higher out of pocket costs to consumers for healthcare services and health insurance; getting the providers involved in determining costs associated with solutions; and minimizing the costs of manufacturing, selling, and purchasing specific healthcare products and services. In a publication by The Centers for Medicare and Medicaid Services (CMS), health spending will continue to increase by 5.5% per year between 2018 and 2027 for a total cost of almost $6 trillion. Driving these costs are prescription drugs, hospitalizations, and physician and clinical services (CMS.gov).

4.6 AN INCREASE IN UNINSURED CONSUMERS

In the year 2000, more than 39 million Americans were without health insurance (H&HN, 2002). Children have relatively low uninsured rates, 11% for those below the age of 12 and 14.1% for ages 13-18 (Holahan, 2006). More than 27% of young adults (ages 19-34) and 12.9% of the elderly are uninsured. The lack of insurance varies by race and ethnicity. Holahan further asserts that the lowest rate is for white non-Hispanics, for whom the rate of the uninsured is 12.5%. The uninsured rate for Hispanics is particularly high (34.1%). The overall lack of insurance also negatively affects the health status of Americans. The uninsured rates are lowest for those in excellent health (13.7%) and increase to 22.9% for those in good health (Holahan, 2006). The rate decreases to 19.5% for those in fair or poor health due to disability coverage by Medicare and Medicaid (Holahan, 2006). By the end of 2018, more than 13.7% of adults were uninsured. Most of these groups included women, households with less than $48,000 annual income, and individuals under the age of 35. As of 2019, the number of uninsured Americans has risen by 3 million individuals or 1.3%. There are many organizations called health insurance marketplaces or health insurance exchanges in each state wherein individuals can purchase health insurance that is in compliance with ACA. Insurers participating in the exchange can offer individuals a range of government regulated and standardized health care plans. Higher insurance premiums; decisions by multiple insurers to withdraw from state ACA exchanges; the end of cost-sharing payments from the federal government to insurers; and adverse policy decisions, such as reducing public messaging and shortening the enrollment period to less than seven weeks, all contribute to the high uninsured rates in the U.S. (Witters, 2019).

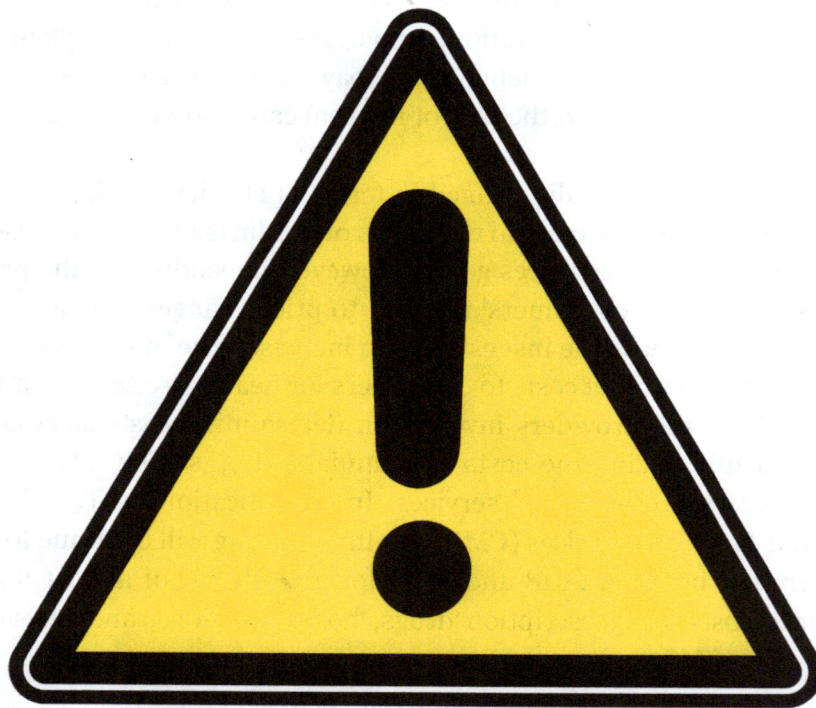

In 2019, 26.1 million Americans did not have health insurance

Figure 4.2: Uninsured Americans

Source: Original Work
Attribution: Corey Parson
License: CC BY-SA 4.0

4.7 HEALTHCARE REFORM

Healthcare delivery in the U.S. is fragmented and disintegrated. This situation inadequately uses resources, which leads to decreased access to healthcare, poor healthcare outcomes, poor patient satisfaction, and increased healthcare costs. Because of these issues, the healthcare system in the U.S. needs restructuring. President Barak Obama attempted to remedy the issue by introducing healthcare reform. Healthcare reform refers to the ability of the government to develop policies to address healthcare delivery and includes expanding health insurance to cover the uninsured, improving access to healthcare providers and specialists, and improving healthcare quality while decreasing costs. The Patient Protection and Affordable Care Act (PPACA), or Affordable Care Act (ACA) or Obamacare of 2010, is the most significant change to the U.S. health care systems since the institution of Medicaid in 1965. The Affordable Care Act was instituted in an effort to increase patient access to healthcare, improve healthcare outcomes, improve quality of care and patient satisfaction with care, and to decrease healthcare costs (Panning, 2014). The ACA sought to address the following initiatives (Panning, 2014):

1. Ensuring that all Americans had access to healthcare,
2. Ensuring that healthcare costs were spread among providers, healthcare facilities, industry, patients, insurance companies, etc.,
3. Reducing the costs associated with healthcare,
4. Financial reimbursement for positive outcomes,
5. Improving quality of services provided, and
6. Increasing the provision of preventive measures.

The Kaiser Family Foundation presents other provisions of the ACA. A few of them are contained in the following list (KFF, 2020):

1. Expanding Medicaid eligibility to adults with incomes up to 138% of the federal poverty level,
2. Income-based subsidies such as pre-tax credits and cost sharing are provided to consumers purchasing insurance through the health exchange or marketplace,
3. Covering dependents up to age 25,
4. Establishing new marketplaces that ensure plans are in compliance with ACA requirements,
5. Protecting and including individuals with preexisting conditions,
6. Prohibiting health plans from placing lifetime or annual limits on the dollar value of coverage for essential health benefits,

7. Requiring private health plans to limit cost sharing for essential health benefits covered in network,

8. Ensuring consumers receive easily understood information regarding their health plan,

9. Requiring employers with more than 50 employees to offer health insurance,

10. Prohibiting employers from imposing wait periods greater than 90 days, and

11. Offering long-term care and mental health services.

Because of the ACA, the insurance market is more accessible, millions of Americans have health insurance and the healthcare industry is moving toward health care value, rather than volume, of services provided. Regardless of its benefits, the ACA continues to face challenges partially due to obstacles associated with the creation of a new insurance market and issues presented by political rivals requesting to repeal the ACA (Rivlin, 2015).

4.8 HEALTH INSURANCE EXCHANGE OR HEALTH INSURANCE MARKETPLACE

The implementation of ACA led to developing the health insurance exchange or health insurance marketplace, which is a comparison-shopping area for health insurance. Private health insurance companies list their health plans with the exchange, then individuals looking for insurance comparisons shop on the exchange from among the available health plan listings. Although private insurance plans are included in the marketplace exchange, because of the ACA, people associate it mostly with public health insurance exchanges developed by the government. Private health insurance exchanges are usually employer-based, wherein employees sign up for their health insurance as part of their benefits (Davis, 2020). Exchanges provide subsidies to help pay for health insurance in the form of premium tax credits designed to make health insurance more affordable. The ACA has helped regulate the sale of insurance policies and made it easier for Americans to have health insurance through the provision of tax credits to individuals with insurance.

4.9 REPEAL OF THE ACA

Currently, Republicans (under the leadership of President Donald Trump) are repealing the ACA with the American Health Care Act (AHCA), which includes changes to Medicaid eligibility expansion and taxes (H.R. 1628, 2017). The AHCA bill as proposed would increase the number of uninsured Americans by 51 million people over a ten-year period and would increase premiums for those who were insured (Brown, 2018). The AHCA does not mandate that individuals purchase health insurance or receive tax penalties for nonpurchase. Also, employers would no longer receive penalties for not offering health insurance to their employees. Under the AHCA, subsidies in the form of tax credits would be offered to families or individuals based on age rather than income. Therefore, older individuals would receive higher tax credits than younger people. The AHCA also covers pre-existing conditions, the 10 essential health benefits, and children up to age 25. Further, annual contributions under HSAs would be increased to allow consumers to save on medical expenses with pre-tax and tax deductions (Brown, 2018).

Butler (2016) suggests that healthcare reform centers on two objectives. The first steps of healthcare reform should include ensuring that all Americans have access to healthcare and health insurance while reducing healthcare costs.

The second objective involves improving health by encouraging the health system to adopt innovation to address the social determinants of health. These determinants include making changes to nonmedical factors that have a bearing on healthcare, such as socioeconomic status and housing, which can be accomplished through developing governmental programs that make provisions for various agencies to come together in partnerships for the common good of affected individuals (Butler, 2016). Additionally, increasing service efficiency through increasing the supply of health resources and decreasing the demand for these resources will improve the healthcare system in the U.S., along with ensuring better coordination of care, ensuring that healthcare practices are patient centered, and allowing the patient to be a part of the decision making process (Brown, 2018).

Stop and Apply

One of the things we discussed in reference to healthcare reform is allowing the patient to play a role in the decision-making process. Mr. Rodriquez made his wishes known that he did not want to be resuscitated. As the hospice manager, consider what measures can be put into place to ensure that patients' wishes are followed. How will you communicate these measures to the employees of your facility?

4.10 THE RISE OF CONSUMERISM

Patient satisfaction is a significant factor in providing quality care. Patients must believe that their needs and requests have been met by the healthcare provider or organization (Haas, et. al, 2000). Williams (2020) asserts that healthcare leaders rate consumerism very highly when it comes to developing strategies for healthcare services. Leaders believe that patient satisfaction, retention, and acquisition, along with support for organizational goals and improving financial performance, drive consumerism. When asking healthcare leaders how they define consumerism, most replied that it was the empowerment of patients with the information they need to make better healthcare decisions. They also believed that patients had a direct bearing on healthcare access and that they were participatory in their healthcare delivery (Williams, 2020). In its simplest terms, consumerism is the desire and ability to freely purchase goods and services in the marketplace, which leads to happiness and wellbeing (Chappelow, 2019). In this respect, consumers want price transparency in order to make fully informed decisions with their resources (Williams, 2020).

Spending has the tendency to fuel the economy. Consumerism also is described as a method of protecting and promoting the interest of the consumer. In healthcare, protecting the consumer appears in the form of a health benefit plan or providing the consumer with the means to support their own health. Consumerism involves placing the employer's health benefit plan, along with economic purchasing power and decision making, into the hands of the plan's participants/employees. However, for this method to be successful, the employees will need managerial support, information, and tools enabling them to engage in healthy behaviors. Healthcare providers also play a vital role in educating, informing, and providing tools to their patients or healthcare consumers so that they can take possession of their health.

Consumers are continuing to experience high health care costs, which increases their desire and need for value-based healthcare services and products. Organizational leaders must be able to meet the needs of these consumers if they truly intend for their organizations to continue to flourish (Volgenberg & Santilli 2018). The purpose of healthcare consumerism, or consumer driven healthcare, is to ensure that healthcare is patient centered. The patient, as the healthcare consumer, dictates the type, quantity, and quality of care they receive. They are technology savvy and assist the physician in determining their healthcare diagnosis based on the presenting symptoms and the best method and cost of correcting the healthcare issue. Healthcare suppliers must focus on keeping the patient happy. In addition, the healthcare system must become proactive in their approach to healthcare delivery. The focus must change to prevention rather than treating symptoms and diseases (Madhavi, 2018). In addition to being more informed, patients are expecting their primary care practitioner to be more attentive to their needs and for the healthcare market to make healthcare services easily attainable and more affordable (Shrank, 2017).

The following trends are on the rise in respect to consumerism. Healthcare is expanding into the retail sector in the form of acute care clinics, such as those in CVS, Walgreens, or Kroger, that treat such conditions as upper respiratory infections. These clinics offer evidenced-based care to the consumer because they adhere to strict evidenced-based guidelines. New strategies related to consumerism are concierge practices payed through insurance companies wherein the patient pays a fee to the practitioners in exchange for twenty-four-hour access to the practitioner. With direct care, the patient has 24-hour access to the practitioner, but the patient pays for all services out of pocket.

Another innovation is home-based diagnostics, which provide an avenue for the patient to self-test and receive the results of these tests within the convenience of their home. The market for home-based diagnostics will yield $37 billion by 2021 (Shrank, 2017). Home-based primary care, in which a healthcare team visits individuals with complex healthcare issues in a home setting, is also receiving increased attention (Shrank, 2017). This is due to the number of elderly patients in the US with chronic illnesses. By 2050, more than 50 million people over the age of 75 will be living in this country (Cornwell, 2107). Many of these individuals will have chronic illnesses and severe disabilities and limitations. Additionally, this population will require more hospitalizations and long-term care services.

Millions of elderly people already are chronically ill, homebound, frail, or have some type of functional limitations that prevents them from accessing healthcare outside of their home (Cornwell, 2017). The current healthcare system is not equipped to care for our aging population. With home-based primary care, patients can receive care from providers who make house calls to diagnose and treat patients using cutting-edge, in-home technology. The patient can have lab tests, EKGs, X-rays, ultrasounds, IVs, etc. in the privacy of their own homes (Cornwell, 2017)

4.11 ADVANCES IN INFORMATION TECHNOLOGY

As new technology emerges, consumers will continue to desire the latest technology. This trend is also true in healthcare. Healthcare consumers desire to be abreast of the latest healthcare technology. In the event of an illness, these consumers request the use of the newest devices in diagnosing and treating their illnesses. Healthcare practitioners and medical facilities will need to ensure they have invested in the latest technology to improve patient access and satisfaction with healthcare providers. The Health Information Technology for Clinical Health (HITECH) Act requires healthcare facilities and providers to implement and use new healthcare technology in the healthcare setting to improve the delivery of healthcare in the U.S. (Paaske, Bauer, Moser, & Seckman, 2017). HITECH was created to promote and expand the adoption of health information technology (such as the use of electronic health records (EHRs) by healthcare providers) by providing incentives to hospitals and physicians who adopted and implemented the EHR. The Act "increased the rate of adoption of EHRs from 3.2% in 2008 to 14.2% in 2015. By 2017, 86% of office-based physicians had adopted an EHR and 96% of non-federal acute care hospitals had implemented certified health information technology" (HIPPA Journal, 2018). It also ensured that healthcare organizations complied with HIPAA standards. We will next discuss several trends in healthcare related technology.

4.12 RADIO FREQUENCY IDENTIFICATION

Historically, radio frequency identification, or RFID, was a system of radio waves that was developed to collect and transfer data for use in industry specifically to track goods as part of supply chain management. The goal of development was to increase efficiency and thereby save money. RFID comprises three parts of an active or passive transponder (tag with or without an energy source), a transponder reader, and a database software application.

The transponder reader uses abstract data from the tag with radio frequency and sends the data to a database through a local area network. Once the data is successfully saved to the server, it can be used as needed.

Recently, RFID usage and benefits have been explored in the healthcare sector. RFID can automatically capture data without human intervention. Neither does it require line of sight to capture information, as is the case with barcodes (Seckman, et. al, 2017). The benefits of RFID in healthcare are numerous. For example, RFID can be useful in reference to patient safety, tracking efficiencies in patient care, and provider satisfaction. It can also provide the ability to reduce misidentification issues in healthcare. Hospitalized patients can be identified and tracked using the Zebra's Z-Band RFID durable thermal printable wristband. Adding the DNR status to the patient's identifying information serves as an alert to the nurse when they scan the patient's armband. The nurse's knowledge of this information can prevent the initiation of an unnecessary code blue. RFID use has also been documented in the evaluation of its efficiency and effectiveness in the preventing medical errors. It has the potential to track wandering patients with elopement risk, particularly with patients who suffer from Alzheimer's and dementia (Seckman, et. al, 2017). For example, Ben is an 89-year-old with Alzheimer's. His daughter went to his room to wake him for breakfast when she discovered that he was gone. As she was about to go outside and begin looking for him, her doorbell rang. It was a neighbor with her dad. The neighbor found him walking down the street. Ann decided to have an RFID implanted in her dad's forearm so that she would be able to tell where he was if he wandered off again. RFID tags provide the ability to reduce misidentification issues in healthcare specifically in relation to medication administration, administration of blood products, surgical procedures, and blood sampling. It has also been successful in matching newborns and their mothers, improving hand hygiene practices, and improving efficiency of care.

Barriers to using RFIDs also exist. These barriers include the following: (1) economic limitations, specifically in response to the high cost of implementation; (2) technical issues, related to system errors, RFID tag readability, interference with medical equipment, and interoperability with other health information technology; (3) organizational challenges, related to lack of buy-in and acceptance; and (4) legal contests, related to privacy and security (Paaske, et. al, 2017).

Stop and Apply

Explain how the use of an RFID might have assisted in the prevention of CPR with Mr. Rodriquez.

4.13 ROBOTICS IN HEALTHCARE

Robotic technology is growing exponentially. Robots can serve many purposes in healthcare, including the following. Service robots perform duties like stock control, cleaning, delivery, and sterilization; Telepresence robots, such as screens on wheels; surgery robots; companion robots; cognitive therapy robots; robotic limbs and exoskeletons that assist staff in lifting patients; and humanoids (Cresswell, Cunningham-Burley, & Sheikh, 2018). Robots serve the following functions: acting on environmental stimuli, sensing, and performing logical reasoning (Wiederhold, 2017). Robots will play a major role in enhancing the quality of life of individuals as they age by increasing independence and social participation. Examples of robotic use include the butler robot called Relay that can transport goods by navigating its surroundings using 3D cameras and laser radar technology, which will make it extremely useful in a healthcare setting. Another example is Paro, which is designed to help patients in either hospital or long-term care settings by improving social interaction and reducing stress. Although technology has come a long way as far as using robots in healthcare, we still have a long way to go in respect to using robots to engage in human functions, such as administering medications, turning a patient in bed or getting a patient out of bed and placing the patient in a chair without incident (Wiederhold, 2017).

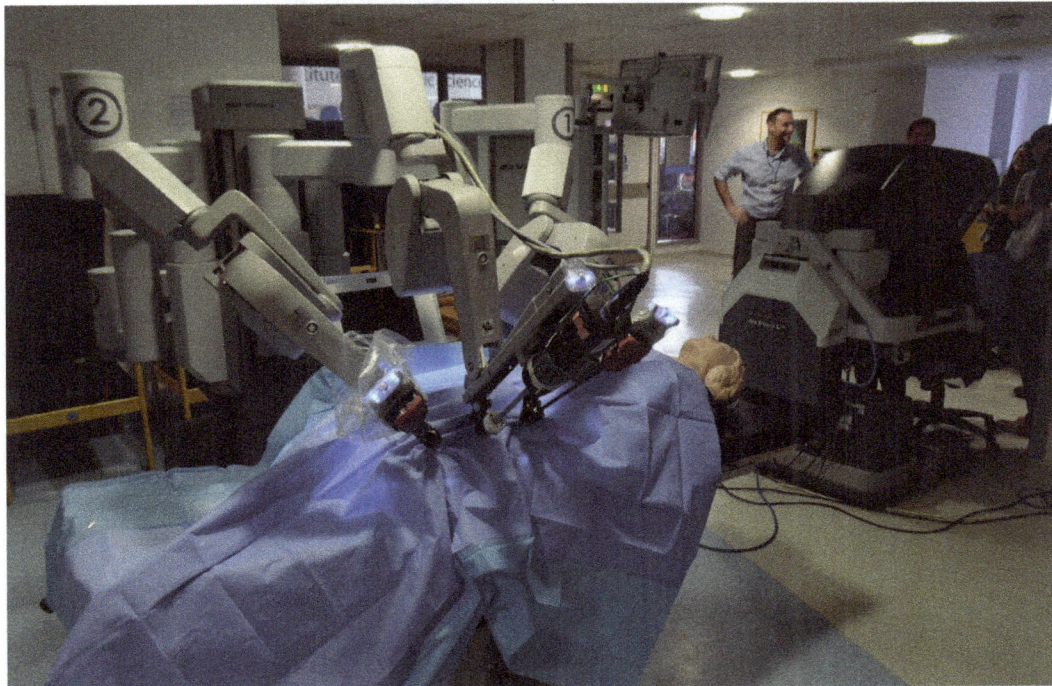

Figure 4.3: Robots in Healthcare

Source: Wikimedia Commons
Attribution: User "Cmglee"
License: CC BY-SA 3.0

We are most familiar with such robotics as the da Vinci ® Surgical System used to assist in the performance of surgical procedures due to their ability to perform small, precise incisions, which speed up the healing process. Robots can assist pharmacists in the following ways: obtaining prescription drug information from the hospital information's system; preparing intravenous solutions; attaining, collecting, and labelling a medication vial or packet; scanning bar codes; and packaging, storing, and dispensing prescriptions. Robots can also assist physicians by monitoring the progress of their patients even when the physician is far away. For example, telerobots with audio/visual and camera capabilities can monitor and care for a patient and communicate or consult with the physician as needed.

One important factor is that robots cannot replace human interaction and should only be used to assist healthcare professionals in the performance of repetitive tasks, data tracking, and extrapolation. Healthcare robotics is in its infancy, and much is still to be learned regarding its full implementation. Using robots in the complex, scientific areas of healthcare is a practice that is still evolving and will be embraced by more healthcare institutions as the costs of such technologies decrease (Fareed, 2019). The use of robots in healthcare also generates legal and ethical concerns. Physical and psychological challenges have been documented. For example, one patient reported that she was run over by a robot that was supposed to be assisting her. In addition, patients may become too emotionally attached to the robots, especially if the patient is from a vulnerable portion of the population, such as people who are mentally challenged, children, or the elderly. Another concern is whether health care professionals should be forced to use a robotic application if this were a safer alternative than human-delivered care. Additionally, the lack of clear, established liability rules surrounding robotics creates a barrier to quicker implementation (Cresswell, Cunningham-Burley, & Sheikh, 2018).

4.14 NURSING HOME TRENDS

As Americans continue to age, so will the need for long-term care settings. By 2040, 4.3 million elderly are expected to require treatment at a long-term care facility as a result of minimal availability of family support and changes in Medicare policies requiring patients to be shifted from acute care facilities to long term care (Institute of Medicine, 1986). Although the need for long-term care services is increasing as the population continues to age, financing these services will continue to be a challenge. The costs associated with nursing home care is increasing at a greater rate than inflation, with the average daily costs ranging from $121.90 to $323.00. Costs are also driven up because of the private sector purchasing of nursing homes (McGrath, 2019). Nursing home users lack the ability to pay for services due to the high cost of institutional care and the lack of insurance coverage. To remedy the problem, many individuals are investing in private long-term care insurance to improve affordability of services in long term care facilities as they are needed (Shi & Singh, 2015). Despite the need for long-term care services, nursing homes are closing. Paula Span of the New York Times reported that 1 in 5 nursing home beds are unfilled and that 200-300 nursing homes are closing each year. This may be due to a lack of Medicare coverage, as Medicare will only cover short-term rehabilitative care following a hospital stay (Span, 2018). Medicaid, however, will cover long-term care.

As the elderly population continues to grow, long-term care facilities are developing services that will draw and retain this population. According to Samantha Stein with the Association for Long Term Care Planning, several trends are forthcoming for nursing home residents. Residents will experience a shift in the dining experience wherein they will have the ability to order their meals as if they are at a restaurant and even invite their families for a pleasurable dining experience. Wellness centers, technology, transportation, spas, and salons will be available on site for their use. They will also be able to enjoy entertainment, such as movie theaters, music, and gardening. Occupational therapists also will be onsite to assist the individuals living in nursing homes improve their physical, social and psychological skills.

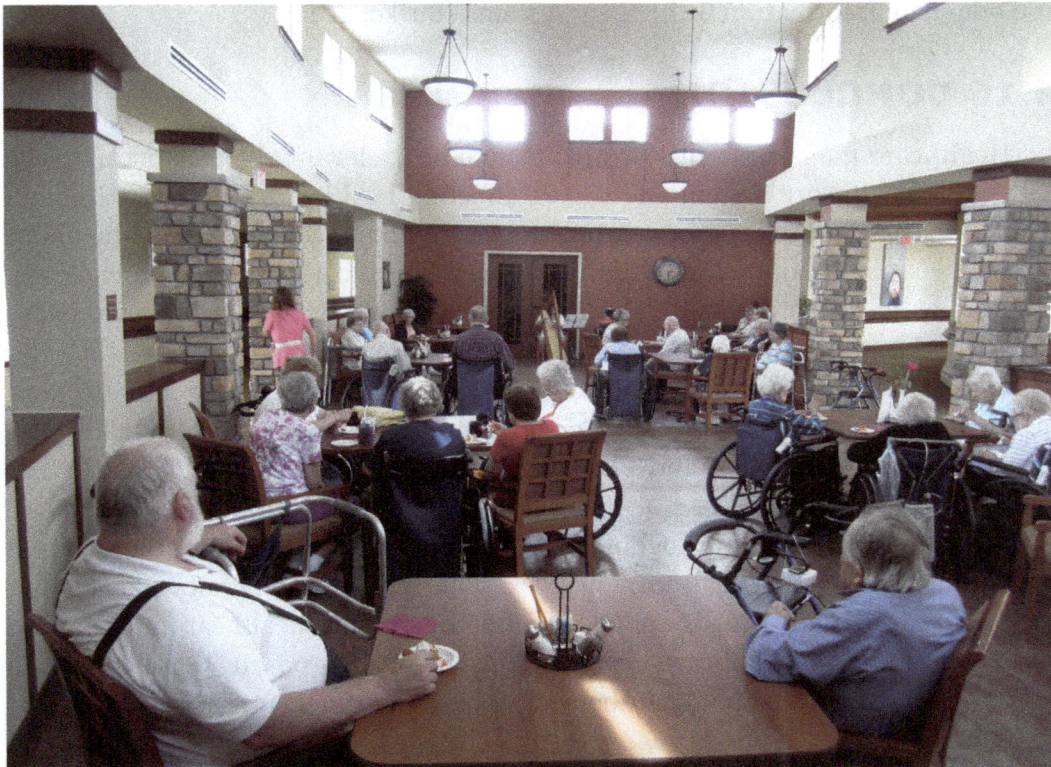

Figure 4.4: LTC Dining and Activities

4.15 ACCOUNTABLE CARE ORGANIZATION TRENDS

Accountable care organizations (ACOs) and integrated delivery systems are a growing trend in the U.S. healthcare system. Integrated delivery systems or networks are a set of organizations that provide various services to a defined population (Buchbinder, Shank, & Kite, 2021). Accountable care refers to an integrated group of providers, such as doctors, hospitals, and other providers, who agree to improve the health, efficiency, and satisfaction of healthcare consumers by providing high-quality, low-cost healthcare services for a specified population, such as Medicare patients (Shi & Singh, 2015). Delivering efficient, low-cost care requires the use of information technology to give physicians access to the patient's medical record (Buchbinder, Shanks, & Kite, 2021). As we have stated, the purpose of an ACO is to integrate and coordinate services from many different providers, reduce costs, and measure improvements and outcomes for the population served (Page, 2017). In order for an ACO to achieve this, they must focus on primary care and early intervention through the implementation of technology that allows data transparency, cost and quality metrics, a focus on the patient when delivering care, and adequate information technology systems (Burke, 2011).

4.16 CONCLUSION

Healthcare managers must be able to monitor relevant changes taking place within the healthcare system and trends affecting healthcare facilities. Although many current trends are affecting healthcare, the manager must stay abreast of methods that incorporate these trends into their specific healthcare organizations. Managers must also recognize that consumerism, driven by costs and quality, is on the rise and that healthcare consumers are demanding higher quality and technology assisted services that will improve their diagnosis, treatment, and healthcare outcomes. Managers must implement systems that will allow the provision of these services and put monitoring systems in place to ensure that quality has been provided.

As we have discussed throughout this chapter, technology will continue to be a significant contender in healthcare organizations for the purpose of ensuring that the quality of patient care is enhanced while decreasing healthcare and patient costs. Additionally, healthcare organizations must incorporate these trends to improve patient satisfaction with their healthcare outcomes.

4.17 KEY POINTS

- Improving the quality of healthcare is a major concern for healthcare providers and one of the initiatives of the many national programs, such as the joint commission, Centers for Medicare and Medicaid Services (CMS), National Committee for Quality Assurance

(NCQA), American Medical Association (AMA), Utilization Review Accreditation Committee (URAC), US Department of Health and Human Services (HHS), The Institute of Medicine (IOM), Agency for Healthcare Research and Quality (AHRQ), the Centers for Disease Control (CDC), and the National Quality Forum (NQF).

- Process refers to the steps that allow us to get from one event to the next. In healthcare, it refers to the sequence of actions that take place while providing healthcare to the consumer.

- Healthcare cost refers to healthcare prices, usually in conjunction with bills, procedures, or medications, or it can refer to how much is spent on healthcare in general by a particular country or globally. It can also refer to the cost of producing healthcare services.

- The increase in insurance coverage through private insurance, Medicare, and Medicaid has increased the demand and usage of healthcare services.

- Healthcare delivery in the U.S. is fragmented and inadequately uses resources, which leads to decreased access to healthcare, poor healthcare outcomes, poor patient satisfaction, and increased healthcare costs.

4.18 KEY TERMS

Healthcare trends, healthcare quality, healthcare costs, healthcare reform, uninsured, affordable care act, consumerism, information technology, e-prescribing, RFID, robotics, nursing home trends, accountable care organizations.

4.19 QUESTIONS FOR REVIEW AND DISCUSSION

1. What is quality of care, and how can it be improved?
2. What does healthcare cost mean?
3. What has increased the demand and usage of healthcare?
4. Why do healthcare costs in the U.S. continue to rise?
5. What is meant by healthcare reform, and why does the healthcare in the U.S. need to be reformed?
6. What is consumerism?
7. Describe reasons for your support or lack of support in regards to implementing Radio Frequency Identification, or RFID, in healthcare.
8. How do you feel about using robots in healthcare?

4.20 REFERENCES

Amadeo, K. (2020). "Universal Health Care in Different Countries, Pros and Cons of Each: Why America Is the Only Rich Country Without Universal Health Care." Retrieved March, 19, 2020; from https://www.thebalance.com/universal-health-care-4156211

Balachandran, M. (2016) 7 "Quality Measure Healthcare Organizations Explained." Retrieved March 19, 2020 from https://datica.com/blog/7-quality-measure-healthcare-organizations-explained/

Brown, B., & Grossbart, S. (2019). "The Top Five 2019 Healthcare Trends". Retrieved March 19, 2020 from https://www.healthcatalyst.com/insights/top-5-2019-healthcare-trends

Brown, D. J. (2018). "Obamacare V. Trumpcare: Challenging the Partisan Politics Sabotaging U.S. Healthcare Reform." University of La Verne Law Review, 40(1), 31–63. Retrieved from https://search.ebscohost.com/login.aspx?direct=true&AuthType=ip,shib&db=lgs&AN=138164207&site=eds-live&scope=site

Buchbinder, S., Shanks, N., & Kite, B. (2021). *Introduction to Healthcare Management*, 4th ed., Burlington, MA: Jones & Bartlett

Burke T. (2011). "Accountable care organizations." Public health reports (Washington, D.C. : 1974), 126(6), 875–878. doi:10.1177/003335491112600614

Butler, S. M. (2016). "Moving to the Next Phase of Reform." Journal of Law, Medicine & Ethics, 44(4), 598–601. https://doi.org/10.1177/1073110516684802

Centers for Medicare and Medicaid Services. "National Health Expenditures Projections 2018-2027." Retrieved October 24, 2019 from, https://www.cms.gov/Research-Statistics-Data-and-Systems/Statistics-Trends-and-Reports/NationalHealthExpendData/Downloads/ForecastSummary.pdf

Centers for Disease Control and Prevention, National Center for Emerging and Zoonotic Infectious Diseases (NCEZID), Division of Healthcare Quality Promotion (DHQP) (2019). Drug Diversion. Retrieved March 22, 2020 from, https://www.cdc.gov/injectionsafety/drugdiversion/index.html

Chappelow, Jim. (2019). Consumerism. Retrieved December 17, 2019, from https://www.investopedia.com/terms/c/consumerism.asp

Cornwell, T. (2017). "Home-Based Primary Care Transforms Health Care for Medically Complex Patients." Today's Geriatric Medicine, 10(6). P. 12. Retrieved March 22, 2020 from, https://www.todaysgeriatricmedicine.com/archive/ND17p12.shtml

Cresswell, K., Cunningham-Burley, S., & Sheikh, A. (2018). "Health care robotics: Qualitative exploration of key challenges and future directions." *Journal of Medical Internet Research, 20*(7). Retrieved from https://search.ebscohost.com/login.aspx?direct=true&AuthType=ip,shib&db=psyh&AN=2018-57213-001&site=eds-live&scope=site

Davis, E., (2020). "What Is a Health Insurance Exchange?" Retrieved March 21,

2020 from, https://www.verywellhealth.com/what-is-a-health-insurance-exchange-1738734

Department of Health. "Electronic Prescribing." Retrieved November 9, 2019 from, http://www.health.ri.gov/medicalrecords/about/eprescribing/

Fareed, A. (2019). Robotics: Changing the Future of Health Care. Retrieved November 11, 2019 from

Haas, J. S., Cook, E. F., Puopolo, A. L., Burstin, H. R., Cleary, P. D., & Brennan, T. A. (2000). "Is the professional satisfaction of general internists associated with patient satisfaction?" Journal Of General Internal Medicine, 15(2), 122–128.

Holahan, John. 2006. "Financing Care for Medicaid and the Uninsured." Ageing International 31 (2): 138–53. doi:10.1007/s12126-006-1009-3.

Hospital Bracelets and Patient ID Wristbands. (n.d.). Retrieved August 25, 2020 from https://www.zebra.com/us/en/products/supplies/hospital-wristband-patient-id-wristband.html

HIPAA Journal (2018). "What is the HITECH Act?" Retrieved March 22, 2020 from, https://www.hipaajournal.com/what-is-the-hitech-act/

H.R. 1628 (115th): American Health Care Act of 2017, Retrieved from https://www.govtrack.us/congress/bills/115/hr1628/summary

"Huge Increase in Uninsured." 2002. H&HN: Hospitals & Health Networks 76 (3): 77. https://search.ebscohost.com/login.aspx?direct=true&AuthType=ip,shib&db=ccm&AN=106054142&site=eds-live&scope=site&custid=ns235467.

Institute of Medicine (US) Committee on Implications of For-Profit Enterprise in Health Care; Gray BH, editor. For-Profit Enterprise in Health Care. Washington (DC): National Academies Press (US); 1986. The Changing Structure of the Nursing Home Industry and the Impact of Ownership on Quality, Cost, and Access. Available from: https://www.ncbi.nlm.nih.gov/books/NBK217907/

Kaiser Family Foundation. (2020). "Potential Impact of Texas v. U.S. Decision on Key Provisions of the Affordable Care Act." Retrieved March 21, 2020 from, https://www.kff.org/health-reform/fact-sheet/potential-impact-of-texas-v-u-s-decision-on-key-provisions-of-the-affordable-care-act/

Madhavi, R. ravulapati_madhavi@yahoo. co. (2018). "A New Era of Healthcare Consumerism: Trouncing Hallucination and High Jinx." IUP Law Review, 8(2), 15–27. Retrieved from https://search.ebscohost.com/login.aspx?direct=true&AuthType=ip,shib&db=lgs&AN=129834962&site=eds-live&scope=site&custid=ns235467

McGrath, L. (2019). "The Future Looks Terrible for U.S. Nursing Home Costs." Bloomberg.com, N.PAG. Retrieved from https://search.ebscohost.com/login.aspx?direct=true&AuthType=ip,shib&db=bth&AN=137548342&site=eds-live&scope=site

National Quality Forum. (2019). Improving healthcare quality. Retrieved October 23, 2019 from, https://www.qualityforum.org/Setting_Priorities/Improving_Healthcare_Quality.aspx

Paaske, S., Bauer, A., Moser, T., & Seckman, C. (Summer, 2017). "The Benefits and Barriers to RFID Technology in Healthcare." Online Journal of Nursing Informatics (OJNI), 21(2). Retrieved from: https://www.himss.org/library/benefits-and-barriers-rfid-technology-healthcare

Panning, R. (2014). "Healthcare Reform 101." Clinical Laboratory Science, 27(2), 107–111. Retrieved from https://search.ebscohost.com/login.aspx?direct=true&AuthType=ip,shib&db=ccm&AN=103892542&site=eds-live&scope=site&custid=ns235467

Page, M.R. (2017). "Analyzing Trends in Accountable Care Organizations: A Nationwide Survey." The American Journal of Managed Care. Retrieved November 11, 2019 from, https://www.ajmc.com/journals/supplement/2017/analyzing-trends-in-accountable-care-organizations-a-nationwide-survey/analyzing-trends-in-accountable-care-organizations-a-nationwide-survey-article?p=7

Parmenter, Eric M. 2004. "Health Care Benefits Crisis: Cost Drivers and Strategic Solutions." Journal of Financial Service Professionals 58 (4): 63–78. https://search.ebscohost.com/login.aspx?direct=true&AuthType=ip,shib&db=bth&AN=13559714&site=eds-live&scope=site&custid=ns235467.

Porterfield, A., Engelbert, K., & Coustasse, A. (2014). Electronic prescribing: improving the efficiency and accuracy of prescribing in the ambulatory care setting. Perspectives in health information management, 11(Spring), 1g.

Quigley, D.D. Wiseman, S.H. & Farley, D.O. (2010). Improving Hospital Inpatient Nursing Care: A Case Study of One Hospital's Intervention to Improve the Patient's Care Experience. Retrieved from, Case Studies of Quality Improvement Initiatives. Content last reviewed April 2020. Agency for Healthcare Research and Quality, Rockville, MD.

https://www.ahrq.gov/cahps/quality-improvement/reports-and-case-studies/Case-Study_QI-Initiatives.html

Rao, G.N. (2002). "How can we improve patient care?" Community eye health, 15(41), 1–3. Retrieved from https://www.ncbi.nlm.nih.gov/pmc/articles/PMC1705904/

Rivlin, A.M., (2005). "What the ACA has achieved and what's next." Retrieved March 21, 2020 from, https://www.brookings.edu/opinions/what-the-aca-has-achieved-and-whats-next/

Sansone, R. A., & Sansone, L. A. (2012). Doctor shopping: a phenomenon of many themes. Innovations in clinical neuroscience, 9(11-12), 42–46.

Santilli, J., & Vogenberg, F. R. (2015). "Key Strategic Trends that Impact Healthcare Decision-Making and Stakeholder Roles in the New Marketplace." American health & drug benefits, 8(1), 15–20.

Sawe, B.E., (2017). "The Biggest Industries in The United States." Retrieved March 19, 2020 from https://www.worldatlas.com/articles/which-are-the-biggest-industries-in-the-united-states.html

Seckman, C. Bauer, A., Moser, T., Paaske, S. (2017). The Benefits and Barriers to RFID

Technology in Healthcare. HIMSS. Retrieved March 22, 2020 from, https://www.himss.org/resources-benefits-and-barriers-rfid-technology-healthcare

Shrank, W. H. (2017). "Primary Care Practice Transformation and the Rise of Consumerism." Journal Of General Internal Medicine, 32(4), 387–391. https://doi.org/10.1007/s11606-016-3946-1

Span, P. (2018). In the nursing home, empty beds and quiet halls. Retrieved November 11, 2019 from https://search.proquest.com/docview/2113638415/fulltext/B46B819D1BF64AA3PQ/1?accountid=12418

Stein, S. (2019). Future of Long Term Care Industry: 10 Long Term Care Trends (To Watch Out For in 2019). Association for Long Term Care Planning. Retrieved November 11, 2019 from http://www.altcp.org/future-long-term-care-industry/

Syed, Ehsan U. 2019. "Will We Ever Bend the Cost Curve in Healthcare?" American Health & Drug Benefits 12 (4): 186–87. https://search.ebscohost.com/login.aspx?direct=true&AuthType=ip,shib&db=ccm&AN=137491480&site=eds-live&scope=site&custid=ns235467.

Vogenberg, F. R., & Santilli, J. (2018). Healthcare Trends for 2018. American health & drug benefits, 11(1), 48–54.

Wiederhold, B. K. (2017). Robotic technology remains a necessary part of healthcare's future editorial. Cyberpsychology, Behavior, and Social Networking, 20(9), 511–512. Retrieved from https://search.ebscohost.com/login.aspx?direct=true&AuthType=ip,shib&db=psyh&AN=2017-41967-001&site=eds-live&scope=site

Williams, J. (2020). Survey: Healthcare leaders say consumerism is top of mind, but barriers to consumer-centric healthcare design still exist. Hfm (Healthcare Financial Management), 74(3), 44–48.

Witters, Dan. 2019. "U.S. Uninsured Rate Rises to Four-Year High." Gallup News Service, January, 1. https://search.ebscohost.com/login.aspx?direct=true&AuthType=ip,shib&db=bth&AN=134272735&site=eds-live&scope=site&custid=ns235467.

PART II

LEADERSHIP

5

THE CONVERGENCE OF LEADERS AND MANAGERS

5.1 LEARNING OBJECTIVES

- Distinguish the difference in competencies between effective leaders and managers
- Identify attributes that are unique to leaders and managers
- Explain the importance of managers who are also strong leaders in today's healthcare industry
- Identify the core functions of management
- Identify styles of leadership

5.2 INTRODUCTION

The terms leader and manager are often used interchangeably. Although leadership and management can overlap, both skills are necessary in order to be an effective supervisor in today's dynamic healthcare system and to navigate the existing healthcare challenges. Leadership is a skill that incorporates effective communication and motivation to influence others to embrace a shared vision while working towards the organization's collective goals. In contrast, management focuses on measuring and monitoring specific tasks related to achieving those goals (Healthcare Leadership Alliance, 2010). Using the hypothetical case of Southern Healthcare Hospice Center, this chapter will illustrate common challenges faced in healthcare management and focus on the core competencies (skills, knowledge, and abilities) of leaders and managers while describing the relationship between both.

The Chapter Case

Amanda is the director of the Southern Healthcare Hospice Center, a long-term care facility that provides assistance to elderly residents. The mission of the facility is "to provide individualized, empathetic long-term care services while helping patients navigate one of the most difficult phases of their lives." The vision of the facility is to provide specialized, transformative care through innovative clinical and administrative strategies. The center has been in operation for over 25 years and mainly serves a largely upper-class, caucasian population until recent demographic shifts took place. The surrounding area now consists of predominantly low-income, Hispanic, Spanish-speaking residents. The director of the facility, Amanda, focuses on staffing, financial management, supervising resident care, community outreach, and evaluating the programs the facility provides to elderly patients and their families. A thorough understanding of federal, state, and local standards are also essential to her position as a healthcare administrator. Amanda is very well organized and motivated; she expects the managers and staff to be self-motivated as well. Recently, the facility has suffered from high staff turnover. Several nurses, administrators, and therapists have quit. Amanda has a demanding schedule and provides oversight and direction to two managers who are responsible for respective staff members in each of the facility's outreach and finance departments. Currently, budget cuts and restraints have occurred, but Amanda has not received adequate information from the finance manager to complete the budgets. Thusly, she is unable to address the concerns identified by the behavior and outreach manager. The managers and staff are increasingly overworked as everyone takes on mounting responsibilities due to the high staff turnover. However, Amanda's optimistic attitude without direction and her expectation of self-motivation among managers leaves her staff feeling dejected. Staff are tired, underpaid, and dissatisfied. As you read through the leadership and management styles and skills in this chapter, identify how the director should address the concerns of her staff using each of the leadership/management's styles described.

5.3 HEALTHCARE MANAGEMENT CHALLENGES

"In its current form, habits, and environment, American health care is incapable of providing the public with the quality health care it expects and deserves."
— *Institute of Medicine*

The only constant in the healthcare system is change, which requires healthcare managers to lead while seamlessly navigating the industry's constantly fluxing state (Buchbinder & Shanks, p. 31, 2012). Growing considerations for healthcare managers include more informed patients, rising healthcare costs, as well as a shift in patient-centered, value-based care as opposed to a fee-for-service system. Value-based care moves beyond the fee-for-service system of diagnosing and treating diseases to addressing the root causes of illnesses, such as patient adherence to medication, access to healthy foods and physical activity, and patients' living and working conditions. The value-based, patient-centered approach attempts to optimize healthcare efforts and costs by delivering cost-effective and quality treatment options based on the unique needs of the patient. Addressing a patient's overall wellness is also associated with greater hospital performance (Brown and Crapo, 2017; Miller, 2019).

Rather than being paid based on the number of patient visits and tests ordered through the fee-for-service system, value-based care models determine payments based on the value and impact of delivered care (Brown and Crapo, 2017). Under value-based care models, providers are incentivized to deliver high-quality, affordable care. Value-based payment contracts are typically structured according to a shared savings model. Shared savings models may differ, but they generally incentivize healthcare providers to reduce spending for a specific patient population by offering providers a percentage of any actualized net savings. The Medicare Shared Savings Program is the most well-known example of the value-based payment model (Brown and Crapo, 2017). Under this model, healthcare organizations must demonstrate how they are meeting quality standards through cost reduction and the provision of patient-centered care. For instance, Medicare requires hospitals to measure and track financial and quality performance by measuring 30-day readmission rates for heart attacks, heart failures, and pneumonia patients (Brown and Crapo, 2017).

Strategic management is key to counterbalancing the initial costs of operating healthcare organizations under value-based models. The ultimate goal of value-based models is to improve quality and cost margins, but shifting to this system may have high initial costs (Brown and Crapo, 2017). A hospital's ability to perform in a value-based care system depends on internal organizational processes. Healthcare administrators must effectively manage shared saving programs to maximize reimbursement, reduce unnecessary costs (e.g., excessive costly treatments and care that results in patient injury), and improve quality and cost-effective care that attracts a large volume of patients, payers, and employers, which is key to operating under new value-based care models (Brown and Crapo, 2017). Healthcare's current shift in focus from fee-for-service to value-based, patient-centered care systems requires strong leadership with innovative approaches that will adapt to and address current healthcare challenges, such as globalization, patient-centeredness, shifting demographics, and advancements in information technology (Cocchi, 2016).

These advancements, specifically regarding information technology, have given rise to new challenges that can compromise regulatory compliance to laws, such as the Health Insurance Portability and Accountability Act, that protect patients, accreditation, and licensing for both hospitals and health care workers (Cocchi,

2016). A 2018 descriptive study examining data breaches among U.S. hospitals found that in recent years the largest percent of data breaches took place within health services, comprising over one-third of all security breaches and affecting the largest number of individuals (Gabriel, et. al, 2018). A retrospective study analyzing HHS OCR Breach Portal data from the years 2013 to 2017 found there were 1,512 data breaches affecting nearly 155 million of patient records (Ronquillo, Winterholler, Cwikla, Szymanski, & Levy, 2018).

The population's shifting demographics, including the growing racial, ethnic, cultural, and religious diversity, in addition to current portions of the population that are aging, also affect health care costs, necessary resources, and the health and social conditions associated with each subpopulation group (National Association of Health Underwriters, 2015). For instance, each population group faces unique socioeconomic factors, such as limited access to insurance or healthcare, and susceptibility to specific diseases. African American women face higher maternal mortality and are more likely to develop diabetes, hypertension, and cardiovascular disease than their caucasian counterparts (Black Women's Maternal Health, 2018; Mullins, et. al, 2005). In addition to racial differences, language barriers, along with cultural and religious diversity, contribute to differences in health outcomes for certain subpopulations. In some cultures, females are not permitted to see male physicians. In other cultures, patients seek alternative herbal remedies before modern healthcare methods, which could be harmful when combined (Juckett, 2013). Some patients may even delay or refuse to seek necessary care as a result of perceived discrimination, distrust, and prior negative experiences with the healthcare system (Thorburn, Kue, Keon, & Lo, 2012; Meuter, Gallois, Segalowitz, Ryder, & Hocking, 2015). Hospitals and health systems must regularly assess their community's makeup to accommodate specific health needs and socioeconomic circumstances. Healthcare providers must also be aware and respectful of the differences present in the patient communities they are serving. As the U.S. population continues to diversify and age, the unique needs and associated conditions (e.g., chronic conditions) of the population will also change. In order to reduce disparities in healthcare, hospitals and healthcare organizations must anticipate change, continually assess, and accordingly respond to the shifting needs of patient populations by addressing barriers, such as healthcare access, language, cultural, and religious diversity (Dall, et. al, 2013).

Moreover, the changes in regulatory policies, including the Affordable Care Act (ACA) and its potential repeal, force healthcare managers to adapt to these ongoing changes. Each change brings new complexities to manage, including shifting expectations and staffing shortages, alongside cost negotiation challenges and coordinating the delivery of quality healthcare services. Health care managers must also consider the internal (e.g., areas of focus that managers address daily) and external factors (e.g., the healthcare organization's resources and activities that directly influence how the organization is run) associated with carrying out their responsibilities. Internal factors include scheduling, billing, maintaining patient satisfaction and quality, facilitating employee relations, achieving high performance, and incorporating innovative technology. External factors include recognizing community demographics and need, enforcing compliance to laws and regulations, keeping up with relevant healthcare laws and licensure requirements, meeting stakeholder demands, evaluating competitors, and managing insurers (Buchbinder & Shanks, p. 31, 2012). Managers with strong leadership skills are needed to effectively address each factor and provide access to safe, reliable, cost-comparative, quality care in a climate of uncertainty (Ambrose & Gullatte, 2011).

Table 5.1 Responsibilities of Healthcare Service Managers by Domain

External Domain	Internal Domain
Recognizing community demographics	Scheduling
Enforcing compliance to laws and regulations	Billing and budgeting
Keeping up with relevant healthcare laws and licensure requirements	Maintaining patient satisfaction and quality care
Meeting stakeholder demands	Facilitating employee relations
Evaluating competitors	Achieving high performance
Managing insurers	Incorporating innovative technology

Source: Buchbinder & Shanks, 2012
Attribution: Whitney Hamilton, Adapted from Buchbinder & Shanks
License: Fair Use

Stop and Apply

What are some of the potential external and internal challenges affecting the Southern Healthcare Hospice Center?

5.4 FUNCTIONS OF MANAGEMENT

Management requires effective navigation of internal and external challenges by measuring and monitoring performance against established goals, following procedures and policies, controlling and organizing systems, adequately allocating resources and maximizing productivity (Gopee & Galloway, 2009). Managers must complete tasks by carrying out essential management functions in teams or individually (Buchbinder & Shanks, 2012, p. 94). Effective management is needed to organize and coordinate the services that are provided within healthcare organizations. An individual healthcare organization's overall performance depends on the healthcare managers' effectiveness and their staff (Buchbinder & Shanks, 2012, p. 9). The healthcare organization cannot fulfill its function of providing safe, satisfactory patient experiences and delivering cost effective and quality healthcare services without effective healthcare managers. **Negotiation, facilitation**, and **delegation** are key skills for healthcare managers. Effective healthcare managers are able to *negotiate* with stakeholders for resources and support to achieve the organization's goals, *facilitate* ongoing communication with staff about organizational goals and how to achieve them, and *delegate* tasks to staff and provide support to achieve organizational goals (World Health Organization, 2008, p. 264).

Managers execute five specific functions in order to achieve organizational goals, including the following:

- **Planning:** setting priorities and performance objectives
- **Organizing:** designating the reporting relationship, determining staff positions, assigning teams, and distributing authority and responsibility
- **Staffing:** recruiting and retaining human resources, strategically developing and supporting the healthcare organization
- **Controlling:** monitoring staff activities, performance and taking appropriate corrective action when necessary, and
- **Directing**: initiating action within the healthcare organization.

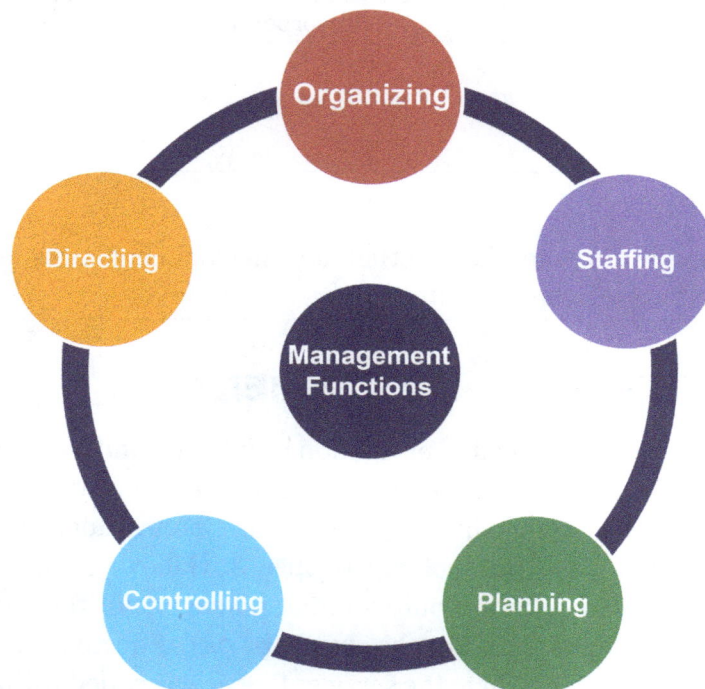

Figure 5.1: Functions of Management

Source: Original Work
Attribution: Corey Parson
License: CC BY-SA 4.0

Stop and Apply

Consider the scenario described at the beginning of this chapter. Amanda supervises the two specific managers described below.

> **Manager 1:** Corinne has a specific background in health administration. She manages staff who provide support to another department that delivers behavioral health and outreach services. Corinne is very motivated and driven. Corinne supports her staff and is very organized; however, she often takes a very black and white view of issues. Upper level leadership values Corinne's latest outreach projects to address the community's shifting needs. Currently, the facility is ill-equipped to handle the largely non-English speaking, Hispanic population. Corinne has also found through her evaluations that there has been an increase in the number of patients with dementia. Due to the lack of available budget information, she is unsure how to address the identified concerns.

> **Manager 2:** Michelle has a strong background in business and finance but has not worked extensively in a long-term care facility. She manages the staff that works on the facility's budgets and finances. She is known as a problem solver and is extremely supportive of her staff. She is very organized and has a wealth of experience in evaluation. However, she is still learning the federal, state, and local repayment options to handle the facility's budget restraints. Michelle is very capable but can sometimes take on too much.

Using the above information and considering the internal and external factors that influence the operations of Southern Healthcare Hospice Center, describe the roles and responsibilities of each of the facility's managers, Corinne and Michelle, as well as the facility's director, Amanda.

5.5 FUNCTIONS OF LEADERSHIP

Leadership describes an individual's behaviors when directing a group's activities towards a shared goal (Al-Sawaii, 2013). Leadership involves influencing other's beliefs, opinions, and actions. It embodies key skills when guiding staff towards a shared vision, including taking and managing risks, creatively solving problems, encouraging innovation, and strong communication.

In the Southern Hospice example, the mission of the facility is "to provide individualized, empathetic long-term care services while helping patients navigate one of the most difficult phases of their lives." The facility was accustomed to serving a wealthy, caucasian population but now serves a predominately non-English speaking, low-income Hispanic community. As a result, the population's needs have shifted, but the vision remains the same.

Nevertheless, the process of fulfilling the vision must shift in order to address the served community's growing needs. Healthcare leadership must also embrace diversity within and outside the organization in order to increase quality and equity in healthcare. For instance, in order to properly provide holistic care for non-English speaking, Hispanic patients mentioned in the case study at the beginning of this chapter, it would be important to consider the community's cultural and religious preferences by hiring staff that represent and reflect the community served (e.g., Spanish-speaking, Hispanic employees). Leadership involves keenly understanding the consumers' needs and defining organizational culture through leading by example.

Healthcare leadership also requires leaders to understand skills and capabilities of their staff in addition to the healthcare system's challenges. This understanding provides valuable insight to leaders on how to effectively motivate subordinates, identify expectations, and overcome challenges and competition. A healthcare institute in New York found an increase in depression among Latino patients. The institute developed an innovative health literacy tool in order to educate patients and reduce barriers to obtaining care for depression. The health literacy tool used Latino soap opera stories, known as "fotonovelas." The organization also enlisted spiritual leaders and patients' family members from the community to help shift negative perceptions about depression (Sanchez, Chapa, Ybarra, & Martinez, 2012). A health organization in Connecticut utilized unique strategies to recruit and retain bilingual and bicultural professionals while also providing training sessions on topics related to Latino health as well as strategies for engagement, interviewing, assessment, cultural values, and the impact of Latino immigration and acculturation. The training sessions were offered to all sectors within the organization, including administrative, management, and clinical divisions, in order to develop higher staff knowledge, skills, and attitudes towards Latino health (Sanchez, Chapa, Ybarra, & Martinez, 2012).

The National Strategy for Quality Improvement in Healthcare (NQS) recommends a three-tier framework for providing optimal care within healthcare organizations, including affordable, accessible, and quality patient care (National Quality Strategy, 2016). Affordability, access, and quality should be the foundation and overarching vision for any healthcare organization. Effective leadership requires the ability to adapt to change and "the capacity to translate vision into reality," as stated by Warren Bennis, an innovator of leadership styles and studies. A healthcare organization's leadership style, ability, and skills enable the organization to flourish during challenging and dynamic times.

5.6 LEADERSHIP STYLES

The most commonly identified leadership methods include autocratic, bureaucratic, Laissez-Faire, transactional, strategic, democratic, and transformational styles. A leader's ability to implement various leadership styles that suit their organization's cultural situation is a crucial skill, especially in the everchanging health-care industry.

Various situations and tasks may require a leader to employ different styles of leadership. For instance, treating and providing safe patient care may require rigid structures and processes, while patient engagement may entail more creative approaches. Healthcare administrators must understand the different types of leadership styles as well as which strategies are the most appropriate in given situations. However, an individual's personality and inherent traits will ultimately influence their overall style of leadership. Despite having a dominant leadership style, leaders can learn and develop a variety of techniques and skills in order to appropriately lead people and manage resources (Ledlow & Coppola, 2014). According to Spaulding (2015), "leadership styles have evolved in the past few decades. The biggest shift has been a move from the 'old school' traits that we have been traditionally been taught to value, such as authoritativeness, strategic thinking, and bottom-line decision-making, to a greater emphasis on humility, vulnerability, transparency, selflessness, and transparency." Not all leadership styles should be adapted to the healthcare industry. As you read the following leadership styles, identify which styles would be most relevant to the scenario presented in this chapter and why.

5.7 AUTOCRATIC LEADERSHIP

Autocratic leadership, or authoritative leadership, is characterized by individual control over all decisions. Unlike democratic leaders, autocratic leaders desire little input from staff members and typically make all decisions based on their own ideas and judgment (Lewin, Lippitt, 1938; Gastil, 1994). They do not encourage creativity and dictate the approaches and processes of achieving organizational tasks.

Some key characteristics of autocratic leaders include the following. They:

- Are rigid and highly structured
- Discourage creativity
- Establish and communicate well-defined rules

Autocratic leadership benefits include quick decision-making processes, clearly defined roles and chains of command, and clear directive systems. This style of leadership works best in settings where accident prevention is critical and project completion follows a set deadline. However, this style of leadership may reduce employee morale, disregard expertise from subordinates, and discourage important input from staff. This style of leadership may also result in a lack of creative solutions to issues that may negatively impact workplace productivity (Gastil, 1994).

Table 5.2 Autocratic Leadership Benefits and Disadvantages	
Benefits	Disadvantages
Quick decision-making	Reduces employee morale
Clearly defines roles and chains of command	Disregards expertise
Clear directive system and procedures	Discourages creativity and input

Source: Original Work
Attribution: Whitney Hamilton
License: CC BY-SA 4.0

5.8 BUREAUCRATIC LEADERSHIP

Bureaucratic leadership is characterized by establishing defined rules and chain of command. Bureaucratic leaders enforce specific rules that focus on the organization's administrative needs. Bureaucratic leaders emphasize consistency and uniformity (Bass & Riggio, 2006).

Key characteristics of bureaucratic leaders include the following. They:

- Establish clear rules
- Are highly structured and rigid
- Are inflexible

The bureaucratic leadership style does not encourage employee creativity and relies on set procedures to produce consistent and accurate results. This form of leadership is inflexible, does not adapt to change, and does not promote employee engagement. This leadership style works in organizations that must ensure a high safety and accuracy levels to complete such tasks as construction or manufacturing.

Table 5.3 Bureaucratic Leadership Benefits and Disadvantages	
Benefits	Disadvantages
Adapts to change and embraces new ways to address challenges	Requires an existing structure in need of change
Addresses current issues and long-term goals	Risky—may lead to unintended consequences
Increases performance, productivity, and morale	Overlooks reality

Source: Original Work
Attribution: Whitney Hamilton
License: CC BY-SA 4.0

5.9 LAISSEZ-FAIRE LEADERSHIP

In contrast to bureaucratic and authoritative leadership, **Laissez-Faire leadership** is characterized by providing the least possible amount of guidance to subordinates (Bass & Riggio, 2006). Laissez-faire leaders entrust all responsibility to their staff. They provide the necessary tools and resources for staff to accomplish organizational tasks but leave the processes and mechanisms to complete the tasks to the staff (Bass & Riggio, 2006).

Key characteristics of Laissez-faire leadership include the following. They:

- Provide staff with the tools needed to complete tasks
- Provide very little guidance
- Entrust staff with decision-making

Laissez-faire leaders encourage creativity and autonomy among staff. This leadership style is most effective when group members are highly motivated and have the knowledge and skills to complete necessary tasks and decisions without micromanagement. This lack of guidance, however, could result in poor performance and a lack of workplace productivity if individuals do not possess the knowledge and expertise to complete tasks. As mentioned above, understanding individual staff members' capabilities is an important leadership function. Further, staff may not have the necessary characteristics, such as self-motivation and dedication to manage tasks, to meet deadlines and make decisions without proper guidance.

Table 5.4 Laissez-Faire Leadership Benefits and Disadvantages	
Benefits	Disadvantages
Encourages creativity and autonomy	Unclear, ambiguous roles
Helps employees feel valued and trusted	Lack of accountability
Enables highly skilled employees to complete tasks without micromanagement	Poor performance and productivity

Source: Original Work
Attribution: Whitney Hamilton
License: CC BY-SA 4.0

5.10 TRANSACTIONAL LEADERSHIP

Unlike Laissez-Faire leadership, **transactional leadership** does not place trust in staff or encourage creative approaches. Transactional leadership promotes subordinate compliance through a system of rewards and punishments (Bass & Riggio, 2006). Transactional leaders focus on results and motivating employees through incentives and penalties. Transactional leadership maintains organizational structure by monitoring and evaluating individual performance against defined requirements. This technique may lead to reduced employee morale and ignoring creative solutions to challenges from well-seasoned staff. Key characteristics of transactional leaders include the following. They:

- Focus on structure and rigidity
- Oppose change

- Define rewards and penalties for workers

Transactional leaders' rigid structure and clear instructions make it easy for staff to complete tasks. Transactional leadership creates consistency and reliability within the organization and ensures staff know what to do during times of pressure. This leadership style works best in situations where structure is essential (e.g., police departments and other first responder positions). Despite the benefits, transactional leadership does not reward creativity and is unable to thrive in the face of change.

Table 5.5 Transactional Leadership Benefits and Disadvantages	
Benefits	Disadvantages
Consistency and reliability	Inflexible
Clearly defined instructions during times of pressure	Does not adapt to change
Rewards and penalties well-defined for staff	Does not reward creativity

Source: Original Work
Attribution: Whitney Hamilton
License: CC BY-SA 4.0

5.11 STRATEGIC LEADERSHIP

Strategic leadership is characterized by applying strategies to manage employees. Strategic leaders motivate their subordinates towards a shared vision. Strategic leadership is characterized by assisting individuals in pursuit of accomplishing the organization's mission and goals. Strategic leaders must also understand the work environment and provide ongoing assistance to subordinates in realizing and completing the organization's vision (Carter & Greer, 2013). They integrate the organization's vision into the organization's culture.

Key characteristics of strategic leaders include the following. They:

- Demonstrate passion for the organization's vision
- Motivate subordinates toward shared goals
- Clearly communicate organizational tasks goals

Strategic leadership benefits include increasing employee morale and workplace productivity by assessing the organization's environment and providing ongoing assistance to identified challenges. Strategic leaders have the ability to assess the environment while identifying and exploring opportunities for advancement. This leadership style works well in organizational settings where change and transformation are impending. Potential strategic leadership disadvantages include overlooking current or developing issues while attempting to address future issues that directly impact the organization's vision. Although strategic leaders plan for the future, plans may go awry and result in unanticipated and costly expenses.

Table 5.6 Strategic Leadership Benefits and Disadvantages	
Benefits	Disadvantages
Increases employee morale	Overlooks developing problems
Explores potential opportunities	Does not address issues unrelated to the vision
Enables highly skilled employees to complete tasks without micromanagement	Potentially risks unwanted, costly expenses

Source: Original Work
Attribution: Whitney Hamilton
License: CC BY-SA 4.0

5.12 DEMOCRATIC LEADERSHIP

Democratic Leadership, also known as participative leadership, is a leadership style that enables individuals within the organization to take a participative or shared role in decision-making (Lewin, Lippitt, 1938; Gastil, 1994). Democratic leaders promote collaboration and encourage creativity among staff.

Some of the primary characteristics of democratic leadership include the following:

- Encouraging creativity
- Promoting collaboration
- Facilitating engagement

Democratic leadership benefits include the increased productivity stemming from creative ideas and team collaboration. Staff may feel more valued because their input is encouraged, resulting in greater dedication and commitment to establishing organizational goals. This leadership style works best in settings such as manufacturing, where accident prevention is critical and projects completion follows a set deadline. Despite the benefits, democratic leadership drawbacks include unclear communication and ambiguously defined roles. Staff may also lack the necessary knowledge and skills to contribute to decision-making. Further, if individuals feel their opinions are not being heard and there is a lack of minority inclusion and individual thought, there may be a reduction in employee morale among staff.

Table 5.7 Democratic Leadership Benefits and Disadvantages

Benefits	Disadvantages
Increases engagement and creativity	Unclear communication and ambiguous roles
Increases staff commitment and dedication	Poor decision-making from less knowledgeable or underqualified staff
Increases workplace productivity	Decreases employee morale due to overridden opinions

Source: Original Work
Attribution: Whitney Hamilton
License: CC BY-SA 4.0

5.13 TRANSFORMATIONAL LEADERSHIP

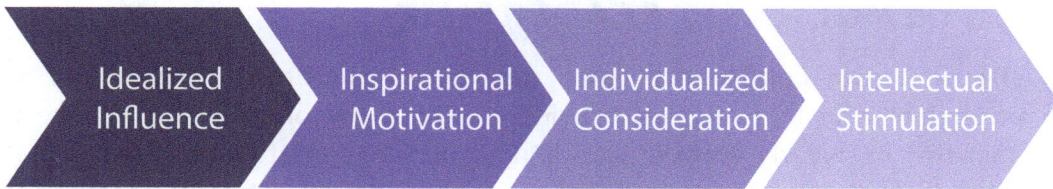

Figure 5.2: The Basic Components of Transformational Leadership

Source: Original Work
Attribution: Corey Parson
License: CC BY-SA 4.0

Transformational leadership is characterized by leaders who encourage and inspire their employees to create change within the organization (Bass & Riggio, 2006). Transformational leaders encourage creativity and out-of-the-box thinking among staff. Leaders who embrace transformational leadership lead by example and use inspiration and empathy to motivate employees. Transformational leadership improves employee morale, workplace performance, and productivity. Key characteristics of transformational leaders include the following. They demonstrate:

- Idealized influence: working to change the organizational system
- Inspirational influence: inspiring and motivating others
- Individualized consideration: maximizing staff expertise, capability, and capacity
- Intellectual stimulation: encouraging creative solutions to current organizational issues

This leadership style works best for revamping outdated, ineffective systems within organizations. For instance, in the Southern Hospice example, the facility was not yet effectively handling the shifting needs of their population.

Transformational leadership works well in organizations (such as this long-term care facility) that are experiencing change yet seeking to fulfill an overarching vision. Transformational leadership uses new solutions to remedy old problems and addresses current issues while upholding a long-term vision. Transformational leadership has also been associated with increased employee performance and increased productivity. Despite this leadership style's many advantages, potential drawbacks include increased risk, in that decisions may be made abruptly and lead to unanticipated consequences. Further, a transformational leader's approach may be too visionary and overlook reality. Their passions and ideas may be too big and not address the real issues in achieving their vision.

Table 5.8 Transformational Leadership Benefits and Disadvantages

Benefits	Disadvantages
Adapts to change and embraces new ways to address challenges	Requires an existing structure in need of change
Addresses current issues and long-term goals	Risky—may lead to unintended consequences
Increases performance, productivity, and morale	Overlooks reality

Source: Original Work
Attribution: Whitney Hamilton
License: CC BY-SA 4.0

Stop and Apply

What transformative strategies could be employed to handle some of the key challenges at Southern Hospice Care?

5.14 THE INTERSECTION OF LEADERS AND MANAGERS

According to Peter Drucker, an influential pioneer of management thinking, "management is doing things right; leadership is doing the right things." A leader's role is to inspire and motivate individuals towards completing shared organizational goals, whereas managers ensure the organization's function. Leaders innovate and focus on individuals, while managers regulate and focus on structure (Ambrose & Gullatte, 2011). However, leadership and management roles intersect, and both are necessary in order to be an effective manager in today's dynamic healthcare system.

Healthcare administrators play an integral role in healthcare organization performance and can adapt many leadership approaches to healthcare organizations in order to optimize management in such a highly complex and ever-changing environment. Leadership and management skills are complementary; both can be learned and developed through experience, and improving skills in one area will enhance abilities in the other. Good managers have strong leadership skills through which they influence staff to get things done efficiently and effectively. The manager's exemplifying qualities—such as sound ethics, mutual respect, and the effective communication skills of a leader while effectively managing cost, care, and staff—will enable the healthcare organization to reach its goals. Healthcare managers will insist on transparency in medical errors, incidents, and patient complaints and on viewing such errors as growth opportunities. Additionally, they will have the necessary leadership skills to effectively handle and address poor staff performance. They will find effective ways to motivate employees (e.g., providing benefits, salary increases, threats to terminate) and ways to improve performance (e.g., more control or increased autonomy).

Both healthcare management and healthcare leadership comprise ongoing and often intersectional learning processes. Applying leadership skills and strategies is crucial to improving organizational performance and patient experience (Austin, McCormick, and Van Puymbroeck, 2016). In the scenario mentioned in this chapter, it is important that Amanda, as the organization's director and leader, clearly communicates the facility's vision to her managers and staff. The director and managers should work together with staff to creatively establish solutions as well as garner the necessary resources and staff to address predominant challenges, such as high employee turnover rates, language and cultural barriers, cost restraints, and shifting health needs (prevalence of dementia).

Within the context of this text, the primary focus of the staff, regardless of individual positions or titles, is on practices that lead to the best possible care for patients. According to the American College of Healthcare Executives, healthcare leadership is defined as "the ability to inspire individual and organizational excellence, create a shared vision and successfully manage change to attain the organization's strategic ends and successful performance" (2011). Through leadership skills, health care managers are able to encourage and motivate employees toward this shared vision of quality, cost-comparativeness, and reliable health care.

5.15 PERSONAL ASSESSMENT: DETERMINE YOUR LEADERSHIP STYLE

Leadership can be thought of as a capacity to define oneself to others in a way that clarifies and expands a vision of the future.

-Edwin Friedman

Leaders and managers must be aware of their personal strengths and weaknesses in order to improve and be successful. In the scenario described throughout this chapter, it would be helpful if the director and each of the managers took a leadership/management assessment. By taking an assessment, each would be able to identify their individual skills and how they can best support employees. The assessment would enable them to figure out how they can work together to use each other's strengths to run the facility. Amanda would benefit from focusing on building her leadership skills and developing her current strengths in order to effectively align staff with the facility's overall mission and clearly communicating the vision to staff in order help improve morale and provide clarity on each of the managers' respective roles and directions. Meanwhile, Corinne and Michelle may want to revisit their positions' roles and responsibilities and how their division's work aligns with the overall organizational mission of Southern Healthcare Hospice Center.

5.16 CONCLUSION

In short, management and leadership are intertwined. Management gets things done, while leadership influences others to get things done. The best managers also have good leadership skills (Ambrose and Gullatte, 2011). Management and leadership skills can be learned and enhanced. Warren Bennis described leadership as a "function of knowing yourself, having a vision that is well communicated, building trust among colleagues, and taking effective action to realize your own leadership potential." In order to influence others, you must know yourself, your own strengths and weaknesses.

https://www.umassglobal.edu/news-and-events/blog/what-type-of-leader-are-you-quiz

5.17 KEY POINTS

- Although the terms leadership and management are often used interchangeably, key characteristics are unique to each.
- This chapter outlined the key competencies of effective leaders and managers.
- The healthcare system requires both, that is, good managers and strong leaders, in order to be effective.
- Good managers have the necessary skills to systematically produce the best results, while strong leaders motivate, inspire, and engender creativity to foster the best working environment to enable such results.

5.18 KEY TERMS

Democratic Leadership, Autocratic Leadership, Laissez-Faire Leadership, Strategic Leadership, Transformational Leadership, Transactional Leadership, Bureaucratic Leadership, Planning, Controlling, Coordinating, Organizing, Commanding

5.19 QUESTIONS FOR REVIEW AND DISCUSSION

1. Define healthcare management.

2. Describe a healthcare manager's functions and provide an example of a task in each function.

3. Compare and contrast functions of healthcare managers and healthcare leaders. How are leadership and management similar? How are they different?

4. Describe the ideal leadership style(s) for healthcare managers.

5. What is your evaluation of the health industry's need for healthcare managers who are also strong leaders in today's healthcare climate? Explain the specific skills, knowledge, and abilities that are important in healthcare management.

5.20 REFERENCES

Agency for Healthcare Research and Quality. "About the National Quality Strategy." 2016 https://www.ahrq.gov/workingforquality/about/index.html

Al-Sawai. (2013). Leadership of Healthcare Professionals: "Where Do We Stand?" *Oman Med J,* 28(4): 285–287. doi: 10.5001/omj.2013.79

Ambrose, D., & Gullatte, M. M. (2011). "Inspiring self and others to leadership." In M. M. Gullatte (Ed.), *Nursing management principles and practice* (2nd ed., pp. 1–19). Pittsburgh, PA: Oncology Nursing Society.

Austin, D., McCormick, B., Van Puymbroeck, M. (2016). "Management functions recreational therapy. Sagamore Publishing." https://www.sagamorepub.com/sites/default/files/2018-07/MngmntFuncRecTherpy-LookInside.pdf

Bass, B., Riggio, R. *Transformational Leadership.* 2006. Mawah, New Jersey: Lawrence Erlbaum Associates.

Bass, B. (1990). *Stodgill's Handbook of Leadership* (3rd ed.). New York: Free Press.

Buschbinder, S. & Shanks, N. (2012). *Introduction to Healthcare Management.* Jones and Bartlett Learning.

Brown, B., Crapo, J. (2017). "The Key to Transitioning from Fee-for-Service to Value-Based Reimbursement." https://www.healthcatalyst.com/wp-content/uploads/2014/08/The-Key-to-Transitioning-from-Fee-for-Service.pdf

Black Women's Maternal Health: "A Multifaceted Approach to Addressing Persistent and Dire Health Disparities." (2018). National Partnership for Women & Families. Black Maternal Health (2018). https://www.nationalpartnership.org/our-work/resources/health-care/maternity/black-womens-maternal-health-issue-brief.pdf

Carter, S., Greer, C. (2013). "Strategic Leadership: Values, Styles, and Organizational Performance." *Journal of Leadership & Organizational Studies.* DOI:10.1177/1548051812471724

Cocchi, R (2016) "Top 10 issues impacting healthcare industry in 2016." Healthcare Business & Technology. Retrieved from: http://www.healthcarebusinesstech.com/issues-impacting-hospitals-2016/

Dall, T., Gallo, P., Chakrabarti, TW., Semilla a., Storm, M. (2013). "An Aging Population and Growing Disease Burden Will Require A Large and Specialized Health Care Workforce By 2025." *Health Affairs.* 32(11): https://doi.org/10.1377/hlthaff.2013.0714

Gabriel, M.H., Noblin, A., Rutherford, A., Walden, A., & Cortelyou-Ward, K. (2018). "Data Breach Locations, Types, and Associated Characteristics Among US Hospitals." Am J Manag Care, 24(2):78-84.

Gastil, John. (1994). "A Meta-Analytic Review of the Productivity and Satisfaction of Democratic and Autocratic Leadership." Small Group Research - SMALL GROUP RES. 25. 384-410. 10.1177/1046496494253003.

Gopee, N. & Galloway, J. (2009). *Leadership and Management in Healthcare.* Sage.

Healthcare Leadership Alliance. "Overview of the HLA Competency Directory." (2010). Retrieved: http://www.healthcareleadershipalliance.org/Overview%20of%20the%20HLA%20Competency%20Directory.pdf; http://www.healthcareleadershipalliance.org/terms.htm--> permission to use definition with citation

Juckett, G. (2013). "Caring for Latino Patients." *Am Fam Physician.* 2013 Jan 1;87(1):48-54.

Lewin. K. '" Lippitt. R. (1938). "An Experimental approach to the study of autocracy and democracy: A preliminary note." *Sociometry, I, 292-300.*

Meuter, R.F., Gallois, C., Segalowitz, N.S., Ryder, A.G., Hocking, J. "Overcoming language barriers in healthcare: A protocol for investigating safe and effective communication when patients or clinicians use a second language." BMC Health Serv Res. 2015 Sep 10;15:371. doi: 10.1186/s12913-015-1024-8.

Miller, K. (2019). "Practitioner Application Strategies for Delivering Value-Based Care: Do Care Management Practices Improve Hospital Performance?" Journal of Healthcare Management: November-December 2019 - Volume 64 - Issue 6 - p 445-446 doi: 10.1097/JHM-D-19-00193

Mullins CD, Blatt L, Gbarayor CN et al. "Health Disparities: A barrier to high-quality care." *Am J Health-Syst Pharm* 2005;62:1873-82.

National Association of Health Underwriters. (2015) *Healthcare Cost Drivers White Paper.* National Association of Health Underwriters. Retrieved from: https://nahu.org/media/1147/healthcarecost-driverswhitepaper.pdf

Ronquillo, J.G., Winterholler, E., Cwikla, K., Szymanski, R., & Levy, C. (2018). "Health IT, hacking, and cybersecurity: national trends in data breaches of protected health information." *JAMIA Open*, 1(1): 15–19, https://doi.org/10.1093/jamiaopen/ooy019

Sanchez, K., Chapa, T., Ybarra, R., Martinez, O. (2012). « Enhancing the Delivery of Health Care: Eliminating Health Disparities through a Culturally & Linguistically

Centered Integrated Health Care Approach." Office of Minority Health. The U.S. Department of Health and Human Services. https://www.integration.samhsa.gov/@ Final_Health_Report.pdf

Spaulding, T. (2015). *The heart-led leader*. New York, NY: Crown Business

Thorburn, S., Kue, J., Keon, K.L., Lo, P. "Medical mistrust and discrimination in health care: a qualitative study of Hmong women and men." J Community Health. 2012 Aug;37(4):822-9. doi: 10.1007/s10900-011-9516-x.

World Health Organization. OPERATIONS MANUAL FOR STAFF AT PRIMARY HEALTH CARE CENTRES -Chapter 10 Leadership and Management. https://www. who.int/hiv/pub/imai/om_10_leadership_management.pdf

6 BUILDING A FOUNDATION IN LEADERSHIP AND MANAGEMENT THEORY

6.1 LEARNING OBJECTIVES

- Summarize leadership and management theory phases
- Identify the most common leadership and management theories' core principles
- Explain leadership and management theories' significance to the healthcare industry
- Develop theory-guided, creative solutions to key healthcare management challenges

6.2 INTRODUCTION

This chapter focuses on major theories as well as leadership and management styles while describing the relationship between leaders and managers. Leadership and management theories, similar to the U.S healthcare system, are dynamic and continue to shift over time. Examining the developing organizational theoretical principles reveals how theories can be adapted in order to optimize leadership and management approaches in the diverse and complex healthcare environment.

This chapter will discuss three distinct categories of leadership theories, including personality/behavioral, contingency/situational, and relational theories. It will also explore the three core phases of management theories: systematic, behavior, and modern management theories. And it will help identify leadership and management approaches you can employ and cultivate throughout your career. As you read through the following theories, refer to the case provided at the beginning of this chapter to determine how the director should approach the situation using each theory.

The Chapter Case

The managers and staff at Southern Healthcare Hospice Center are increasingly overworked as everyone takes on mounting responsibilities and longer workdays due to the high staff turnover. Amanda, the director of the facility, has devised a set of organizational policies. One of the policies specifically states that staff members are not allowed to sleep while on duty. A staff member made a complaint to the long-term care manager that several night-shift workers were taking naps and sleeping in beds in unoccupied patient rooms. These staff members were violating the night shift policy as well as neglecting their responsibilities. As you read through the various leadership and management theories, consider how a manager would address this scenario using concepts from each of the listed leadership or management theories.

*Adapted from Xu, J. (2017). Leadership theory in clinical practice. Clinical Nursing Research 4: 155-157

6.3 THE EVOLUTION OF LEADERSHIP THEORIES

Leadership theories have evolved in three phases, like building blocks developed on top of each other over time. Early leadership theories dating as early as 450 B.C focused on leaders' specific attributes and behaviors. Situational leadership theories prevailed in the 1960s and 1970s to provide a more integrative approach to leadership, and examined where leadership skills were mainly being adapted and put into context—the workplace environment. Currently, modern leadership theories examine the leader's interactive relationships and their workplace dynamics, where interactions occur. Studying leadership theories and how they have evolved provides leaders with an understanding of how the field has developed over time, and will help them develop their own competencies in practice and not repeat mistakes or adhere to outdated leadership philosophies (Ledlow & Coppola, 2014).

6.4 PERSONALITY/BEHAVIORAL LEADERSHIP THEORIES

Personality or behavioral theories focus on the specific traits or actions that make individuals effective leaders. Trait and behavioral based theories reflect the era in which they were developed and studied. Most early leaders were born into class, privilege, and authority, and thus were appointed through birth for their leadership roles. Personality and behavioral leadership theories include the Great Man Theory and Trait Theory.

6.4.1 Great Man Theory

Description:

Developed approximately around 450 B.C.E., the Great Man theory is as old as history itself; it postulates leadership traits as intrinsic. In other words, great leaders are destined for success from birth (Ledlow & Coppola, 2014). Undoubtedly, great men have had a hand in charting our civilization's course. The admiration for some of those great men—such as Alexander the Great and Julius Caesar—were some of the most prominent leaders through birth entitlement and contributed to the belief that leadership skills are intrinsic assets, as opposed to skills that can be developed over time (Zaccaro, 2007).

Main Assumption:

- Leaders are born with specific inherited skills that cannot be developed or acquired over time.

Limitation:

- The Great Man theory does not acknowledge the external or contextual factors that may influence leadership.

6.4.2 Trait Theory

Description:

Similar to the Great Man Theory, the Trait Theory identifies specific traits that are associated with effective leaders. Leadership research from the 1840s to approximately 1880 examined certain behaviors and characteristics of great men. According to the influential historian Thomas Carlyle (1849), leadership is an innate and unique characteristic of extraordinary individuals. Influenced by the work of Carlyle, statistician Francis Galton (1869) elaborated on the notion of intrinsic, extraordinary traits and postulated such traits were passed down from generation to generation and could not be developed (Zaccaro, 2007). It wasn't until 1948 that the Trait Theory of leadership was challenged by psychologist Ralph Stogdill. Stogdill argued that leadership was not solely the result of innate traits but instead the result of the interaction between an individual and the social situation (Stodgill, 1974). However, Stogdill did recognize specific characteristics that were consistent among successful leaders (see table below).

Table 6.1 Stogdill's Traits and Skills of Successful Leaders	
Traits	Skills
Adaptable to Situations	Clever (intelligence)
Ambitious and Achievement-Oriented	Conceptually skilled (abstract to operational)
Assertive	Creative
Cooperative	Diplomatic and tactful
Decisive	Fluent in speaking
Dependable	Knowledgeable about group tasks
Dominant	Organized
Energetic	Persuasive
Persistent	Socially skilled
Self-confident	
Tolerant of stress	
Willing to assume responsibility	
Alert to social environments	

Source: Stogdill, 1974
Attribution: Whitney Hamilton, Adapted from Stogdill 1974
License: Fair Use

Main Assumptions:

- Specific traits are associated with effective leaders.
- Leadership skills are the unique characteristics of extraordinary individuals.

Limitation:

- The Trait Theory does not acknowledge the influence of social environments on leadership.

6.4.3 Machiavellian Leadership

Description:

Niccolo Machiavelli in his notable book, *Il Principe,* or *The Prince* (1532), outlined key leadership principles necessary to be successful, including ruthlessness and malevolence. He also posited leaders must be feared, not loved. This approach is an authoritarian form of leadership that controls and regulates subordinates through fear and punishment. Machiavelli did, however, acknowledge that the subordinate's capabilities are a reflection on the leader (Calhoun, 1969). Machiavellian leadership seeks to build strong and structured teams. The major assertion of Machiavellian leadership was that "the end justifies the means." Despite the focus on fear and malice as a motivational tool in leadership, Machiavelli's underlying premise views leadership as noticeably similar to the Great Man and

Trait Theories in that they all state strong leaders must possess certain unique, innate traits (Ledlow & Coppola, 2014).

Main Assumptions:

- Leaders are to be feared, not loved.
- The end justifies the means.

Limitations:

- A leader who motivates strictly from fear may cause disengagement, workplace dissatisfaction, and decreased retention among staff.
- Ideas and creativity from qualified staff may be overlooked, staff may feel a disconnection from the organization, and full capacities may not be reached by individuals or the organization.
- Machiavellian leaders will do anything it takes to reach their ultimate goals; however, the processes may not always be ethical.

6.4.4 Lewin and Likert's Leadership Styles

Description:

In 1939, Kurt Lewin and a group of psychologists conducted leadership experiments and identified three main leadership styles: autocratic, democratic, and laissez-faire. In an autocratic leadership style, the leader makes decisions without consulting subordinates. In a democratic leadership style, the leader involves subordinates in the decision-making, although the final decision may rest solely on the leader. To the contrary, laissez-faire leadership minimizes the leader's involvement in decision making and permits subordinates to make their own decisions. Lewin and colleagues found that autocratic leadership caused the highest levels of dissatisfaction, while the democratic style was the most effective in accomplishing tasks (Lewin, Lippitt, & White, 1939). Later, psychologist Rensis Likert identified four additional leadership styles based on his research studies at the University of Michigan: exploitative, benevolent authoritative, consultative, and participative. The exploitive leadership style uses fear methods, such as punishment and threats, to motivate subordinates. The benevolent leader may also use fear methods to gain conformity but may incorporate rewards and incentives to encourage compliance as well. Consultative leaders attempt to listen to subordinate ideas; however, the leader will still make the ultimate decisions. Leaders who follow the participative leadership style will fully engage subordinates in decision-making and carry out their ideas and opinions (Likert, 1967).

Main Assumptions:

- Lewin and colleagues conducted leadership experiments and identified three types of leadership styles: autocratic, democratic, and laissez-faire.

- Likert identified four additional styles of leadership: exploitative, benevolent authoritative, consultative, and participative.

Limitation:

- The situation and context in which leadership occurs is not considered in the Lewin or Likert leadership models.

6.5 CONTINGENCY/SITUATIONAL LEADERSHIP THEORIES

Contingency/situational leadership theories provide an integrative approach to examining effective leadership attributes within the work environment, where such tactics can be adapted to suit various situations. These theories incorporate situations, context, and environments into leadership approaches. Contingency/ situational theories acknowledge that there is no single strategy for structuring, organizing, and leading a team. Unlike trait and behavioral theories that suggest leadership skills result from genetics and innate capabilities, contingency/ situational theories examine the influence of external and social factors that impact leadership (Hunt, 2019).

6.5.1 Hersey and Blanchard's Situational Leadership Theory

Description:

Blanchard and Hersey developed the Situational Leadership Theory in 1969, which focuses on a manager's ability to adapt their leadership style to fit an organization's needs. Under this leadership approach, leaders must select the best leadership style that fits the people being led, the context, and the relevant organizational situation. Blanchard and Hersey identify four leadership styles and four corresponding maturity levels (the level of a worker's experience) that describe the staff in a ranking system ranging from 1 to 4 (see table below). Telling is the most direct leadership style, by which the leader assigns tasks to the subordinates and tells them how to complete them. Under this form of leadership, the maturity level of workers is a 1, indicating workers are the least experienced and will need continual, direct instructions in order to complete responsibilities. Selling is less direct than the telling leadership style and requires more engagement between the leader and the subordinates. Leaders who demonstrate the selling leadership style may collaborate and engage with group members when trying to convince them to complete tasks a certain way. Workers under this form of leadership have a maturity level of 2 but still lack the necessary skills and experience to complete tasks despite their willingness and eagerness to do so. The participative leader will fully engage with team members and include members in decision-making (Graeff, 1983).

Staff under participative leadership have the willingness and necessary skills to complete their responsibilities. The delegative leader will impart most responsibilities to the group. Staff under delegative leadership have a maturity level of 4 and possess the skills and confidence to handle tasks completely on their own (Graeff, 1983).

Table 6.2 Hersey and Blanchard Situational Leadership	
Leadership Style	Maturity Level
Telling: *the most direct form of leadership, where the leader assigns tasks and instructions for completion to staff.*	**M1.** The least experienced staff, who will need continual, direct instructions in order to complete responsibilities.
Selling: *less direct than the telling leadership style and requires more engagement between the leader and the subordinates.*	**M2.** Inexperienced staff who have the willingness to complete tasks before they are fundamentally ready.
Participative: *fully engages with team members and includes the group in decision-making.*	**M3.** Staff at this level have the willingness and skill to complete their responsibilities with little guidance.
*The **delegative** leader will cast most responsibilities on the group.*	**M4.** Individuals at this level possess the skills and confidence to handle tasks completely on their own.

Source: Hersey and Blanchard, 1969
Attribution: Whitney Hamilton, Adapted from Hersey and Blanchard 1969
License: Fair Use

Main Assumptions:

- Focuses on a leader's ability to be flexible and adapt their leadership style to meet the needs of the organization.
- Based on variable leadership styles depending on the people being led and the situation.

Limitation:

- The concept of staff maturity is not fully defined in this model (e.g., emotional or positional).

6.5.2 Fiedler Contingency Model

Description:

Scientist Fred Fiedler developed the Fiedler Contingency Model in the mid-1960s. Similar to the Blanchard and Hersey Situational Leadership Model, Fiedler's model posits there is not a single best style of leadership; rather, the most effective leadership style depends on the situation (Hosking & Schriesheim, 1978). Unlike Blanchard and Hersey's model, Fiedler's model posits a leader's style depends upon their innate personality and does not change; instead, leaders must be placed into positions that suit their leadership style. Fiedler identified three factors that affect a leader's effectiveness: (1) leader-member relations, (2) task structure, and (3) the leader's position of power and ability to reward and/or reprimand staff (Fiedler, 1976). The leader-member relations refer to the degree the staff trusts and respects the leader and is willing to comply with instruction. Task structure refers to the extent at which a task has been defined. Position power refers to the amount of power the leader has within the organization. In Fiedler's model, a leader's effectiveness depends upon the work group performance, which depends upon the three aforementioned situational factors. The work group performance also depends on the leader's style and the situational favorableness (e.g., the degree of control the leader has over the situation) where the relationship occurs.

Fielder developed a tool called the Least Preferred Coworker (LPC) for individuals to determine their leadership style. The scale identifies the person with whom the leader least prefers to work with among the group members. The evaluation categorizes three groups of people: (1) Relationship oriented: satisfied by strong interpersonal relationships and considers these relationships critical to accomplishing tasks; (2) Task oriented: individuals focused on completed tasks rather than interpersonal relationships; and (3) The middle-LPC people who were adaptable and not overly consumed by relationships or the completion of tasks (Fiedler, 1976). According to Fiedler's model, the more favorably the leader rates the individual they least prefer to work with, the more relationship oriented the leader is. To the contrary, the less favorably the leader rates the individual they least prefer to work with, the more task-oriented the leader is. To put it simply, a high or more favorable LPC, the more relationship-oriented the leader. The lower or less favorable the LPC, the more task-oriented the leader. Task-oriented leaders have the most success with either strongly favorable or unfavorable situations. In contrast, relationship-oriented leaders have the best results with situations of mixed favorability (Fiedler, 1976; Hosking & Schriesheim, 1978).

Main Assumptions:

- Leaders have only one leadership style which is fixed and can be scored on the Least Preferred Coworker scale which identifies whether the individual is a relationship-oriented or task-oriented leader.

- A leader's effectiveness is contingent upon how well their leadership style matches the situation (situational favorableness) and/or how much control they have over the situation. Fiedler identified 3 situational factors: (1) leader-member relations, (2) task structure, and (3) the leader's position of power (Fiedler, 1976; Hosking & Schriesheim, 1978).

Limitation:

- The model posits a leader's effectiveness as dependent upon the situation; however, leaders may have varying degrees of effectiveness in certain situations.

6.5.3 Vroom and Yetton's Normative Leadership

Description:

In 1973, Vroom and Yetton elaborated on previous situational theories, noting how situational factors led to unpredictable leadership behavior. In this model, decision quality is the best solution or alternative for such behaviors. Decision acceptance is the extent to which subordinates accept the decisions made by leaders. Leaders focus more on decision acceptance when the decision quality is significant (Vroom and Yetton, 2007). Their theory on normative leadership identified five procedures for decisions: Autocratic (A1 and A2), Consultative (C1 and C2), and Group based (G2) (see table below):

Table 6.3 Vroom and Yetton's Normative Leadership Procedures for Decision-Making
A1: the leader obtains information and decides alone.
A2: the leader gains some input from subordinates then makes the final decision alone.
C1: the leader shares problems with individual subordinates and listens to their ideas and then decides alone.
C2: the leader shares problems with subordinates as a group, listens to ideas, and then decides alone.
G2: the leader shares problems with subordinates and seeks both a consensus agreement and decision acceptance from the group.

Source: Vroom and Yetton, 2007
Attribution: Whitney Hamilton, Adapted from Vroom and Yetton, 2007
License: Fair Use

Main Assumptions:

- Acceptance of a leader's decisions increases effectiveness.
- Participation in decision making increases decision acceptance.

Limitation:

- The model works best when the importance of decision quality and decision acceptance are clear; however, the importance of each factor may not always be known or clearly established.

6.5.4 Path-Goal Theory

Description:

The path-goal theory was introduced in 1970 by Martin Evans and later advanced by House. The path-goal theory identifies the ideal behaviors that are most suitable for team members and the organizational environment in order to best lead staff through a **path** in completing daily organizational activities (**goals**). This model assumes managers will change their leadership style based on their employees and workplace environment. House and Mitchell (1974) identified four types of leadership styles (directive, supportive, participative, and achievement) based on a previous study at Ohio State University analyzing two leadership behaviors referred to as initiating structure and consideration (Stogdill, 1974; House, 1971; House, 1996). The **initiating structure** refers to the leader's behavior in defining their relationships with subordinates and establishing well-defined organizational patterns and task behaviors, including planning, organizing, scheduling, and overseeing work completion. **Consideration** refers to relationship behaviors between leaders and employees indicating friendly emotions, such as trust and respect (Hersey and Blanchard, 1969; House, 1971; Stogdill, 1974; House, 1996).

Table 6.4 Four Types of Path-Goal Leaders
Initiating Structure
• **Directive:** The leaders tells employees exactly what needs to be done and how to do it.
Consideration
• **Achievement:** The leader sets difficult goals for subordinates and expects the highest level of workplace performance, illustrating confidence in their ability to accomplish the expectation (technical, scientific, and achievement environments) • **Participative:** the leader includes employees in the decision-making process. • **Supportive:** the leader creates strong relationships with employees by creating a positive and welcoming workplace environment.

Source: Hersey and Blanchard, 1969
Attribution: Whitney Hamilton, Adapted from Hersey and Blanchard 1969
License: Fair Use

Main Assumption:

- Managers will change their leadership style based on their employees and workplace environment.

Weakness:

- The theory posits that the manager's leadership style is contingent upon the staff's characteristics, which could be difficult to understand and maintain when managing a large and diverse employee base.

6.6 RELATIONAL LEADERSHIP

Relational leadership theories focus on the dynamics of an effective leader's relationships (e.g., interpersonal communication and interactions) and the context and environment in which leadership relations are constructed and enabled (Uhl-Bien, 2006). These theories move beyond the hierarchal roles and relationships between managers and subordinates and examine the interactive process in which subordinates are viewed as partners and collaborators rather than as mere followers (Uhl-Bien, 2006). Relational leadership theories focus on the leader's ability to provide a positive working environment.

6.6.1 Transformational v. Transactional Leadership

Description:

The transformational and transactional leadership concepts were developed by political scientist James MacGregor Burns (1978) through his research on political leaders. The transformational leadership theory refers to the relationships between leaders and subordinates in which the leader motivates and inspires subordinates to reach organizational goals. Transformational leadership involves both leaders and subordinates working together to elevate one another to achieve higher levels of morale and motivation. Transformational leaders are able to connect with subordinates through empathy, trust, and honesty. Transformational leadership creates meaningful individual and organizational change that realigns the perceptions, expectations and values of employees to the organization's vision. Transformational leaders are able to clearly articulate organizational goals and possess personality traits that motivate and energize subordinates to align with their revitalizing vision (Burns, 1978). Bernard M. Bass later expanded Burns' ideas on leadership, revealing the following four behaviors of transformational leaders:

- **Individualized consideration:** the leader listens and addresses the needs and concern of each subordinate.

- **Intellectual stimulation:** the leader encourages creativity in their subordinates and supports subordinates to take innovative approaches to complete tasks. The leaders' views challenge any unforeseen difficulties as opportunities to learn.

- **Inspirational motivation:** the leader is able to communicate and convey a vision that is motivational and appealing to subordinates.

- **Idealized influence:** the leader is a model of ethical behavior and gains the respect and trust of subordinates. (Bass and Riggio, 2006).

Conversely, transactional leadership encourages subordinate compliance through a system of rewards and punishments. Bass believed transactional leaders outlined two elements of exchange, including contingent rewards and management by exception. Contingent rewards are the exchange of employee efforts for a monetary or non-monetary reward (e.g., bonuses, salary increases, recognition). Management by exception refers to correction and criticism when an employee does not meet outlined expectations. While transformational leaders motivate and encourage subordinates, transactional leaders depend on self-motivated employees whom they encourage to comply through short term rewards (Avolio & Bass, 1999). Transactional leadership is an exchange of work performance and rewards. Further, transactional leaders operate within the existing organizational culture, while transformational leaders seek to positively shift the organizational culture (Bass and Riggio, 2006; Avolio & Bass, 1999; Burns, 1978).

Main Assumption:

- Transformational leaders convey an inspiring vision that motivates and inspires subordinates to align with organizational goals, while transactional leaders motivate subordinates through a system of incentives (Bass and Riggio, 2006; Burns, 1978).

Weakness:

- Under transactional leadership, employees may not be motivated to accomplish organizational duties unless there is an incentive offered.

6.6.2 Leader-Member Exchange Theory

Description:

The leader-member exchange theory was developed in the 1970s and examines the relationship between managers and their subordinates. This theory posits that all managerial-staff relationships follow these three distinct phases (Linden, Sparrowe, Wayne, 1997):

1. **Role-Taking:** managers assess the competence (e.g., skill and capability) of new employees.

2. **Role-Making:** the new team employees begin to work with the team, and managers subconsciously sort new team members into one of two groups, which are:
   ◊ **In-Group**—team members who have proved themselves dedicated and skilled. The manager trusts this group the most and provides them with attention and opportunities for advancement. Often, the in-group has similar traits and work ethic as the manager.

   ◊ **Out-Group**—team members who did not meet the manager's expectations, possibly due to a lack of motivation or incompetence. This group is given less challenging tasks and opportunities for advancement.

3. **Routinization:** routines are established between the managers and employees. The in-group team will work hard to maintain the good opinion of their managers while the out-group members may start to dislike or distrust their managers. It is very difficult to be accepted in

the out-group after negative perception has been established (Linden, Sparrowe, Wayne, 1997).

Main Assumption:

- Assumes the relationship between managers and their subordinates moves through 3 distinct phases that leads to lasting positive or negative perceptions of managers and their employees.

Limitation:

- The manager's perception of loyal or disloyal employees may be inaccurate. Employees in the out-group may be talented and dedicated but overlooked and not given a chance to demonstrate their skills. On the contrary, individuals in the in-group may not be dedicated or equipped with the necessary skills to do their jobs effectively.

6.6.3 Authentic Leadership

Description:

In 2003, Bill Georgia, a business management professor, developed the authentic leadership concept. Authentic leadership refers to the ethical behavior and awareness of a leader that enables the construction of positive workplace relationships. Like transformational leaders, authentic leaders motivate and inspire subordinates. Authentic leadership creates an open and "authentic" workplace environment. Authentic leaders acknowledge their inherent strengths and limitations. They share the success of the organization and realize that success is a team effort. They are empathetic and able to connect with subordinates while still engendering respect (Shamir, Eilam, 2005; Avolio & Gardner, 2005). Authentic leaders demonstrate the following behaviors:

- **Transparency:** the leader is transparent and encourages open communication. The leader discusses success in addition to failure. The leader motivates but also corrects unacceptable behavior.
- **Integrity:** the leader handles all situations with integrity and strong ethics.
- **Consistency:** the leader consistently inspires subordinates.
- **Listening:** the leader listens to the ideas and concerns of subordinates.
- **Vision:** the leader communicates a clear vision.
- **Motivate:** the leader encourages and motivates employees to reach higher levels of success (Shamir, Eilam, 2005).

Main Assumption:

- Authentic leaders create an open, positive working environment through their honesty and transparency.

Limitation:

- Authentic leadership requires true authenticity, which may not always be inspirational and positive—especially during tumultuous times.

6.6.4 Distributive, Collaborative, and Shared Leadership

Description:

Distributive, collaborative, and shared leadership refer to different leadership theories and approaches that explain the functions of sharing and distributing leadership roles. Collaborative leadership entails a cooperative process of leaders and employees working together towards completing organizational goals. Collaborative leaders enhance organizational performance by encouraging dialogue between various groups within the organization, sharing information and experience, and reducing challenges within the organization. After communicating organizational information and goals to employees, collaborative leaders enable subordinates to make their own informed decisions on how to carry out tasks. Collaborative leadership promotes including different cultures and perspectives while facilitating integration and interdependency among multiple departments within the organization. Employees and departments are unified by the shared organizational vision. Shared leadership refers to team-level leadership that empowers staff to share decision-making and reach organizational goals. Shared leadership focuses identifying core team values and optimizing team efficiency to achieve organizational tasks. Distributed leadership refers to distributing leadership functions throughout an organization where organizational roles are less hierarchical and more collaborative.

The distributed leadership approach has 4 key characteristics:

1. **sense-making**: the ability to understand complex, shifting workplace environments
2. **relating**: the ability to build strong, honest relationships
3. **visioning:** creating an inspiring and appealing vision that employees will strive to work towards
4. **inventing:** creating new ways of reaching organizational goals.

Leaders distribute responsibility in order to maximize individual's strengths and balance weaknesses in order to most effectively reach organizational goals (Al-Sawai, 2013).

Main Assumption:

- Leaders and employees will synergistically work together to complete organizational goals.

Limitation:

- Collaborative, distributive, and shared leadership requires diverse individuals and teams (e.g., various backgrounds, experiences, perspectives, and fields) to work together, which may disrupt productivity and lead to conflict and objections on how to reach organizational goals.

Stop and Apply

Which leadership theory or trait(s) would you employ to address staff who were in violation of the night-time policy in the scenario described at the beginning of this chapter?

Table 6.5 The Leadership Theory Chronicles

Personality/Behavioral Leadership (450B.C-1960s)	Contingency/Situational Leadership (1970s)	Relational Leadership (Late 1970s-Present)
Focuses on the specific traits or actions that make individuals effective leaders.	Focuses on adaptable leadership approaches to workplace situations, contexts, and environments	Focuses on the leader's interactive relations and dynamics in the workplace where interactions occur
<ul><li>Great Man Theory</li><li>Machiavelli</li><li>Trait Theory</li><li>The Leadership Grid</li><li>Lewin's Leadership Styles</li><li>Likert's Leadership Styles</li></ul>	<ul><li>Hersey and Blanchard's Situational Leadership Theory</li><li>Fiedler Contingency Model</li><li>Vroom and Yetton's Normative Leadership</li><li>Path-Goal Theory</li></ul>	<ul><li>Path-Goal</li><li>Transformational</li><li>Transactional</li><li>Leader-Member Exchange</li><li>Authentic Leadership</li><li>Distributive, Collaborative, and Shared Leadership</li></ul>

Source: Original Work
Attribution: Whitney Hamilton
License: CC BY-SA 4.0

6.7 MANAGEMENT THEORY PROGRESSION

Leadership theories focus on the processes by which an individual influences subordinates to achieve common organizational goals. In contrast, management theories focus on the creation of organizational order and structure. Similar to leadership theories, management theories also developed over three core phases: systematic, behavior, and modern management. The earliest management theories, dating to the early 1900s, focused on the regulation and control of organizational procedures. Behavioral theories, developed later in the 1960s, examined the specific behaviors of individuals within the organization that contributed to workplace productivity. Contemporary management theories are more integrative in their approach to management and integrate systematic processes with an understanding of workplace interpersonal relationships.

6.8 SYSTEMATIC MANAGEMENT THEORIES

Systematic management theories focus on regulating and controlling organizational processes and procedures.

6.8.1 Scientific Management

Description:

Frederick Winslow Taylor, an American engineer, introduced a mechanical perspective to increase workplace productivity by applying engineering principles to factory workers. Taylor's scientific management theory attempts to identify the most efficient way to perform any job. The goal of scientific management is to optimize workplace productivity by finding one specialized, "best" way for workers to complete tasks and rewarding employees for the quality and amount of work completed. Taylor developed three principles of scientific management (Taylor, 1919):

1. Incorporate work methods based on a scientific observation and study of the job tasks

2. Methodically select and train each worker

3. Ensure methods are being followed by working with each worker

Managers must apply strategic principles to plan work tasks, and workers must actually perform the tasks in the manner set by the manager.

Main Assumption:
- Each job task has a best method for completion and heightened productivity.

Limitations:

- Scientific management principles may lead to workplace dissatisfaction and even reduced productivity by overlooking creative, new approaches to completing workplace tasks.

- Workers may focus more on the quantity or amount of work produced, neglecting the quality.

6.8.2 Administrative Management

Description:

After years studying managerial processes that maximize organizational efficiency, Henri Fayol introduced the administrative management theory by outlining five basic functions of managers, including planning, organizing, commanding, coordinating and controlling, in addition to the 14 principles of management (Wren, Bedeian, and Breeze, 2002; table below).

Table 6.6 14 Principles of Management	
Division of work:	Organizations comprise individuals who are specialized in different areas and possess varying levels of expertise and knowledge. Personal and professional development supports increasing knowledge and specialization among staff, and staff specialization increases organizational efficiency and productivity.
Authority:	Management has the authority to give orders to staff in order for organizational tasks to be completed.
Discipline:	Managers must uphold good conduct and respectful interactions within the organization.
Unity of Command:	A clear chain of command exists wherein employees receive orders and responsibilities from a specified manager.
Unity of Direction:	Managers monitor employee progress and ensure all employees are delivering assigned activities that align with the organizational objectives/mission.
Subordinate interests:	Personal/individual interests are subordinate to the interests of the organization.
Remuneration:	Staff efforts should be rewarded either monetarily e.g., bonuses, extra compensation, etc., or non-monetarily e.g., praise, rewards, etc.
Centralization:	Decision-making must be a balanced process that depends on the organization's size hierarchy.
Scalar chain:	Clear chain of command/organizational structure exists. Each employee should have a manager they can contact in case of an emergency.

Order:	Employees must have the appropriate resources needed to carry out organizational duties. Additionally, the work environment must be safe.
Equity:	Employees must be treated justly, fairly, and equally.
Stability of tenure:	Managers should aim to reduce employee turnover and adequately recruit and retain appropriate staff members.
Initiative:	Employees should be able to freely express new ideas.
Espirit de Corps:	Managers are responsible for employee morale in the workplace and must create and sustain an atmosphere of shared trust and understanding.

Source: Wren, Bedeian, and Breeze, 2002

Attribution: White Hamilton, Adapted from Wren, Bedeian, and Breeze, 2002

License: Fair Use

Main Assumption:

- There are five basic management functions and 14 ways managers can effectively accomplish the five basic functions.

Weakness:

- Administrative management aims to maximize workplace efficiency but may not consider unintended consequences that may arise, such as overlooking creative approaches, ignoring rising or current problems while trying to reach end goals, and employees' feelings of dissatisfaction due to an overreliance on specific rules, functions, and procedures.

6.8.3 Weber's Bureaucratic Theory

Description:

Weber's bureaucratic theory of management provides a systematic structure to organizations in order to ensure efficiency. Bureaucratic management seeks to ensure consistency and precision by structuring the organization to operate within a specific power structure in a top-down manner where decisions are made at the top, with middle managers providing oversight to lower-level employees who carry out specific tasks (Lutzker, 1982). Weber outlined 6 key characteristics of bureaucracy:

Table 6.7 Weber's Bureaucratic Theory	
Characteristic	Description
Hierarchical Management Structure	Hierarchical levels of authority where each level controls the level below and is governed by the level above. The highest level has the greatest authority and power.
Division of Labor	Tasks and responsibilities are clearly defined
Formal Selection Process	Staff hiring and promotion is based on meeting requirements, including experience, competence, examinations, education, and/or training.
Career Orientation	Staff are designated to fill specific roles based on their expertise and competence.
Formal Rules and Regulation	Rules and regulations are set to ensure reliability and compliance.
Impersonal	Rules are uniformly and consistently applied to all staff, preventing nepotism and favoritism.

Source: Lutzker, 1982
Attribution: Whitney Hamilton, Adapted from Lutzker, 1982
License: Fair Use

Main Assumption:

- Bureaucracy will establish a formal structure enabling efficiency and consistency from all staff within the organization.

Limitation:

- Bureaucratic management's hierarchical nature may cause lower-level employees to feel devalued and may limit such employees from sharing innovative ideas and contributing to decision-making.

6.9 BEHAVIORAL MANAGEMENT THEORIES

Behavioral management theories examine individual organizational behaviors, including such aspects as motivation, negotiation, conflict resolution, expectations, and group dynamics that contribute to workplace productivity.

6.9.1 The Leadership Grid

Description:

The leadership grid, also known as the management grid, was developed in the 1960s by Robert Blake and Jane Mouton and focuses on the attitudes that determine behavior. Blake and Mouton identify five different styles of leadership that drive a manager's behavior based on concern for people and concern for results (Hersey and Blanchard, 1969). Concern for people refers to the extent leaders consider team members' needs in decision-making. Concern for results refers to the extent managers emphasize organizational goals in decision-making. The five management/leaderships styles include:

- **Impoverished management:** refers to a self-centered managerial style primarily concerned with self-preservation and ensuring issues are not the manager's fault. This type of manager shows indifference toward staff as well as the overall organizational mission.

- **Produce or perish management:** refers to the disciplinarian manager who does not consider their staff's needs.

- **Country club management:** this type of manager values the staff's needs first above everything else with the assumption that the staff's happiness will lead to optimal productivity.

- **Team management:** this type of manager is committed to empowering staff and encouraging staff to work as a team in an effort to increase productivity. This form of management is often considered the most effective form of leadership.

- **Middle of the road management:** this manager is able to balance the staff's needs as well as the organization's needs for production, without, however, fully fulfilling either aspect (Hersey and Blanchard, 1969).

6.9.2 Human Relations Theory

Description:

In the 1920s, Elton Mayo attempted to improve workers' satisfaction at Western Electric Company by changing the environmental conditions (e.g., changing the lighting, altering break time, and changing the temperature) in the factory—through studies commonly known as the Hawthorne Studies. The Hawthorne Studies sought to examine the physical conditions and factors that enable employees to work most efficiently, but instead found that socio-psychological factors increased workers' productivity. The attention from researchers made the workers feel valued, thereby increasing their motivation and productivity. The human relations theory stemming from the Hawthorne Studies assumes individuals prefer to work for organizations where they are valued, supported, and able to develop over time. Thus, when managers demonstrate the significance and value of each worker and provide them with encouraging feedback and support, staff are motivated to achieve organizational goals (Mayo, 1933; Roethlisberger & Dickson, 1939).

Main Assumption:

- Encouragement and support stemming from positive workplace manager-staff relationships increase employee productivity.

Limitation:

- The theory assumes workers are highly motivated by social factors (e.g., relationships and attention); however, human behavior is complex and multifaceted. A variety of factors may contribute to workplace motivation and behavior.

6.9.3 Theory X Y

Description:

As a result of the Hawthorne Studies, Douglas McGregor, a social psychologist, also examined the influence of motivation on productivity and, in 1960, introduced Theory X Y. This theory's basic assumption is that the average person, the X type individual, does not like work and will avoid it if possible; thus, employees must be motivated through incentives, coercion, and control. The model also assumes that most people are not ambitious and desire ongoing supervision in order to avoid responsibility. In contrast, theory Y workers and individuals are self-motivated and happy to work. Theory Y individuals accept responsibility for work tasks and find satisfaction through completing organizational goals. Encouragement, rather than punishments and rewards, are used to motivate theory Y employees (Heil, Bennis, & Stephens, 2000; McGregor, 1960).

Main Assumption:

- The average person dislikes work and will avoid it if possible; thus, employees must be motivated through rewards or punishment.

Limitation:

- Each individual is different, and creating an organizational environment that meets the needs of both types of workers can be challenging.

6.10 MODERN MANAGEMENT THEORIES

Modern management theories are an integrative approach to management that incorporate systematic processes and an understanding of workplace interpersonal relationships.

6.10.1 Systems Theory

Description:

In the 1960s, Katz and Kahn were the first to apply a systems approach to organizational behavior. The systems theory measures workplace effectiveness based on the interaction between the organization and its environment. In systems theory, the organization can be an open or closed system. Closed systems are unaffected by the environment, while open systems are affected by changes in the environment. Most organizations are open systems that depend on the environment for several reasons: customers who purchase the product/service, suppliers who provide the resources, employees who provide the labor, investors who endow the finances, and governments that regulate. Successful organizations are able to adapt to the changes in the environment and continue to grow. Organizations that face dynamic and ever-changing environments can encounter uncertainty when figuring out how to survive and thrive. Pfeffer and Salancik defined effectiveness as "how well an organization is meeting the demands of the various groups and organizations that are concerned with its activities" (1978, p. 11).

Systems theory involves a process of input, throughput, feedback, and output. Input refers to the organization's ongoing monitoring of any changes of environment. Feedback lets the organization identify whether the organization is operating correctly or identify the adjustments they should make in order to correct potential issues as a result of environmental shifts. The input (environmental information) is used to respond to environmental changes, and the adjustments are made accordingly (throughput). The adjustments may affect the structure and/or processes of the organization. The organization then tailors its strategies to align with the organization's overall goals and mission (output). The organization then measures the effectiveness by seeking feedback. The process is repeated until the proper solution is found. The systems approach focuses on the methods to maintain the organization's long-term success rather than accomplishing short-term goals.

Main Assumption:

- Most organizations are open systems that depend on the environment for (1) customers who purchase the product/service, (2) suppliers who provide the resources, and (3) employees who provide labor, investors who endow finances, and governments that regulate.

Limitation:

- The theory focuses on the external factors that influence the organization's long-term goals and mission but may overlook the internal, day-to-day operations and processes that impact organizational effectiveness.

6.11 HEALTHCARE MANAGEMENT AND LEADERSHIP THEORY IN PRACTICE

6.11.1 Patient Centered Management

Many health care organizations have been prompted to take a systems-based approach to healthcare management, moving patient-centered care from theory to practice (Institute for Patient and Family-Centered Care, 2012). Chronic conditions—such as diabetes, hypertension, and heart disease—are widely prevalent and costly yet avoidable illnesses that claim thousands of lives and consume nearly 90% of the nation's annual healthcare spending (CDC, 2020). Moving to a patient-centered approach moves beyond approaches that merely treat disease but instead address the root causes of disease, which will ultimately save overall health expenditures and lives (Sweeney & Waranoff, 2007; Stewart, et. al, 2000). Due to their rising costs and prevalence, managing chronic diseases is an urgent concern. Healthcare administrators and physicians must work to engage and educate patients by addressing their patients' unique needs and developing personalized plans. For instance, failure to adhere to treatment and medication plans may be associated with non-clinical factors, such as affordability or cultural preferences for traditional, natural remedies rather than prescription medications.

The social determinants of health, or the conditions in which people live, work, and play, that influence health outcomes, must be addressed in order to enable preventing chronic disease and achieving optimal health (CDC, 2020). Providers have used predictive analyses from the Electronic Health Record (EHR) to target high-risk individuals who may benefit from lifestyle changes and specialized treatment methods. Integrating predictive analyses and tailoring medications and treatment solutions to specific high-risk groups can improve patient adherence to medical treatment and eventually improve individuals' overall health and wellness while reducing healthcare costs. Personalized interventions can also be implemented to prevent and delay chronic disease (Ye, et. al, 2018).

The shift in focus integrates patients into practicing quality improvement and moving beyond an individual, practitioner approach to more of a patient-centered and interdisciplinary approach to healthcare management. Incorporating more than just the doctors, practitioners, and involving patients, utilizing health information technology and coordinated care practices has been shown to maximize efficiency and improve health outcomes (Sweeney, et. al, 2007, Lorig, 1999; Lorig, et. al, 2001; Coulter, 2007; Edgman-Levitan, 2003; Bechel, 2001). As mentioned in the previous chapter, the shifting attitudes—from the costly, ineffective system of diagnosis and treatment towards a cost-effective, individualized healthcare focus—has led many health organizations to adopt a patient-centered approach to healthcare management.

Patient-centered care approaches have often included implementing infrastructural changes, such as electronic health records and advanced access to scheduling. Patient centered care strengthens the patient-clinician relationship, promotes communication about things that matter, helps patients know more about their health, and facilitates their involvement in their own care (Epstein & Street, 2011).

The Institute of Medicine defines patient-centered care as "care that is respectful of and responsive to individual patient preferences, needs, and values" (2001). True patient-centered care integrates the patient's culture, personal opinions, values, and lifestyle, as well as their families, into care. The patient and family collaborate with health care professionals in the decision-making process regarding the patients' health in order to provide quality care and improve the patient's overall experience.

The traditional, bureaucratic, top-down approach to healthcare is shifting towards a patient-centered model that enables collaboration and interdisciplinary approaches to healthcare delivery. Healthcare managers oversee and ensure providers are using the most valuable healthcare options, which are also the most cost-effective. Patient-centered healthcare practices enhance patient satisfaction; ensure patients understand their condition, prognosis, and treatment options; and fully involve patients in decision-making. Surveying patients on their care experiences provides the unique patient perspective and can shed light on changes that may be necessary to improve health care access, such as, for example, revised appointment policies, hours of operation, and patient-centered changes to care and treatment options. A neuroscience center redesigned its approach to integrate a focus on patient and family engagement. Within three years, the facility experienced a 50% decrease in hospital length of stay and a 62% reduction in medical errors. Patient satisfaction also increased from the 10th to the 95th percentile, and the staff retention rates also increased. Studies show patient-centered care results in fewer complications, deaths and helps to reduce costs (Institute for Patient and Family-Centered Care, 2012).

Involving patients and their families will increase engagement in patient care and improve their overall experience within the healthcare system. In 2011, the clinical and executive leadership team of an independent practice in Humboldt County, California re-designed its healthcare system to focus on providing patient-centered care. The team developed easy-to-read patient brochures and evaluated the online system patients use to access their electronic medical records. They identified and addressed potential challenges the patients may face using the online portal and suggested ways to rewrite office policies in a way that patients would understand. The facility also developed a survey to better understand why patients objected to childhood immunizations. In 2011, seven practices in south-central Pennsylvania introduced similar programs as a collaborative to implement patient-centered care. These practices focused on patient communication and active involvement in their care. The patients would bring all of their medication to the provider in order to review proper dosing. One practice implemented an alert system to notify patients of the provider wait time. The staff assessments illustrated not only improved patient-provider interactions but also increased patient satisfaction with the new team approach to healthcare (Institute for Patient and Family-Centered Care, 2012).

Sharing education and knowledge, involving family and friends, collaborating with other care teams, considering spiritual and non-medical aspects of health care, respecting patients needs and preferences, and making health information accessible are the core elements associated with providing quality and truly patient-centered care. In order to successfully ensure a patient-centered health care environment, the healthcare leader must demonstrate true leadership skills by engaging every member of the healthcare organization; clearly and continually communicating the vision; involving patients and their families; creating a supportive work environment for staff; monitoring, measuring, and evaluating process outcomes; and considering and addressing feedback provided by patients and staff.

Stop and Apply

Which management theory would you employ to address or prevent staff policy violations, such as the nighttime policy described at the beginning of this chapter?

Table 6.8 The Development of Management Theories

Systematic Management Theories (early 1900s)	Behavioral Management Theories (1960s)	Modern Management Theories (1960s-current)
Examines the regulation and control of organizational processes and procedures.	Examines individual organizational behaviors, including such aspects as motivation, negotiation, conflict resolution, expectations, and group dynamics that contribute to workplace productivity.	Examines the integrative approach to management that incorporates systematic processes and understanding workplace interpersonal relationships.
• Scientific Management • Administrative Management • Weber's Bureaucratic Theory	• Human Relations • Behavioral Science • McGregor's Theory X Y • Leadership Grid	• Systems Theory

Source: Original Work
Attribution: Whitney Hamilton
License: CC BY-SA 4.0

6.12 CONCLUSION

This chapter has provided an overview of core management and leadership theories that have evolved over time. It emphasized the significance of leadership and management to the healthcare environment. Understanding and establishing a strong foundation in the principles of leadership and management is key to producing effective leaders and managers with the necessary skills to successfully lead people and manage resources in the dynamic healthcare system.

6.13 KEY POINTS

- Leadership's role is essential to managing the healthcare industry's complexities.

- Leadership theories should serve as a guide to effective leadership by focusing on the dynamic relationship between the leader's values and capabilities to the organization's culture and context.

- Early leadership theories focused on leaders' specific traits and suggested leaders were born, not made. Later situational leadership theories were developed to consider organizational context and the environment where the leader's skills were applied. Currently, modern leadership theories examine the leader's interactions as well as the dynamics of the workplace where the interactions occur.

- Management theories evolved in three phases. Early management theories examined systematic ways of increasing workers' productivity, seemingly treating humans as machines rather than acknowledging the influence of social factors and interrelations on productivity, which were concepts later introduced in human relations management theories. Modern management theories examine an even more integrative approach to management that incorporate an understanding of workplace interpersonal relationships as well as systematic procedures.

6.14 KEY TERMS

Democratic Leadership, Autocratic Leadership, Laissez-Faire Leadership, Strategic leadership, Transformational leadership, Transactional leadership, Bureaucratic leadership, Planning, Controlling, Coordinating, Organizing, Commanding

6.15 QUESTIONS FOR REVIEW AND DISCUSSION

1. Explain the importance of effective leadership in the health industry and the challenges in the healthcare system that require strong leadership.

2. Describe the 3 phases of leadership and identify unique characteristics associated with each of the phases.

3. Distinguish the 3 phases of management and identify unique characteristics associated with each of the phases.

4. What distinguishes the phases of leadership theory from ancient to modern times, and what are the differences within each phase?

5. What is leadership, and why is leadership vital to successful health organizations? Write a paragraph that supports your definition and another paragraph explaining it.

6. Upon considering the trait, behavioral, and situational leadership phases of research, which phase seems most relevant today in the health industry? Are there underlying constructs from each phase that can work together to form a coherent leadership model that explains leadership and can predict organizational outcomes? Break down each phase and relate the underlying constructs to leadership in health organizations today, paying particular attention to organizational outcomes.

7. Which attributes do you (or would you) look for in a manager? Which attributes do you look for in a leader? In your answers to these questions, is there a theoretical link to your responses? Compile a list of managerial attributes and a list of leadership attributes. Categorize each managerial and leadership attribute as a "trait," a "behavior," or a "situational" attribute, and summarize the major themes of your lists in one to two paragraphs.

8. Distinguish the phases of leadership theory from ancient to modern times, and identify unique characteristics associated with each of these phases.

9. Relate the phases of leadership theory to modern leadership practices and research.

6.16 REFERENCES

Al-Sawai, A. (2013). "Leadership of Healthcare Professionals: Where Do We Stand?" *Oman Med J,* 28(4): 285–287. doi: 10.5001/omj.2013.79

Avolio, Bruce J. and Bass, Bernard M. (1999). "Re-examining the components of transformational and transactional leadership using the Multifactor Leadership Questionnaire." Journal of Occupational and Organizational Psychology. 72, 441-462.

Avolio, T., Bruce, J., Gardner, W.L. (2005). "Authentic leadership development: Getting to the root of positive forms of leadership." The Leadership Quarterly 16 (2005) 315 – 338 https://www.mcgill.ca/engage/files/engage/authentic_leadership_avolio_gardner_2005.pdf

Bechel DL , Myers WA , Smith DG . "Does patient-centered care pay off?" *Jt Comm J Qual Improv* . 2000 ; *26* (7): 400 – 9 . Crossref, Medline, Google Scholar

Calhoun, Richard P. "Niccolo Machiavelli and the Twentieth Century Administrator." *The Academy of Management Journal* 12, no. 2 (1969): 205-12. http://www.jstor.org/stable/254816

Coulter A , Ellins J . "Effectiveness of strategies for informing, educating, and involving patients." *BMJ* . 2007 ; *335* (7609): 24 . Crossref, Medline , Google Scholar

Edgman-Levitan S , Shaller D , McInnes K , Joyce R , Coltin K , Cleary P . *The CAHPS improvement guide: practical strategies for improving the patient care experience.*

Boston (MA) : Harvard Medical School ; 2003 . Google Scholar

Fiedler, EF, Chemers, MM., Mahar, L. (1976) *Improving Leadership Effectiveness: The Leader Match Concept.* New York: John Wiley, 1976. 219 pp., paperbound. *Group & Organization Studies, 2*(2), 254–255.

Graeff, Claude L. (1983). "The Situational Leadership Theory: A Critical Review." Academy of Management Review, Vol. 8, 285-291. https://doi.org/10.5465/amr.1983.4284738

Hersey, P., & Blanchard, K. (1969). "Life cycle theory of leadership." Training and Development Journal, 23, 26-35.

Hersey, P. and Blanchard, K. H. *An introduction to situational leadership. Training and Development Journal,* vol. 23 (1969). pp. 26–34.

"Health and Economic Costs of Chronic Diseases." Centers for Disease Control. 2020. https://www.cdc.gov/chronicdisease/about/costs/index.htm

Heil, G., Bennis, W., & Stephens, D. C. (2000). *Douglas McGregor, revisited: managing the human side of the enterprise.* Wiley.

Hickman, GR. (2009). *Leading Organizations: Perspectives for a New Era.* Sage Publications- Cambridge University Press.

~Burns, JM. (1978). *Leadership* (Excerpts). New York: Harper & Row.

~Bass, BM, Riggio, RE. (2006). The Transformational Model Leadership

Hosking, D., & Schriesheim, C. (1978). "Reviewed Work: Improving Leadership Effectiveness: The Leader Match Concept." Administrative Science Quarterly, 23(3), 496-505. doi:10.2307/2392426 http://bus.lsu.edu/management/faculty/abedeian/articles/Fayol.pdf

House, R.J. (1971). "A Path-Goal Theory of Leader Effectiveness." *Administrative Science Quarterly.* 16, 321-328.

House, R.J., Mitchell, T.R. (1974). "Path-goal theory of leadership." *Journal of Contemporary Business.* 3: 1–97.

House, R.J. (1996). "Path-goal theory of leadership: Lessons, legacy, and a reformulated theory." *Leadership Quarterly.* 7 (3): 323–352.

Hunt, Thaddeus & Fedynich, Lavonne. (2019). "Leadership: Past, Present, and Future: An Evolution of an Idea." 8. 22-26. 10.18533/journal.v8i2.1582.

Institute of Medicine. *Crossing the quality chasm: a new health system for the 21st century.* Washington (DC): National Academies Press; 2001

Institute for Patient- and Family-Centered Care. *Profiles of change: MCGHealth (MCG Medical Center and MCG Children's Medical Center)* [Internet]. Augusta (GA): MCGHealth ; [updated 2012 Aug 13 ; cited 2012 Sep 29]. Available from: http://www.ipfcc.org/profiles/prof-mcg.htmlGoogle Scholar

Jackson, C. 1997. "Behavioral science theory and principles for practice in health education." *Health Education Research Theory Practice*, Vol 12, no. 1, 143-150.

Klein S. "Issue of the month: bringing patients to the center of hospital care." *Quality Matters* [serial on the Internet]. 2007 Mar/Apr [cited 2013 Jan 7]. Available from: http://www.commonwealthfund.org/Newsletters/Quality-Matters/2007/March-April/Issue-of-the-Month-Bringing-Patients-to-the-Center-of-Hospital-Care.aspx Google Scholar

Leadership: Current Theories, Research, and Future Directions. Available from: https://www.researchgate.net/publication/51425324_Leadership_Current_Theories_Research_and_Future_Directions [accessed Sep 30, 2019].

Lewin, K., Lippit, R. and White, R.K. (1939). "Patterns of aggressive behavior in experimentally created social climates." *Journal of Social Psychology, 10,* 271-301

Likert, R. (1967). *The human organization: Its management and value,* New York: McGraw-Hill

Linden, R., Sparrowe, R.T., and Wayne, S. (1997). "Leader-Member Exchange Theory: The Past and Potential for the Future." *Personnel and Human Resources Management.* 15: 47-119. https://www.researchgate.net/profile/Robert_Liden/publication/232504779_Leader-member_exchange_theory_The_past_and_potential_for_the_future/links/543e7c430cf2e76f02228137.pdf

Lorig KR, Sobel DS, Stewart AL, Brown BW, Bandura A, Ritter P, et al. "Evidence suggesting that a chronic disease self-management program can improve health status while reducing hospitalization: a randomized trial." *Med Care.* 1999; *37* (1): 5-14. Crossref, Medline, Google Scholar

Lorig KR, Ritter P, Stewart AL, Sobel DS, Brown BW, Bandura A, et al. "Chronic disease self-management program: 2-year health status and health care utilization outcomes." *Med Care.* 2001; *39* (11): 1217 – 23. Crossref, Medline , Google Scholar

Lutzker, MA. 1982. "Max Weber and the Analysis of Modern Bureaucratic Organization: Notes Toward a Theory of Appraisal." American Archivist. 45(2): 119-130.

Mayo, E. (1933). "The human problems of an industrial civilization." New York: The Macmillan Company.

McGregor, D. (1960). *The human side of enterprise.* New York.

McGregor, D. (1960). *Theory X and theory Y.* Organization theory, 358-374.

Roethlisberger, F.J. & W.J. Dickson (1939). *Management and the worker.* Cambridge, Mass: Harvard University Press.

Stogdill, R.M. (1974). *Handbook of Leadership: A Survey of Theory and and Research.* New York: Free Press.

Shamir, B., Eilam, G. "What's your story?": A life-stories approach to authentic leadership development." The Leadership Quarterly (2005), 10.1016/j.leaqua.2005.03.005

Stewart M, Brown JB, Donner A, McWhinney IR, Oates J, Weston WW, et al. "The impact of patient-centered care on outcomes. *J Fam Pract.* 2000; *49* (9): 796 – 804. Medline , Google Scholar

Sweeney L, Halpert A, Waranoff J. "Patient-centered management of complex conditions can reduce costs without shortening life." *Am J Manag Care.* 2007; *13* (2): 84 – 92. Medline, Google Scholar

Taylor, F.W. *The Principles of Scientific Management.* 1919. New York, Harper and Brothers http://strategy.sjsu.edu/www.stable/pdf/Taylor,%20F.%20W.%20 (1911).%20New%20York,%20Harper%20&%20Brothers.pdf

Uhl-Bien, M. "Relational Leadership Theory: Exploring the social processes of leadership and organizing." https://doi.org/10.1016/j.leaqua.2006.10.007

Vroom, V.H. and Yetton, P.W. (2007). *The Role of Situation in Leadership.* American Psychological Association. Doi: http://dx.doi.org/10.1037/0003-066X.62.1.17

Vroom, V.H. (1964). *Work and motivation.* New York: Wiley.

Wren, D. A., Bedeian, A. G., & Breeze, J. D. (2002). "The foundations of Henri Fayol's administrative theory." *Management Decision, 40*(9), 906-918.

Ye C, Fu T, Hao S, Zhang Y, Wang O, Jin B, Xia M, Liu M, Zhou X, Wu Q, Guo Y, Zhu C, Li YM, Culver DS, Alfreds ST, Stearns F, Sylvester KG, Widen E, McElhinney D, Ling X. (2018). "Prediction of Incident Hypertension Within the Next Year: Prospective Study Using Statewide Electronic Health Records and Machine Learning." J Med Internet Res 2018;20(1):e22

Zaccaro, SJ. (2007). "Trait Based Perspectives of Leadership." George Mason University. American Psychological Association. 62(1): 6-16. DOI: 10.1037/0003-066X.62.1.6 http://citeseerx.ist.psu.edu/viewdoc/download?doi=10.1.1.475.9808&rep=rep1&type=pdf

7 THE ROLE OF LEADERS AND MANAGERS IN ESTABLISHING ORGANIZATIONAL ETHICS

7.1 LEARNING OBJECTIVES

- Distinguish the role of leaders and managers in influencing organizational culture, performance, and change while establishing organizational ethics
- Describe key challenges facing today's healthcare leaders
- Explain the role of leaders in addressing the current dynamic complexities within the healthcare industry
- Identify the leadership skills necessary to navigate organizational change

7.2 INTRODUCTION

Chapter seven further distinguishes how important leadership and management skills are by defining the roles of leaders and managers when influencing organizational culture, performance, and change. Many challenges exist within today's healthcare industry that directly affect the way leaders run their organizations. This chapter will examine the current challenges within the health industry and indicate the main factors health leaders and managers need to understand in order to strategically and effectively lead people and manage resources in the midst of turbulence. In order to keep up with the current trends in the U.S. healthcare system, health managers must understand how change occurs and create settings that encourage innovation. Organizational culture is influenced by the characteristics leaders and managers value, which influence the organization's outcomes. This chapter will describe the key elements necessary to sustain an organizational culture, thereby ensuring high organizational performance.

The Chapter Case

As previously outlined, The Southern Healthcare Hospice facility has been facing several challenges following recent demographic shifts. The surrounding area now consists of predominately low-income, Hispanic, Spanish-speaking residents and is experiencing an increase in the number of patients exhibiting symptoms of dementia. The facility currently lacks linguistic services, and the staff are also not fully trained to handle patients exhibiting symptoms of dementia. Patients and their families are highly dissatisfied, and overall health outcomes and on-site accidents have been worsening as a result of miscommunication. Further, the manager, Corinne, has been coming into work very late, yet she reprimands other staff for being tardy. Patients are also complaining about the rudeness of staff, which has not yet been addressed. The facility is also suffering from high staff turnover and staff dissatisfaction. Several nurses, administrators, and therapists have quit. The managers and staff are increasingly overworked as everyone takes on mounting responsibilities as a result of the high staff turnover. As you read through this chapter, identify the steps the director and healthcare managers should take in order to improve the facility's organizational culture and adapt to the external and internal changes.

7.3 ORGANIZATIONAL CULTURE

Organizational culture refers to the beliefs, values, and ways of interacting that contribute to an organization's environment (Schein, 2010). The culture encompasses the organization's shared beliefs and values that are established, shared, and reinforced by the organization's leaders. As defined by the American College of Healthcare Executives Code of Ethics, the professional health leader's responsibility is "to maintain or enhance the overall quality of life, dignity and wellbeing of every individual needing healthcare service and to create a more equitable, accessible, effective, and efficient healthcare system" (ACHE, 2011). The organization must have a foundation that follows the 4 basic pillars of biomedical ethics, which are to have respect for patients, maximize benefits, avoid harm, and provide fair and equitable treatment (see figure below). Building on these basic ethical healthcare principles will determine the organization's culture and the way the organization fulfills its commitments to the staff, patients, and community. The leaders of the healthcare organization create and convey the culture, establishing the manner in which healthcare is planned, delivered, and evaluated. As stated by the organization theorist Edgar Schein, culture and leadership "are two sides of the same coin and neither can really be understood by itself." The healthcare leaders establish the organization's culture and exemplify and convey the values of the organization to its constituents (Donnellan, 2013). The healthcare leader must nurture and sustain an ethical culture, which results in staff who are committed and dedicated to practicing the ethical values of the organization.

The healthcare organization's leadership is key to achieving quality care and patient satisfaction. The leaders and all staff within the healthcare organization, despite job titles or roles, share a part in providing the best quality care to patients. Leaders must be able to clearly communicate the facility's commitment to serve its community, meet its patients' unique needs, and create an organizational culture that is conducive to this commitment. For example, implementing an ethics training program to inform all staff, ranging from clinical practitioners to department administrators, on how to maintain ethical and moral standards when faced with potential ethical dilemmas. Such exercises can help establish a strong ethical and high performing culture. Health care administrators must also encourage staff to report unethical behavior by reminding staff of the importance of maintaining an ethical and professional work environment for patients. Building rapport with staff to ensure staff members feel safe to express their concerns and report unethical behavior is another vital role of healthcare administrators. Creating a culture that fosters open communication and feedback provides administrators with the opportunity for continual improvement. Healthcare managers must establish an ethical culture of safety, accountability, transparency, teamwork, negotiation, communication, and ongoing learning. Establishing this culture begins by recruiting and retaining staff who share the organization's values.

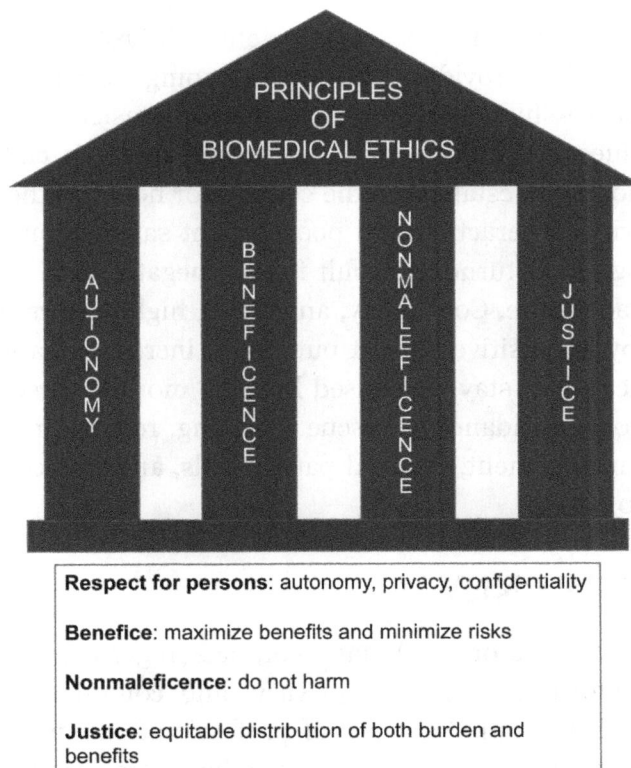

Figure 7.1: Basic Biomedical Principles

Source: Original Work
Attribution: Whitney Hamilton
License: CC BY-SA 4.0

7.4 SAFETY

Healthcare administrators engage with the doctors and nurses who are on the ground providing patient care in addition to other healthcare staff and patients. In order to enable the delivery of safe care, health administrators must have the ability to work collaboratively with teams of healthcare professionals, plan ahead, and anticipate outcomes. Similar to the effects of distracted driving, healthcare administrators who overlook critical processes due to distractions can cause unintended yet life-threatening consequences. For instance, failing to remind and ensure all staff properly wash their hands can contribute to the spread of infection and death. In long-term care facilities, infections represent an excess of $1 billion in annual healthcare costs (Murray, 2018). A randomized research study assessing the impact of a hand hygiene intervention program implemented in 26 nursing homes found the facilities that implemented the hygiene training experienced a 21% decline in mortality rates and a significant decline in antibiotic prescriptions in contrast to the nursing homes that did not implement the training program (Temime, et. al, 2018). Health care administrators must have the capability to think proactively, because reacting to complications rather than anticipating potential challenges can be fatal.

7.5 ACCOUNTABILITY

Healthcare managers must also clearly define the roles and responsibilities of all staff. Additionally, providing staff with ongoing training and support will help the staff to successfully and accurately complete tasks while reinforcing the organization's values and mission. The healthcare facility's culture, set by the organization's leadership, establishes the context for how healthcare is delivered. Poor patient-provider interaction and poor patient satisfaction, negative health outcomes, and high staff turnover result from a negative and ineffective health care organizational culture. Conversely, an ethical, high performing organization is characterized by its positive patient outcomes, increased patient satisfaction, shorter hospital length of stay, decreased hospital mortality, reduced healthcare associated infections, avoidance of rescue rationing, reduced medication errors, inadequate pain management, reduced patient falls, and reduced medical errors (Sfantou, et. al, 2017).

7.6 TRANSPARENCY

Healthcare administrators may face conflicts regarding the protection of personal health information, patient privacy, and compliance to government rules, regulations, laws, and standards of professional conduct. However, staff must be transparent with patients and their families, even admitting to fault when accidents happen. A healthcare organization built on strong ethical principles and guided by ethically sound leaders results in better patient care, efficient healthcare delivery, and satisfied staff and patients. Healthcare leaders and all working in the healthcare system need to make ethically sound decisions—especially during times of ethical uncertainty, like doing the wrong thing when it feels morally "right."

7.7 NEGOTIATION

Conflict is unavoidable and almost inevitable whenever people are involved. However, conflict does not have to be negative. When addressed appropriately, conflict can lead to innovative and creative solutions to even the most challenging problems. Health care administrators must be able to work collaboratively with internal staff (among hospital organizational units) and external partners (e.g., stakeholders and regulators) and be able to negotiate. Individuals may disagree on how to reach end goals; however, the goal and mission to promote patient safety and satisfaction should always be paramount. Health administrators must effectively and collaboratively work with teams in order to cultivate a culture and staff dedicated to ensuring patient safety.

7.8 COMMUNICATION AND ONGOING LEARNING

The necessary ingredients for developing and sustaining a culture and system that delivers safe and quality care are strong, effective leaders who establish a culture of safety, open communication, and a system of learning. Figure 7.2 shows the components of that framework. The leader must demonstrate their commitment to the healthcare organization's mission by creating an open and welcoming environment that encourages input and feedback from patients and staff. The leader creates and maintains the organizational culture by this ongoing interaction with the organization's staff, patients, and surrounding community. Through this interaction, in addition to their behaviors and skills, the leader influences the effectiveness of the healthcare organization.

A strong culture that is centered on patients can similarly increase patient satisfaction, patient engagement and patient adherence to medical regimes, resulting in positive health outcomes and overall reduced healthcare costs. Healthcare managers must also be role models for the organization's beliefs and reinforce organizational values. Providing ongoing feedback and enabling two-way communication will help ensure organizational missions and tasks are clearly defined, understood, and implemented. Open communication will also recognize and address the concerns and needs of staff and patients. Applying principles of key leadership and management theories by encouraging staff and balancing systems of rewards, constructive criticism, and recognition can further motivate employees toward fulfilling organizational tasks.

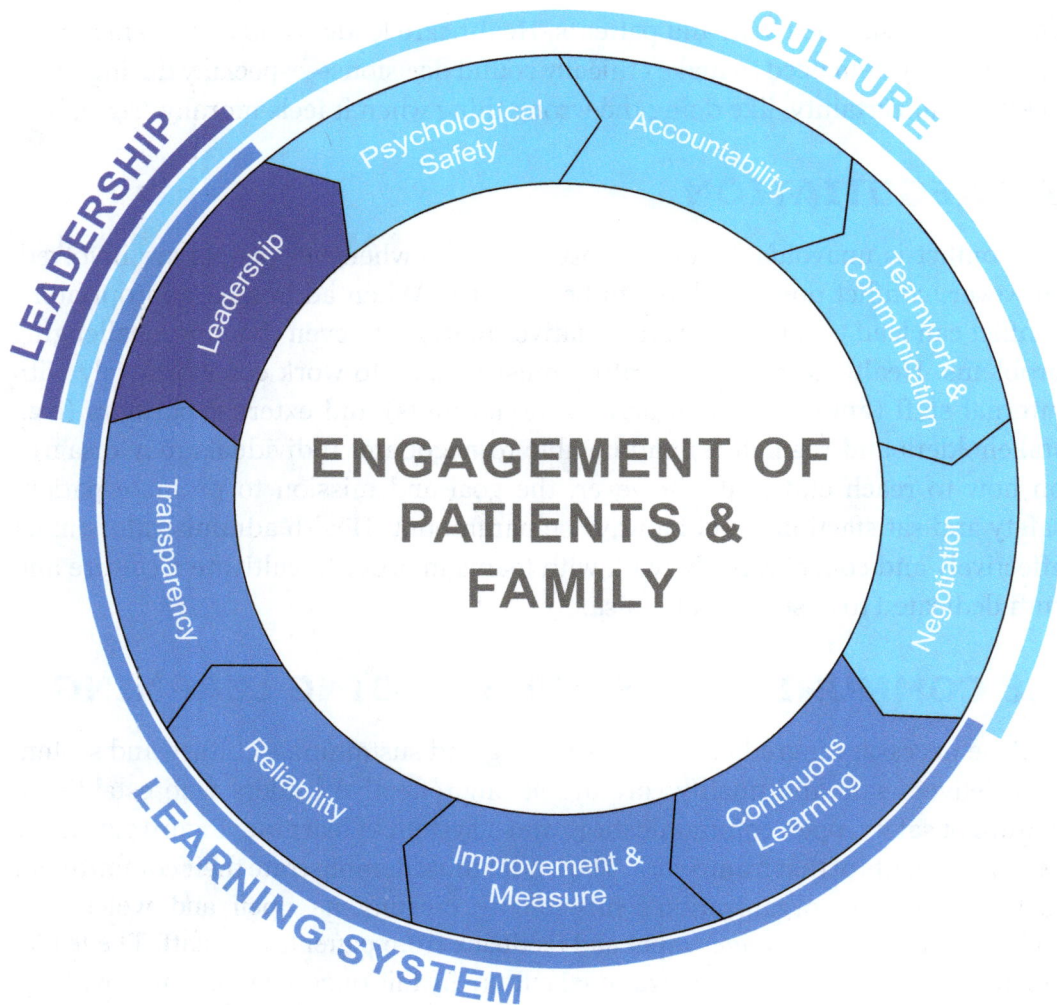

Figure 7.2: Framework for Safe and Reliable Care

Source: Frankel, Harden, Federico, and Lenoci-Edwards, 2017
Attribution: Corey Parson, Adapted from Frankel, Harden, Federico, and Lenoci-Edwards, 2017
License: Fair Use

Effective leadership is the critical component of an effective, thriving healthcare organization. Healthcare leaders must be able to adapt to change by responding to and addressing the community's shifting needs while ensuring that all staff members have the necessary resources and support to provide care that focuses on individual patients' care. Effective healthcare leaders incorporate a communication system among staff with timely feedback, promote staff and patient engagement, foster organizational learning, implement a process of interaction and engagement, and remain dedicated to patient safety and quality improvement.

Stop and Apply

Describe the current organizational culture at Southern Healthcare Hospice Center. How would you, as the healthcare administrator, address the current issues related to the organization's culture?

7.9 CODE OF ETHICS

The National Association for Healthcare Quality (NAHQ) publishes the Code of Ethics for Healthcare Quality Professionals as a guide for specialists and administrators. Health care professionals must promote organizational participation in maintaining ethical standards and maintain a formal system to address ethics complaints. NAHQ publishes the Code of Ethics for Healthcare Quality Professionals as a guide for specialists and administrators. Healthcare administrators may face the following key ethical challenges: (1) aiming to balance cost and the provision of quality, (2) adhering to legal orders and protecting patient privacy, (3) avoiding harm and reducing risk, and (4) maintaining a professional healthcare environment (described in further detail below).

7.9.1 1. Balancing Costs and Quality Care

As stated, Ms. Gonzales was uninsured. However, in an attempt to control costs, patients should be encouraged not to forgo treatments and tests based solely on costs but to consider the relationship of the cost and expected health outcome. High costs without an actual benefit would waste resources; however, health care professionals must balance the relationship of cost and quality of care in order to avoid offering non-standard care and committing billing violations.

Physicians are unlikely to encounter legal difficulties providing uncompensated care to uninsured patients because current laws are structured to reduce fraud and abuse pertaining to arrangements involving third-party payers; there is no violation associated with reducing or waiving a fee when the patient is self-pay. However, the medical coder should have consulted the doctor, who may have been willing to grant permission to waive fees through an adjustment. Although the medical coder wanted to help a friend, she may have unknowingly violated the law. The under coding example in this case study, where Ms. Camilla was billed for a minor visit when the patient received an extended visit, misrepresents the services that were actually provided and so violates the law. When working with federal programs such as Medicare, physicians must bill for the services they provide and report accurate claims. Inaccurate coding can lead to inaccurate assumptions that have serious consequences for other patients. For example, future coverage of services by Medicare and Medicaid could be withheld, based on empirical studies of forged databases showing good health outcomes for patients receiving low-intensity care (Weiner, 2001).

7.9.2 2. Adhering to Legal Orders and Protecting Patient Privacy

Healthcare administrators must understand and adhere to state and federal legal regulations in order to ensure compliance and provide safe healthcare to all patients. Proper health care regulations, reviews, and audits ensure the care being provided by health care practitioners and health care facilities is safe and effective. Health care regulatory agencies monitor health care practitioners and facilities, provide information about industry changes, promote safety and ensure legal compliance and quality services. Federal, state, and local regulatory agencies often establish mandatory rules and regulations for health care organizations. Other agencies have voluntary participation but are important because they provide rankings and demonstrations of quality. In the following table are several examples, but not nearly an exhaustive list, of laws and agencies regulating patient care.

Table 7.1 Regulations and Agencies Related to Patient Care	
Laws/Regulations/Acts	
The Health Insurance Portability and Accounting Act (HIPAA)	The HIPPA law, enacted in 1996, regulates federal guidelines and standards pertaining to electronic health records. HIPPA pertains to specific laws that govern the release of a patient's medical information and clearly states which patient information can be released to third parties and which information must be kept confidential. The HIPAA Privacy Rule comprises national regulations for Protected Health Information (PHI) in healthcare treatment and payment (CDC, 2018).
Affordable Care Act (ACA)	The ACA (2010) was set up to change the way people are insured and aims to lower healthcare costs and increase healthcare coverage and accessibility to previously uninsured individuals. The law was predicated on prevention and essential health benefits. The law is continually undergoing major changes as issues regarding its implementation are encountered, which also leads to ongoing changes in the way healthcare is delivered (CMS, 2020).
Food and Drug Administration Safety and Innovation Act (FDASIA)	The FDASIA of 2012 promotes safe and effective information technology by advancing the development of a regulatory framework for Health Information Technology to improve applications to promote patient safety and innovation in healthcare delivery (FDA, 2018).

The Health Information Technology for Economic and Clinical Health Act **(HITECH Act)**	The HITECH Act, passed in 2009, ensures the quality, safety, and secure exchange of health information. The Act requires practices to notify patients of any security breaches and has several provisions that enforce HIPAA rules (HHS, 2017).
The False Claims Act	The False Claims Act was enacted in 1863 to eliminate fraudulent healthcare claims (Department of Justice, 2020).
Federal Anti-Kickback Statute	The Federal Anti-Kickback Statute of 1972 is a federal fraud and abuse statute that forbids the exchange of anything of value in an effort to encourage (or reward) business referrals that are reimbursed by federal healthcare programs. The law is intended to protect against overutilization, increased costs, and poor-quality services (American Society of Anesthesiologists, 2020).
Physician Self-Referral Law/ Stark Law	The Stark Law was enacted in 1989 as an anti-fraud law that prohibits physician self-referral. The law bans physicians from referring patients for specific health services paid for by Medicare or any other entity in which the provider has a fiscal relationship (American Society of Anesthesiologists, 2020).
Healthcare Organizations/Agencies	
The Joint Commission on Accreditation of Healthcare Organizations (JCAHO)	JCAHO, founded in 1951, seeks to ensure healthcare organizations provide quality care by employing a system in which health care organizations are examined based on their compliance and improvement activities and then are granted a seal of approval after earning accreditation. These seals are important to health care organizations, as they are a factor when determining reimbursement from Medicare (JCAHO, 2020).
Centers for Medicare and Medicaid Services (CMS)	CMS, enacted in 1965, provides information regarding the quality, safety, and security of health care organizations to consumers and provides government-subsidized medical coverage through a number of programs, including the following: • **Medicare:** for the elderly and disabled • **Medicaid:** for lower-income individuals and families • **State Children's Health Insurance Program (SCHIP):** for health insurance coverage for children under 19 (CMS, 2020).

Agency for Healthcare Research and Quality (AHRQ)	The AHRQ, established in 1999, conducts research aimed at improving the quality of health care, by reducing health care costs, addressing patient safety, reducing medical errors, and ensuring healthcare is equitable, accessible, and affordable.
National Committee for Quality Assurance (NCQA)	The NCQA, established in 1991, accredits healthcare organizations. The NCQA also ensures the quality of managed care plans and requires HMOs to provide standard and objective information. The NCQA has a quality improvement framework that bases results on clinical performance and patient experience (NCQA, 2020).
Accreditation Commission for Healthcare (ACHC)	ACHC is a non-profit accreditation organization that has accredited hospital organizations, including home health, hospice, and renal dialysis organizations since 1986 (ACHC, 2020).

Source: Original Work
Attribution: Whitney Hamilton
License: CC BY-SA 4.0

Steady advancements in information technology and the availability of practical applications that support the delivery of coordinated care, provide performance reviews, and enhance communication are invaluable resources to hospital administrators. However, such technological advancements also raise concerns in regards to patient privacy and protection. Healthcare administrators can overcome these challenges by investing in reputable systems that have the capability to prevent fraudulent activity and establish processes that monitor and log all activity that is conducted on such electronic health record systems.

Healthcare administrators also face ethical dilemmas regarding patient's friends and family. When a patient's relatives and loved ones do not understand confidentiality and attempt to intervene in their loved one's care, patients must be aware that their family does not have to be involved in their medical care and decisions. Health care leaders must also be prepared to handle end-of-life issues that may arise with terminally ill and elderly patients. Toward the end of life, cardiopulmonary resuscitation (CPR) attempts are often performed; however, there are some cases where resuscitation is unwarranted by patients. As discussed in the example illustrated in chapter 4, Mr. Rodriquez requested that he not be resuscitated. A Do Not Resuscitate (DNR) refers to allowing a natural death and is a legal order indicating a patient does not want to receive CPR if they stop breathing. During end-of-life events, practitioners must act quickly, based on available information and records which could be faulty or incomplete. When making resuscitation orders, many factors must be considered, including the potential benefit (e.g., patient quality of life) and the potential risks (e.g., financial, worsened health condition).

7.9.3 3. Beneficence and Maleficence

Beneficence is defined as the moral obligation to show compassion to patients. Non-maleficence refers to avoiding causing harm to patients. All healthcare professionals are obligated to honor the principles of beneficence and maleficence in order to uphold the well-being of all patients. Leaders in the health care field must embody high ethical standards and have a moral obligation to strive towards achieving the greatest good for all patients (Kinsinger, 2009). For instance, all procedures and treatments must be recommended with the intent of doing the most good for the patient. Hospital staff, including practitioners and administrators, must develop and maintain a high level of skill and expertise, making sure they are trained on the most up-to-date practices. Healthcare leaders must acknowledge a one-size-fits-all approach to healthcare does not exist and consider individual patient needs.

7.9.4 4. Maintaining a Professional Environment

The medical coder in the case study was already instructed to heighten costs; therefore, she may not have considered her behavior unethical when attempting to lower costs for a patient who was struggling financially. An ethical culture must be established, especially during times of such uncertainty. The organization's ethical standards must be not only established but also shared by all staff in order to guide uniform decision-making.

Healthcare leaders establish an organization's culture, which determines how the group functions as well as how staff behave and interact with patients and each other. Misconduct can range from unprofessional interactions with patients and other staff members, to HIPPAA violations, to expense padding through extra charges, to violating confidentiality regulations, and to discrimination. Insubordination can include excessive tardiness, talking back to managers, taking excessive breaks, ignoring requests, and using profanity. The American Nurses Association has developed a trifold framework for preventing and addressing unprofessionalism and uncivility in the workplace, including primary, secondary, and tertiary prevention methods (MacLean, Coombs, Breda, 2016). Primary prevention includes educating and communicating a strong organizational culture that promotes respect and professionalism. Healthcare leaders must develop policies and procedures to safeguard professional practices that do not tolerate workplace violence and incivility. Leaders should provide ongoing staff education as well as a method for reporting and investigating alleged incidents and employing consequences for noncompliance to policies (MacLean, Coombs, Breda, 2016). Developing mottos and slogans to reinforce positive professional relationships can serve as an organizational campaign to educate and remind staff to uphold professional standards and reinforce positive workplace norms. Videos demonstrating potential workplace misconduct scenarios with examples of code words and ways to address such instances can also be a part of educational training. Secondary prevention focuses on reducing harm once an unprofessional incident has occurred. After misconduct is reported, health care leaders should initiate an investigation and enforce proper consequences in order to correct behaviors to prevent further incidents, copycat behavior, or retaliation. Tertiary prevention efforts aim to reduce escalating a misconduct situation in the workplace. Under tertiary prevention, leaders maintain detailed records of misconduct and monitor behaviors in case patterns develop. Leaders also institute performance improvement plans for individuals who have engaged in unprofessional behaviors (MacLean, Coombs, Breda, 2016).

The manner in which managers address incidents of misconduct will establish their respect and credibility with staff and determine their management style and their ability to effectively lead (MacLean, Coombs, Breda, 2016). The way the leader responds to behaviors and the mechanisms they use to motivate employees largely shapes the organizational culture. The ethical culture affects the staff's morale and productivity, shaping the values and beliefs that influence their decision-making. Recognizing and rewarding staff for ethically carrying out organizational tasks can motivate and create a positive organizational culture. The healthcare leader must determine which actions will be rewarded, praised, or even criticized and challenged. Are rules justly applied and followed? Is negative behavior overlooked or challenged immediately? Are leaders and management open to suggestions or close-minded? The ethical healthcare leader must be open to criticism and feedback. A healthcare leader should also embody the organization's ethical values in their personal lives. A leader can run the risk of discrediting the values of the organization and losing the trust and respect of constituents if they are professional at work but behave unprofessionally outside the workplace and/or show a lack of scruples on social media.

Stop and Apply

As a leader, have you witnessed toxic workplace behaviors, such as eye rolling, sarcasm, or threats? What about aggression; withholding pertinent patient information/sabotage; disrespectful, rude, or condescending comments; or scapegoating? How was it handled?

Using the trifold framework for preventing and addressing workplace misconduct, let's return to the case study outlined at the beginning of the chapter. How should the organization's leadership address Corinne's management? How can the healthcare organization, in the case study presented in this chapter, be transformed into one which shares an ethical culture?

Table 7.2 Consequences of Poor Organizational Culture	
Operational	• Decreased workplace productivity and morale • Increased staff burnout and turnover
Legal	• Expenses for a risk management expert • Increased legal fees, malpractice costs, and settlement costs
Public Affairs	• Negative public image and perception • Decreased referrals and philanthropic support

Source: Original Work
Attribution: Whitney Hamilton
License: CC BY-SA 4.0

Stop and Apply

Let's take a look at the case of Ms. Camila Gonzales. She is a 76-year-old, self-employed housekeeper with no health insurance. Prior to being admitted to Southern Healthcare Hospice Center, she visited the neighboring hospital after experiencing sporadic episodes of chest pain that typically followed her evening meals. Occasionally, she experienced pain after her daily walk to work. She also had experienced a rapid weight loss, which further increased her concern regarding her health.

The physician carefully listened to her and performed a physical exam. He explained her symptoms were most likely a result of heartburn which had nothing to do with the heart but were due to acid from the stomach regurgitating into the esophagus. He knew she should undergo a cardiac stress test and endoscopy to rule out coronary artery disease and cancer, especially considering her age, weight loss, and family history. However, the costs of the tests would amount to thousands of dollars, and Camilla had already explained she had no health insurance and could not afford expensive treatment. Although the physician knew the standard approach involved ruling out cardiac disease and gastrointestinal cancer, he also recognized the likelihood that she had neither. Her reported history suggested her condition would most likely be gastrointestinal, not cardiac, because she is a non-smoker and engages in frequent physical activity, making cancer and heart disease unlikely. However, a delay in diagnosis could compromise her care. Ultimately, the physician only treated her for heartburn and prescribed a proton pump inhibitor which would cost over $100/month.

In an attempt to control the financial costs of the hospital and maximize revenue, the medical coder had been ordered by her supervisor to pad cost by consistently assigning Evaluation and Management (EM) codes at a higher level than what is supported by documentation. The medical coder, a close friend of Ms. Camila, is aware of her financial standing. Therefore, she reduced the office visits costs by undercoding the visit by stating the visit lasted only 15 minutes rather than the 45 minutes she was seen. She also provided the patient with samples of the proton pump inhibitor that was supplied by a pharmaceutical representative.

*Adapted from Weiner, 2001 'I Can't Afford That!'

Identify the ethical dilemmas presented in this scenario. How would you address the medical coder who did the wrong thing but possibly felt she was doing the "right" thing by making adjustments in the billing of a patient who couldn't afford care? How can the Southern Healthcare Hospice Center be transformed into a healthcare organization in which a shared ethical culture is apparent in all situations, that is, an organization that provides staff and associates with a moral compass?

7.10 ORGANIZATIONAL PERFORMANCE

Organizational culture plays an integral role in the success of a healthcare organization. Thus, health administrators and leaders should foster an organizational culture that is not only ethically driven but also set on high-performance. Establishing a culture of high-performance requires an emphasis on increasing health care quality and access while decreasing healthcare costs. Organizational performance analyzes the healthcare organization's performance against its mission and goals. The performance evaluation illustrates whether the healthcare organization is fulfilling its overall mission. Clinical and economic assessments of hospital performance are valuable to not only the hospital and physicians, but also to payment systems as well as policymakers, because it provides an indicator of the organization's performance quality. The results of a performance evaluation can translate into actionable improvement items. Hospital performance assessments typically report on six distinct characteristics which are described by the Institute of Medicine as the indicators of high-quality healthcare organizations. These include practices that are (1) safe, (2) effective, (3) reliable, (4) patient-centered, (5) efficient, and (6) equitable (Ohama, 2009; Sfantou, et. al, 2017). Measuring the organization's structure, process, patient health outcomes, and patient satisfaction are central components of assessing the care quality provided by a healthcare organization. The goal of assessing hospital performance is to create a system that provides optimal quality patient care through transparency, accountability, and credibility (Tooker, 2005). All of the healthcare organization's members should be involved and participating in creating an organizational culture that is transparent, involves continual communication, and uses multisource feedback. Multisource feedback includes evaluations from physicians, non-physicians, patients, and peers with timely feedback on quality indicators and target improvement areas (Kaye, Okanalwon, & Urman, 2014). In order to ensure high organizational performance, health care administrators must focus on communicating a shared vision that is operationalized at every level, that clearly aligns objectives for all staff members, teams, and departments supporting and enabling management; engages staff from various levels; creates a system of ongoing learning; stays abreast of innovation and quality improvement; and effectively working and collaborating with all healthcare staff (West, Lyubovnikova, Eckert & Denis, 2014).

Healthcare administrators' duties are vast and entail tasks that range from policy making to scheduling. However, no matter the task, a healthcare administrator's goal is to provide efficient coordination and delivery of quality healthcare services. A health organization's quality of care is defined as the extent to which the expected health outcomes are achieved and concurrent with the latest professional knowledge and skills within health services. The healthcare organization's leadership, whether it's an inpatient care facility, in-home care unit, or long-term care facility, is vital to developing an organizational culture committed to high performance and quality assurance. Employing appropriate leadership styles, as mentioned in previous chapters, enhances the manner in which healthcare leaders coordinate delivering quality health care.

Table 7.3 The Institute of Medicine's (IOM) Six Characteristics of High-Quality Healthcare Organizations

Safe	Avoid injuries to patients resulting from the care that is intended to help them.
Effective	Match care to science, avoid overuse of ineffective care and underuse of effective care.
Patient-Centered	Honor the individual and respect choice.
Timely	Reduce waiting for both patients and those who give care.
Efficient	Reduce waste.
Equitable	Close racial and ethnic gaps in health status.

Source: "Six Domains of Health Care Quality," 2018
Attribution: Whitney Hamilton, Adapted from "Six Domains of Health Care Quality," 2018
License: Fair Use

Stop and Apply

What specific steps can Laura take to create a culture of high-performance at Southern Healthcare Hospice Center? Which aspects of the facility must first be understood and/or evaluated?

7.11 ORGANIZATIONAL CHANGE

Organizational change is the process by which an organization changes its structure, strategies, and/or culture to adapt to internal or external pressures. Organizational change also entails the effect of the changes on the organization. Key drivers of organizational change within the healthcare environment include economic conditions; patient characteristics and behaviors; advancements in information technology; new government policies, such as the Affordable Care Act; and a fundamental shift to value based, patient-centered care. With recent demographic shifts, changing social norms, and an aging population, these changes have been occurring rapidly. In order to thrive during internal or external fluctuations, the organization must learn to adapt by operating more efficiently and cost-effectively. Delivering clear communication, delineating staff roles and responsibilities, and effectively coordinating care are key skills for health administrators to embody when navigating organizational change. Healthcare administrators must focus on the following key aspects: shifting the structure of the healthcare organization, establishing and conveying the organization's mission, understanding current policies and political trends, establishing the organization's culture, staying abreast of technological advancements, and recruiting and maintaining a qualified hospital staff.

Structure: The healthcare administrator can shift the structure (the hierarchy within an organization) to include more than just the physicians in planning and decision-making while shifting focus to provide integrative, quality, and value-based care.

Mission: The healthcare administrator must establish and exemplify the organization's commitment and mission to providing patient-centered, high-quality, low-cost care by replacing practices that incentivize providing expensive treatments that do not produce optimum health outcomes.

Policies: Health administrators must have a thorough understanding of current policies and legal agreements.

Culture: Health care leaders must ensure an ethical, high-performing culture that emphasizes quality, low-cost care.

Technology: Successful healthcare organizations integrate information technology, telemedicine, and keep up with technological advancements.

Workforce: Healthcare administrators must also recruit and retrain staff who align with the organization's culture.

7.12 BEST PRACTICES

Despite medical advancements, the U.S. stills faces issues over ever-increasing health care costs, limited health care access, and a lowering healthcare quality (Robert Wood Johnson, 2018; Berwick, 2002). In 2016, the U.S. spent nearly twice as much as 10 high-income countries on medical care yet did not perform as well as those countries on many population health outcomes. In 2016, the U.S.

spent 17.8% of its gross domestic product on health care, while spending in other high-income countries ranged from 9.6% (Australia) to 12.4% (Switzerland). Life expectancy in the U.S. was the lowest of the countries at 78.8 years, while the mean of all the countries was 81.7 years. Infant mortality was also the highest in the U.S. at 5.8 deaths per 1000 live births, while the mean was 3.6 per 1000 for all of the countries. The U.S. spent approximately twice as much as other high-income countries on medical care, yet mortality rates in the U.S. were overall lower than the other nations (Papanicolas, 2018).

Moreover, millions of individuals in the U.S. are underinsured or lack health insurance altogether. The Institute of Medicine (IOM) describes three dimensions of this health care crisis (2000): underuse, overuse, and misuse of care (Berwick, 2002).

- Underuse refers to standard health care practices that are not followed. For example, the physician in the case study knew that standard procedure would be to provide the patient with a stress test and endoscopy to rule out heart disease and gastrointestinal cancer, but he did not offer the treatment based on costs. Another example of underuse would be the fact that only 55-65% of women over the age 40 are receiving annual breast exams (Kohn, Corrigan, & Donadlson, 2000; Berwick, 2002; CDC, 2020).

- Overuse refers to implementing costly health care procedures and treatments even when they may not be the most efficient or best option to help the patient. An example of such overuse is if a physician unnecessarily prescribes antibiotics for simple infections (Kohn, Corrigan, & Donaldson, 2000).

- Misuse refers to medical errors that result from failure to properly perform appropriate treatment or provide inappropriate treatment. An instance of misuse would be patients' experiencing adverse reactions to drugs, surgical accidents, and/or other serious or fatal harm inflicted upon them. As mentioned in chapter 3, according to the IOM reports *To Err is Human* and *Crossing the Quality Chasm*, as many as 98,000 individuals die in hospitals every year as a result of preventable medical errors (Berwick, 2002).

The underuse, overuse, and misuse of healthcare results in the expensive, fragmented care system that is currently prevalent in the U.S. In contrast to other developed countries, such as Canada, Germany, and Australia, the U.S. underperforms in critical areas, such as quality, safety, patient centered care, and satisfaction, while providing more expensive care (Papanicolas, 2018). The U.S. healthcare system clearly needs a redesign that integrates quality and the patient experience. The IOM recommends a re-design that is systems-minded, builds knowledge, and is patient-centered.

So, how does a poor, inefficient system adapt to change and transform into a high-quality, high performing healthcare system? A research team from the Boston University School of Public Health conducted an evaluation of the most successful components of a health care system redesign (Ohama, 2009). The team examined over 20 hospitals that re-designed an inefficient and costly hospital system. They found the hospitals that successfully re-designed their system focused on patient integration and coordination, while also emphasizing healthcare access, cost, and quality. The first step each hospital management team recognized was the need for change in order to avoid closure. The realization that change must occur and be sustained within the organization was the first step to motivate and engage staff to participate in the ongoing change efforts. The research team also found a clear vision and strategy for change was established and implemented within each of the healthcare organizations. Healthcare administrators and leaders drive organizational change by providing a consistent direction and demonstrating an authentic passion, commitment to change, and quality improvement. Hospitals developed and distributed print brochures that identified internal and external challenges in addition to potential solutions. Health care staff across all disciplines were engaged and involved in planning and implementing the healthcare system's changes. Additionally, the vision, processes, and overall mission were clearly and persistently communicated to staff. A successful hospital system re-design consisted of including all staff in planning and implementation, decentralizing authority, and evenly distributing decision making. Evaluations and focus groups were also used to monitor patient outcomes, satisfaction, and employee satisfaction. The researchers found the most transformative healthcare systems that profoundly improved patient health outcomes and satisfaction were highly innovative and integrative. Successful hospital systems integrated information technology, specifically electronic health records, that stored data, provided support for decision-making and scheduling, and measured performance outcomes (Ohama, 2009).

Tips for Healthcare Administrator's to Establish an Ethical Culture of High Performance and Successfully Navigate Organizational Change:

1. *Clearly embody, convey, and communicate a compelling, ethical organizational vision that encourages staff to ethically fulfill organizational tasks and missions.*

2. *Establish hiring practices that will recruit and retain staff that directly align with the organization's vision, mission, and values.*

3. *Provide ongoing training and support programs that build knowledge and reinforce the organization's ethical values and mission.*

4. *Employ a system of reward, constructive criticism, and recognition to motivate employees to carry out the organization's mission.*

5. *Clearly establish well-defined structures, processes, and systems, and*

delineate staff roles and responsibility that are clearly aligned with the organization's vision, goals, strategic plan, and overall mission.

6. *Provide feedback channels to notify employees of their performance.*

7. *Create open and continual communication and establish a welcoming environment with a strategy for handling conflict.*

8. *Evaluate the organizational culture through ongoing evaluation with surveys and/or focus groups containing staff and patients.*

9. *Connect the organization's values to the community served by addressing the identified concerns and needs of patients and staff.*

10. *Demonstrate the organization's values by being a strong leader and ambassador of the healthcare organization.*

7.13 CONCLUSION

This chapter described the key challenges facing today's healthcare leaders and examined the role of healthcare administrators in navigating such challenges to influence organizational culture, performance, and change. In order to keep up with the shifting U.S. healthcare system, health managers must understand how change occurs and create adaptable organizational settings. This chapter outlined the key elements that enable a workplace culture that results in high organizational performance.

7.14 KEY POINTS

- This chapter develops the distinction between leadership and management skills by outlining the roles of leaders and managers to influence organizational culture, performance, and change.

- This chapter also describes the key leadership skills that are necessary to sustain organizational cultures that ensure high organizational performance.

- In order to keep up with the ever-changing healthcare system, healthcare leaders must create an environment that fosters innovation and creativity.

7.15 KEY TERMS

Organizational culture, Ethics, Biomedical ethics, Organizational performance, Organizational change

7.16 QUESTIONS FOR REVIEW AND DISCUSSION

1. Describe the healthcare leader's role in establishing organizational culture and navigating organizational change. What key skills and aspects of leadership and management theory should be applied to establishing organizational culture and navigating change?

2. Describe what is meant by a culture of high-performance.

3. Why is the healthcare manager's role in ensuring high performance critical? Explain.

7.17 REFERENCES

Accreditation Commission for Healthcare. (ACHC). "Empowering Providers to Enhance Patient Care." (2020). https://www.achc.org

Agency for Healthcare Quality and Research. (AHRQ). "Healthcare Research and Quality Act of 1999." 2014.

American Society of Anesthesiologists. "Anti-kickback Statute and Physician Self-Referral Laws (Stark Laws)." (2020). https://www.asahq.org/quality-and-practice-management/managing-your-practice/timely-topics-in-payment-and-practice-management/anti-kickback-statute-and-physician-self-referral-laws-stark-laws

Berwick DM. "A User's Manual for The IOM's 'Quality Chasm' Report." Health Affairs, 21(3): 80–90, 2002.

Centers for Disease Control and Prevention. CDC. "Health Insurance Portability and Accountability Act of 1996 (HIPAA)." (2018). https://www.cdc.gov/phlp/publications/topic/hipaa.html

Centers for Disease Control. (2020). "Mammography." https://www.cdc.gov/nchs/fastats/mammography.htm

Centers for Medicaid and Medicare Services. "CMS' program history." (2020). https://www.cms.gov/About-CMS/Agency-Information/History

Department of Justice. (2020). "The False Claims Act." https://www.justice.gov/civil/false-claims-act

Donnellan, John J. Jr. "A Moral Compass for Management Decision Making: A Healthcare CEO's Reflections, Frontiers of Health Services Management: (2013)." Volume 30 - Issue 1 - p 14–26

Frankel A., Haraden C., Federico F., Lenoci-Edwards, J. *A Framework for Safe, Reliable, and Effective Care*. White Paper. Cambridge, MA: Institute for Healthcare Improvement and Safe & Reliable Healthcare, 2017.

Kaye, A. D., Okanlawon, O. J., & Urman, R. D. (2014). "Clinical performance feedback and quality improvement opportunities for perioperative physicians." *Advances in medical education and practice, 5*, 115–123. doi:10.2147/AMEP.S62165

Kinsinger F. S. (2009). "Beneficence and the professional's moral imperative." *Journal of *chiropractic humanities, 16*(1), 44–46. doi:10.1016/j.echu.2010.02.006

Kohn, L. T., Corrigan, J., & Donaldson, M. S. (2000). *To err is human: Building a safer health system*. Washington, D.C.: National Academy Press.

MacLean, L., Charmaine, C., Breda, K. (2016). "Unprofessional workplace conduct... defining and defusing it." Nursing Management. 2016; 47(9): 30-34.

Ohama, DiAnn. (2009) "What Makes for Successful Health Care System Redesign? Team at Boston University's School of Public Health Identifies Five Critical Factors." Robert Wood Johnson Foundation. Retrieved from: https://www.rwjf.org/en/library/research/2009/08/what-makes-for-successful-health-care-system-redesign--.html

Papanicolas I, Woskie LR, Jha AK. "Health Care Spending in the United States and Other High-Income Countries." *JAMA*. 2018;319(10):1024–1039. doi:10.1001/jama.2018.1150)

Schein, E. (2010). *Organizational Culture and Leadership*. San Francisco, CA: Jossey-Bass.

Sfantou, D. F., Laliotis, A., Patelarou, A. E., Sifaki-Pistolla, D., Matalliotakis, M., & Patelarou, E. (2017). "Importance of Leadership Style towards Quality-of-Care Measures in Healthcare Settings: A Systematic Review." *Healthcare (Basel, Switzerland), 5*(4), 73. doi:10.3390/healthcare5040073

https://www.ncbi.nlm.nih.gov/pmc/articles/PMC5746707/

"Six Domains of Health Care Quality." 2018. Agency for Healthcare Research and Quality. https://www.ahrq.gov/talkingquality/measures/six-domains.html

"The State of Health Care Quality in America." (2018). Robert Wood Johnson Foundation.

Temime, L., Cohen, N., Ait-Bouziad, Denormandie, P., Dab, W., and Hocine, M. (2018). "Impact of a multicomponent hand hygiene–related intervention on the infectious risk in nursing homes: A cluster randomized trial." American Journal of Infection Control, 46(2): 173 – 179.

The Joint Commission. Accreditation and Certification. (2020). https://www.jointcommission.org/accreditation-and-certification/

The National Committee for Quality Assurance. (NCQA). A QUALITY IMPROVEMENT FRAMEWORK. https://www.ncqa.org/programs/health-plans/health-plan-accreditation-hpa/

Tooker, J., & Ambulatory Care Quality Alliance (2005). "The importance of measuring quality and performance in healthcare." *MedGenMed: Medscape general medicine, 7*(2), 49.

U.S Centers for Medicare and Medicaid Services. "Health Affordable Care Act (ACA)." (2018). https://www.healthcare.gov/glossary/affordable-care-act/

U.S Department of Health and Human Services. "HITECH Act Enforcement Interim Final Rule." (2018). https://www.hhs.gov/hipaa/for-professionals/special-topics/hitech-act-enforcement-interim-final-rule/index.html

U.S Food and Drug Administration. "Food and Drug Administration Safety and Innovation Act (FDASIA)." (2018). https://www.fda.gov/regulatory-information/selected-amendments-fdc-act/food-and-drug-administration-safety-and-innovation-act-fdasia

Weiner, S. 2001. "I Can't Afford That!" Dilemmas in the Care of the Uninsured and Underinsured J Gen Intern Med. 2001 Jun;16(6):412-8. https://www.ncbi.nlm.nih.gov/pmc/articles/PMC1495228/

8 CORE LEADERSHIP AND MANAGERIAL PROCESSES

8.1 LEARNING OBJECTIVES

- To describe the roles of leaders and managers in influencing organizational culture and performance.
- To discuss such core leadership and managerial methods as (A) Motivating people, (B) Guiding teams, (C) Designing teams, (D) Coordinating work, (E) Communicating effectively, (F) Exerting influence, (G) Resolving conflict, (H) Negotiating agreements, (I) improving performance, and (J) Managing innovation and change
- To describe elements of motivation and compare and contrast concepts of motivating people
- To describe stages of team design and apply techniques and strategies for coordinating work in teams
- To discuss characteristics of effective communication
- Investigate skills on exerting influences on teams effectively
- To examine techniques beneficial to resolving conflict and negotiating agreements
- To discuss concepts involved in managing innovation

8.2 INTRODUCTION

The chapter explores critical managerial functions, including motivation, effective communication, team coordination, influence exertion, performance improvement, negotiation, and conflict resolution management. This chapter will focus on the case study section of influencing organizational culture and the code team at the hospice center's performance. This chapter will also focus on the role of identifying core leadership and managerial methods as this relates to thehospice center's employees.

8.3 UNDERSTANDING THE DIFFERENCE BETWEEN GROUP AND TEAM

In order to function cohesively in the workplace, individuals must know that working in a group or team is necessary. There are distinct differences between groups and teams. To be considered a **group**, two or more individuals are interacting and interdependent and have come together to achieve an objective or goal. Groups share common interests or characteristics. On the other hand, a **team** generates positive energy and is evolved with effective task alignment, purpose, structure, and social awareness (Walston, 2017).

Table 8.1: Understanding the Difference Between Group and Team

GROUP	TEAM
Focused leadership	Shared leadership
Individual accountability	Individual and team accountability
Individual work outcomes	Teamwork outcomes
Desire for efficient meetings	Desire for open discussion and problem solving
Effectiveness measured by indirect influence	Effectiveness measured by collective work output
Discussion, decision, delegation	Discussion, decision, and working together on output

Source: Walston, 2017
Attribution: Melissa Jordan, Adapted from Walston, 2017
License: Fair Use

8.4 ROLES OF INFLUENCE FOR LEADERS AND MANAGERS

In order for individuals to be willing to share in the responsibilities of the organization's success, one must understand the role of leaders and managers when influencing others.

8.4.1 Goals, Mission, Vision

Communication is key when it comes to leaders and managers motivating, building, clarifying, and affirming shared values of the organization. **Motivation** comprises the processes that account for an individual's intensity, direction, and persistence of effort toward attaining a goal. Leaders and managers should set the example by aligning their actions with these shared values and goals. According to Kouzes and Posner (2002), employees are more motivated and loyal when they believe their own values and goals and those of the organization are cohesively aligned.

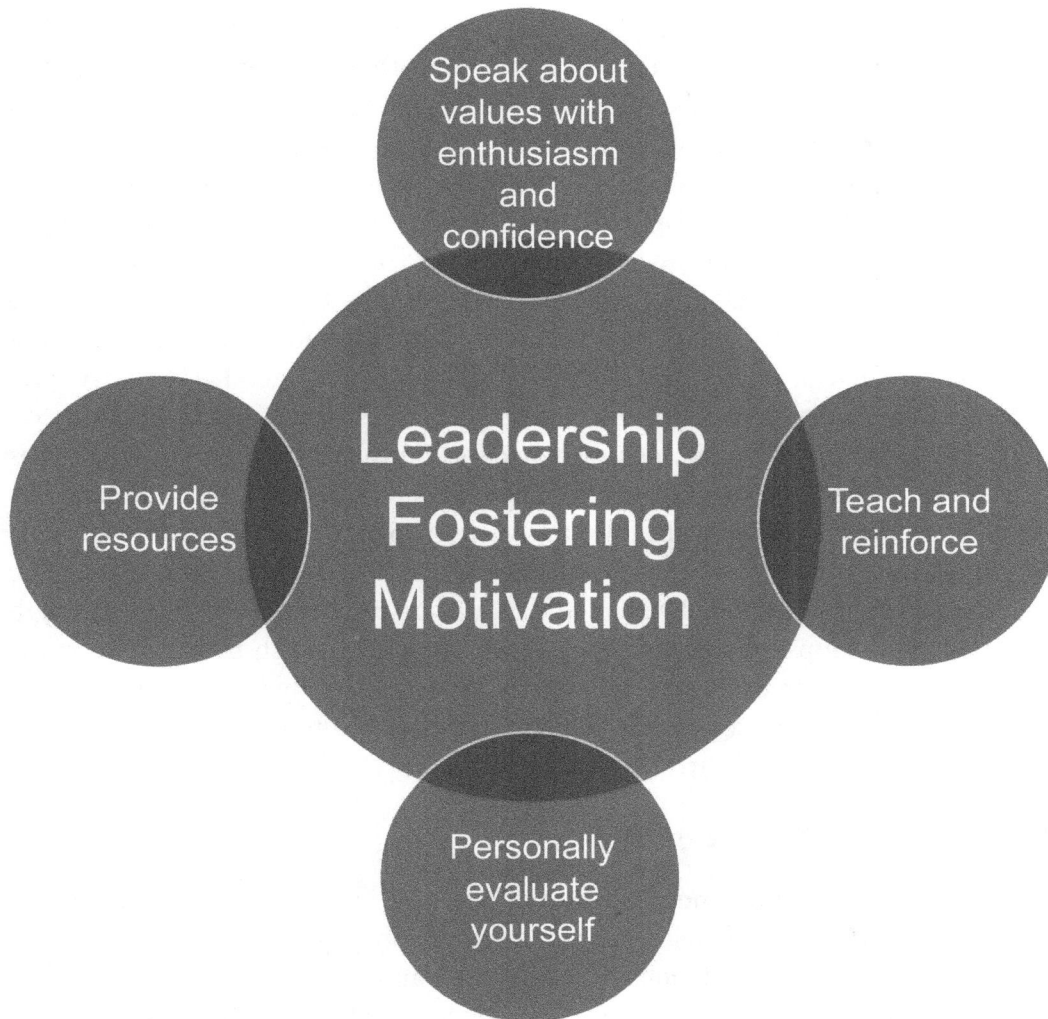

Figure 8.1: Leadership Fostering Motivation

Employees must also have a thorough understanding of the company's mission and vision. As noted previously, a **mission** is simply what an organization represents through good, clear, sound ethical guidelines, agendas, and focuses on what the company is firm on accomplishing. A vision is, in a sense, futuristic because it is what the company hopes to become and wants to accomplish that no one else has yet achieved. Leaders and managers must create these meaningful climates by first personally believing in themselves before they have the ability to motivate and inspire others.

Employees who are not familiar with a company's core values, mission, and vision are not engaged in their job. A lack of job engagement will lead to an increased amount of absenteeism in productive workforce days, high turnover rates, decreased job productivity, and poor customer service (Goestch & Davis, 2015). Leaders and managers can speak enthusiastically and confidently about their shared values, missions, and visions. If employees see leaders excited about the organization, they are more likely to consider their own emotional response toward's the organization's overall vision and goals. Leaders and managers should also teach and reinforce positive behaviors in the workplace. Doing so can be as simple as posting pictures on walls, sending positive and helpful emails, and providing training and development services as needed. Leaders and managers may become so focused on the administration of leading others that they forget to evaluate themselves. Doing a personal audit sets the example for others to do the same. Consequently, leaders and managers should audit their daily routines and evaluate their priorities. Auditing daily calendars and agendas is also helpful in determining what topics are important, how much time should be spent on that topic, and when one should come back to reevaluate. Providing employees with the resources they need to have a better understanding of the organization's values, mission, and vision will allow employees to explore their environment. This opportunity will also allow employees to understand how they can participate in the organization's performance. Leaders and managers can provide resources though webinars, workshops, ebooks, websites, and many other such means. The key is to ensure that resources are readily and easily available. By implementing these action, leaders and managers can determine if they are moving their employees and organization forward through motivation.

8.4.2 Various Types of Teams

Teams have several functions, from providing excellent service to making innovative products. Various types of teams in organizations are available to choose from in getting these jobs done. Leaders and managers must understand how to get the best performance from individuals who bring their talents together in order to accomplish the common goal efficiently and effectively. **Team design** includes an understanding of how to define the roles and responsibilities for the team's tasks. Collaboratively identifying working agreements will allow the team to realize its purpose and goal. This chapter discusses three types of team design: self-managed work teams, cross functional teams, and virtual teams.

Self-managed teams consist of, typically, 10-15 employees. These individuals take on high skill-related jobs and sometimes take on responsibilities from their former supervisors. Their tasks include scheduling work assignments, scheduling members assigned to do those tasks, problem solving actions, and decision making.

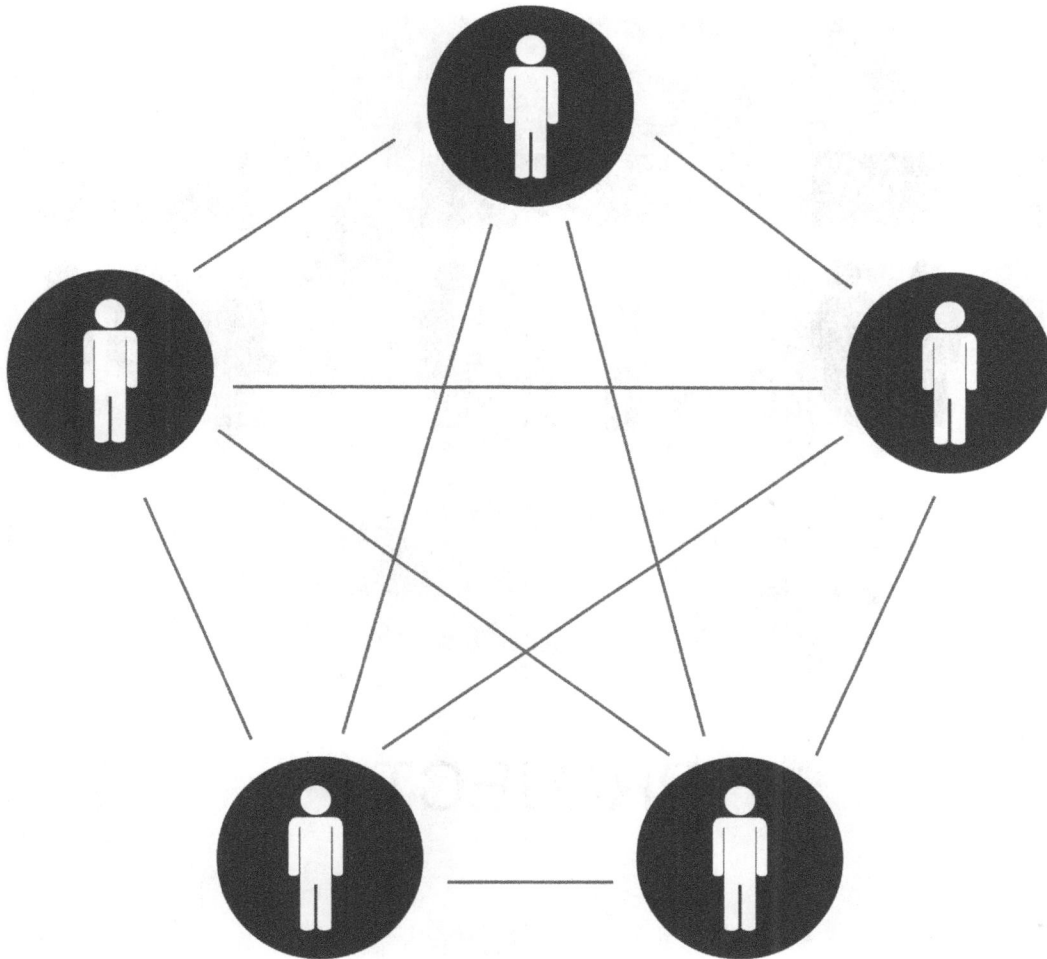

Figure 8.2: Self-Managing Teams

Source: Original Work
Attribution: Corey Parson
License: CC BY-SA 4.0

Cross functional teams comprise employees from the same tiered level, but they have different work areas and come together to complete a specific task. These teams are highly effective, allowing people from different areas to come together and exchange information, learn and develop new ideas, and analyze complex projects.

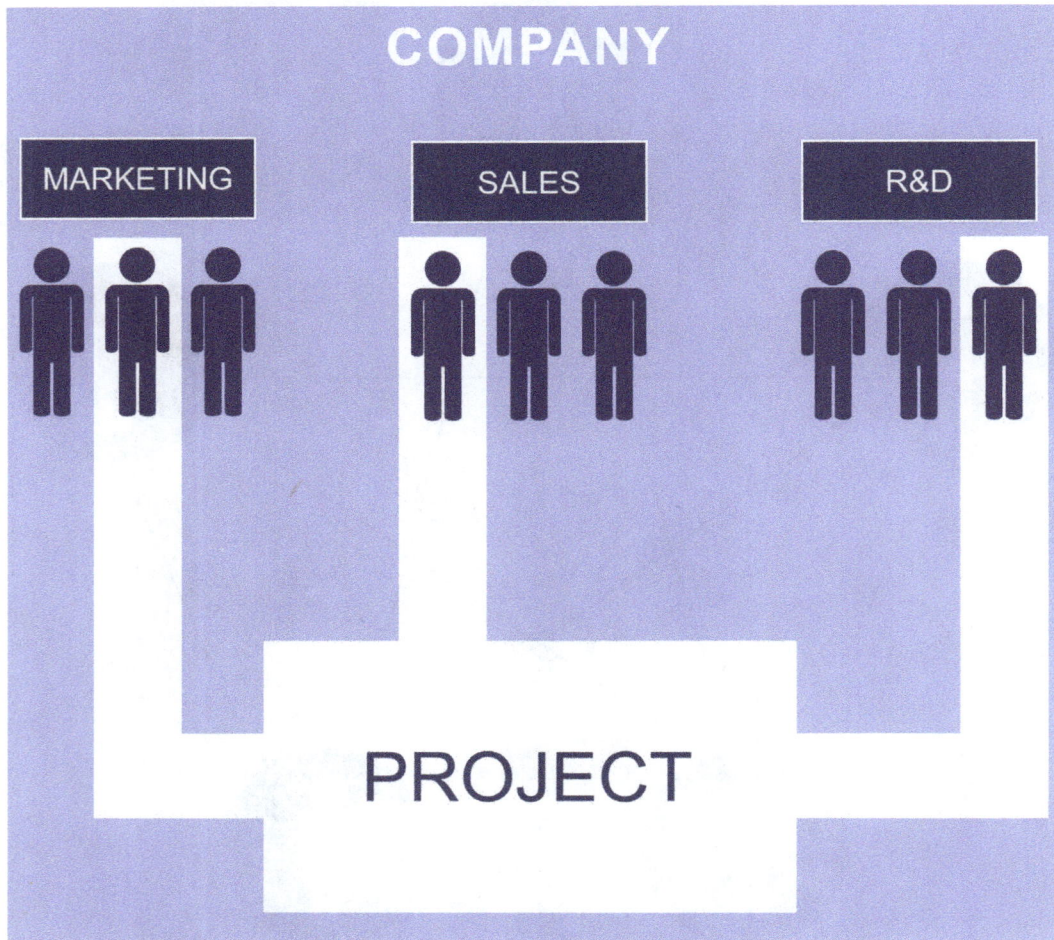

Figure 8.3: Cross-Functional Teams

Source: Original Work
Attribution: Corey Parson
License: CC BY-SA 4.0

Virtual teams use technology to come together to complete a certain task. These members are usually dispersed, and collaborate most of the work online through wide area networks, video conferencing, email, and various other means of technology. These teams face unique challenges because they do not have the social rapport as do the other teams described in this chapter. Because they do not meet in person for face-to-face discussions, virtual teams tend to exchange less social and/or emotional information (Robbins & Judge, 2011). Leaders and managers, therefore, must ensure that trust is established among these members and progress is monitored closely so as to not get off track.

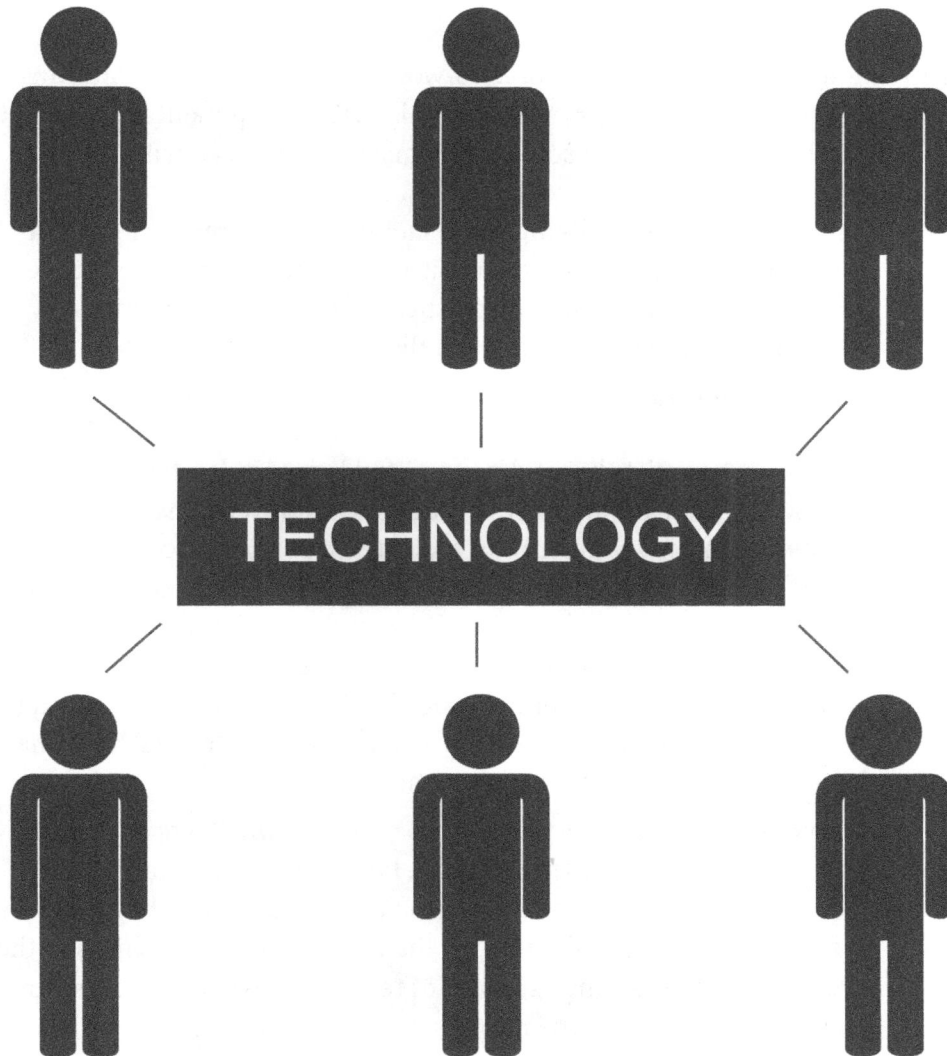

Figure 8.4: Virtual Teams

Source: Original Work
Attribution: Corey Parson
License: CC BY-SA 4.0

Stop and Apply

Review the emergency code at the beginning of this chapter to answer these questions:

What went smoothly and what needed improvement?

1. Is there a code/medical response team where you work?

2. What are the steps to activating the code team?

3. What emergency equipment is available to you?

8.4.3 Creating Effective Teams

Bringing together a group of people to work together can be a daunting task for anyone. Leaders and managers must organize vital components that will allow individuals to do a job better and solve problems efficiently as a team.

- *Team context* is identifying those factors that are most important in the performance of the team with adequate resources, effective leadership and structure, the trust climate, and performance evaluation and reward systems in the organization.

- *Team composition* is identifying all abilities and skills of team members. Team leadership abilities also matter, as effective team leaders assist those who may need help. Understanding the personality of team members influences employee behaviors. The diversity of team members can affect team performance. Diverse teams benefit from each other's differing perceptions, opinions, and points of view. Managers and leaders must also determine the teams' size. Much smaller teams have five-to-nine people function under the assumption that a smaller number of people should be employed to do the task. Members of larger teams can have trouble with coordinating, leadership issues, and communication.

- *Team process* relates to the process variables which correlate with team members' commitment levels, how well team members get along with each other as a group, the understanding of how the team manages conflict, and decreasing the number of social loafers in the group. Process is an integral part of team effectiveness because any deviation or loss from the process decreases productivity and task completion.

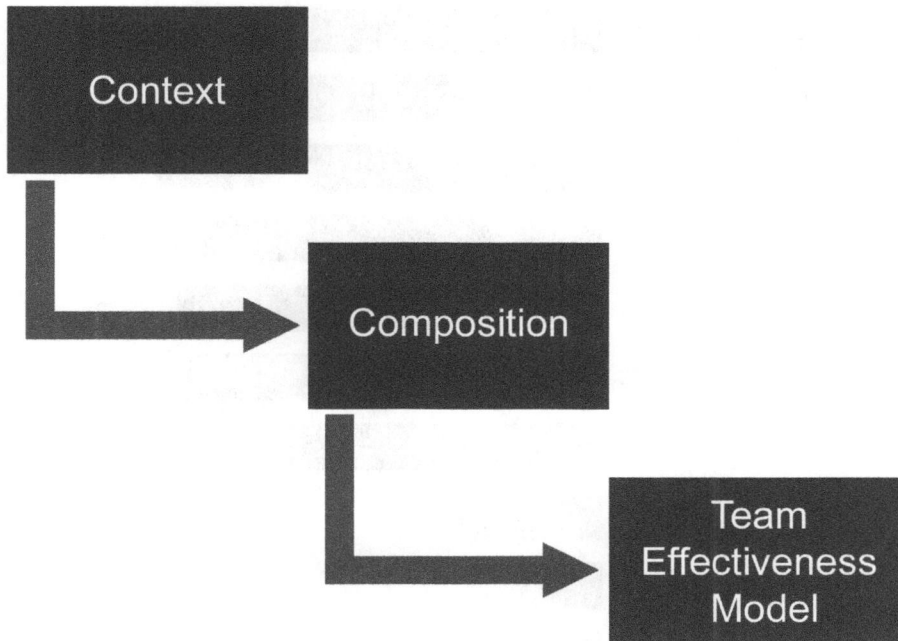

Figure 8.6: Creating Effective Teams

Source: Original Work
Attribution: Melissa Jordan
License: CC BY-SA 4.0

Stop and Apply

Review the case study at the beginning of the chapter. You have learned about creating effective teams. As the manager of the hospice center, how could individuals in the code team function more effectively in this situation? Brainstorm ways to educate hospital staff about how to activate code teams.

In today's information technology driven world, we believe children should gain a good understanding of science and math in order to compete with other countries that outperform the U.S. economically. The Pew Research Center asked a national sample of adults to select a list of 10 skills needed for children to get ahead of the global competition. According to Goo (2015), children need to acquire several skills to succeed in life, but the most important skill that tops the list is effective communication. Likewise, two of the top five most important skills are reading and writing, which are also communication skills components.

Communication — 90
Reading — 86
Math — 79
Teamwork — 77
Writing — 75
Logic — 74
Science — 58
Athletic — 25
Music — 24
Art — 23

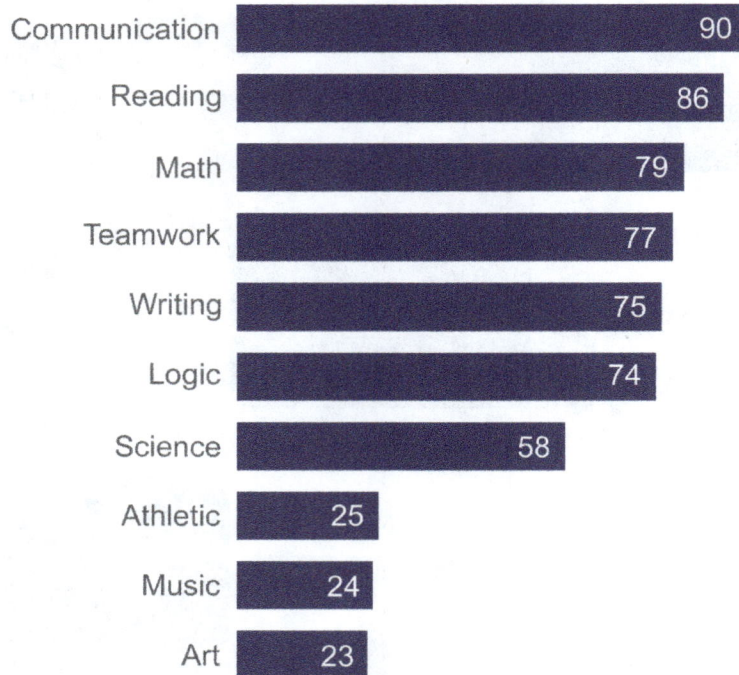

Figure 8.5: The Skills to Succeed

Source: American Trends Panel, 2014
Attribution: Corey Parson, Adapted from American Trends Panel, 2014
License: Fair Use

8.4.4 Effective Communication Process

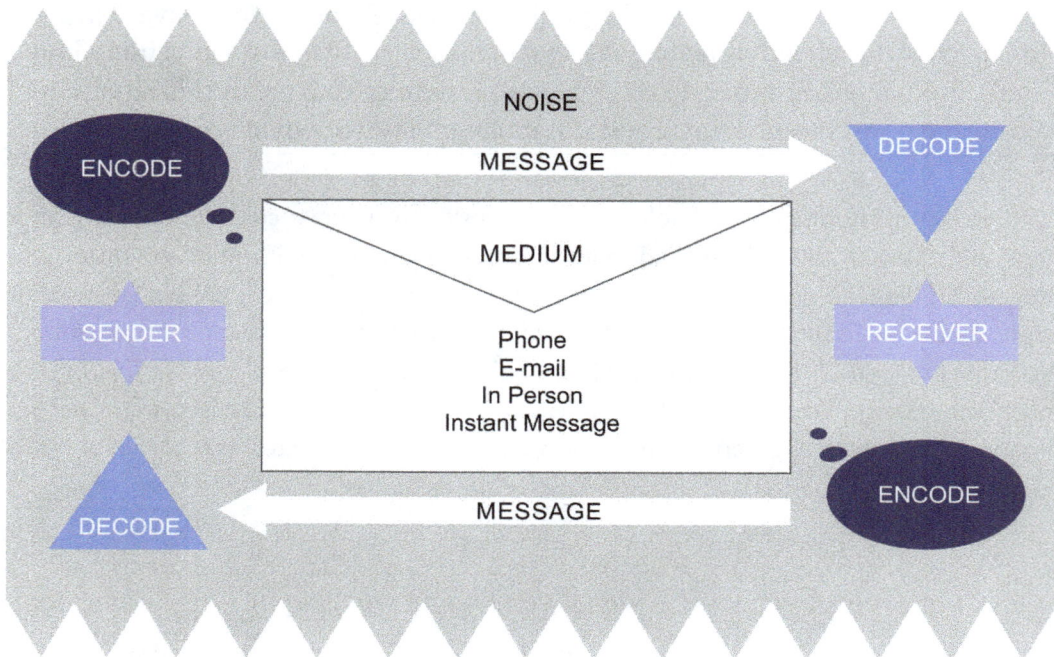

NOISE

ENCODE

MESSAGE

DECODE

SENDER

MEDIUM

RECEIVER

Phone
E-mail
In Person
Instant Message

DECODE

MESSAGE

ENCODE

Figure 8.7: Effective Communication Process

Source: Original Work
Attribution: Corey Parson
License: CC BY-SA 4.0

Communication is a two way process of transmitting information and understanding from one individual or group (sender) to another individual or group (receiver). Communciation starts with the sender having a thought or idea which is then encoded and transmitted through a selected mode of communication to the receiver. The receiver then decodes the message and gives it meaning, encodes a response, and then delivers feedback to the sender, who then decodes that response. Often during the process, communication may be surrounded by noise that can hinder, impede, or effect misconstructing an accurate exchange of the information.

8.4.5 Barriers to Effective Communication

As important as it is for leaders and managers to understand what makes communication effective, they must also be aware of the barriers to effective communication. Barriers to communication involve anything that can distort effective communication. Leaders and managers must consider how information can be misconstrued, lost, or misrepresented.

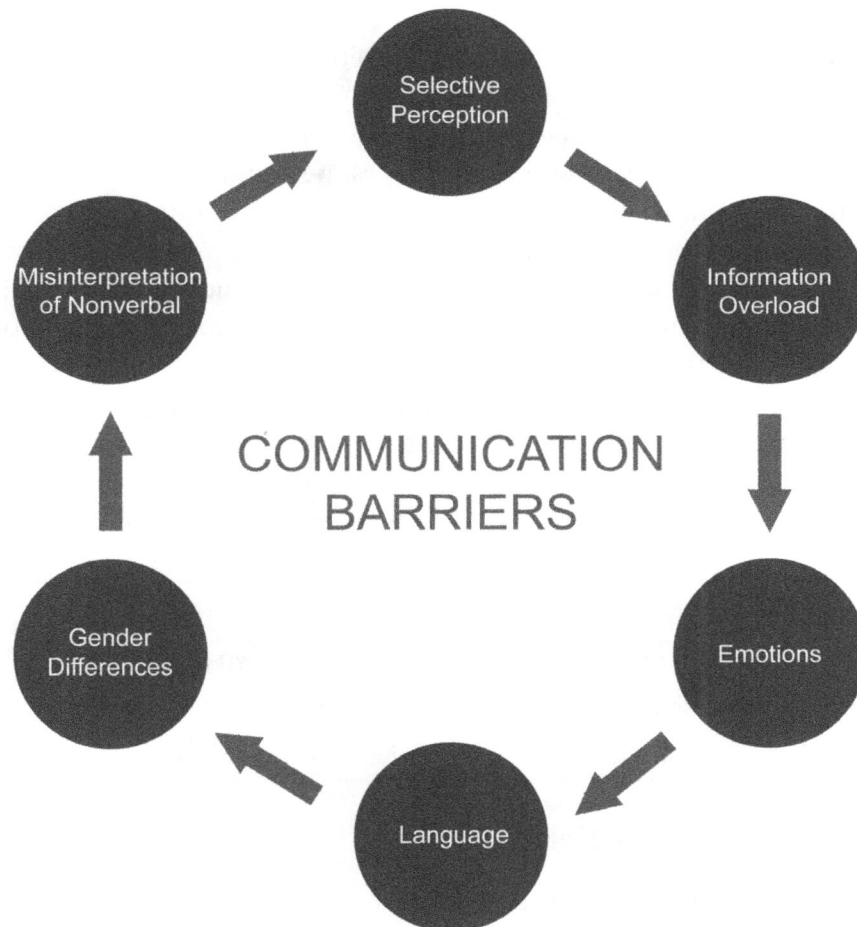

Figure 8.8: Barriers to Effective Communication

Source: Original Work
Attribution: Melissa Jordan
License: CC BY-SA 4.0

Selective perception happens when the receivers in the communication process selectively choose to hear and see what they want to, based on their needs, emotions, motivations, or any other personal characteristics.

Information overload is when the information, once received, has overloaded the processing capacity. In this situation, people often tend to ignore, select, forget, or pass over information. How much information is disseminated to employees is important in relation to what you are trying to effectively communicate.

Emotions can change a discussion and how the receiver perceives the information. When one is emotional, the message may be interpreted differently. If one is angry or depressed, for example, then these emotions can hinder effective communication, and the thinking processes will likely lead to emotional responses.

Language is not the same for everyone when communicating, even when you speak the same language. One may find the workplace extremely diverse in language today. Words can mean different things to different people, no matter the language, age, or gender. Language is not standardized, and one need not assume that words and terms they use in the workplace mean the same to the person on the receiving end.

Gender differences can be a barrier to effective communication. Women and men can talk in socially enculturated and particular ways to each other and hear each other from different perspectives. If individuals do not understand how to communicate effectively with different genders, people may distance themselves from each other. Culturally and stereotypically, women often are expected to focus on connecting with others and building relationships, while men often are expected to emphasize status and dominance in communication (Walston, 2017). Leaders and managers must develop strategies in overcoming these types of communication modes and expectations.

Misinterpretation of nonverbal communication can be a barrier. Silence can speak volumes and thus overshadow the meaning behind the message. For example, someone standing with their arms crossed can be perceived by the receiver as being upset, frustrated, or even disinterested in the receiver.

Stop and Apply

- Where is communication likely to break down at the code site?
- Who should be notified in the event of a patient code?
- How can you make Do Not Resuscitate orders available and effective?

8.4.6 Managing Conflict

Conflict and negotiation are present in our everyday lives no matter what industry we work in. Anyone who may have a different perception from another person can create an environment of conflict. If conflict is managed swiftly and correctly, an organization can move forward in accomplishing its core values, mission, and vision. If conflict is managed ineffectively or poorly, conflict can result in a toxic environment for everyone. **Conflict** is defined as a "competitive or opposing action of incompatibles; mental struggle resulting from incompatible or opposing needs, drives, wishes, or external or internal demands; the opposition of persons or forces that gives rise to dramatic action." (Merriam-Webster, 2015).

Types of Conflict

Leaders and managers can resolve conflict effectively and efficiently by first understanding the different types of work-related conflict. These include task conflict, process conflict, relationship conflict, and non-task organizational conflict.

Task conflict is when different opinions or viewpoints arise about details that are related to work and the task goals. Questions arise about what has to be accomplished and what one has to do to get the task accomplished.

Process conflict involves disagreements on how to do the job or the various ways the job can get done.

Relationship conflict develops from personal beliefs, political beliefs, values, personality differences, and individual work style.

Non-task conflicts develop disagreements and disputes that have nothing to do with the job task, including company policies, hiring decisions, organizational leaders, power, and personal influences.

Effective Management of the Conflict Process

The conflict management process must be done swiftly and effectively before the conflict starts to escalate and creates an unhealthy environment for everyone involved in the workplace. Not addressing conflict quickly and efficiently can decrease job productivity, create job stress, diminish communication, decrease job performance, increase resistance to change, and diminish employee retention and loyalty (Robbins & Judge, 2011; Walton, 2017). Effective conflict management involves defining acceptable behavior, addressing conflict proactively, understanding the involved parties' motivations, and using the conflict as an opportunity for growth.

Leaders and managers can use several conflict resolution techniques in the workplace. Communication is the first step in the conflict resolution process, and moving forward to resolve the conflict will get all parties involved back on track with quality performance.

Table 8.2: Conflict Resolution Techniques	
Problem Solving	Face-to-Face meeting with conflicting parties for the purpose of problem-solving resolution
Expansion of Resources	Conflict caused by scarcity of resources; an expansion of the resources can create a win-win.
Avoidance	Isolation or withdrawal from or suppression of the conflict.

Compromise	Each person involved in the party of the conflict gives up something of value.
Authoritative Command	Management uses formal authority to resolve the conflict and communicates decisions and desires to the individuals involved in the conflict.
Superordinate Goals	Creating and developing a shared goal that cannot be obtained without cooperation from both conflicting parties.
Accommodating	An individual in the conflicting party who seeks to appease the other conflicting party will be willing to place the opponent's interest above their own. They support someone else's desires despite their own reservations.

Source: Original Work
Attribution: Melissa Jordan
License: CC BY-SA 4.0

Stop and Apply

Identify Task Conflict in this case scenario.

1. What could have been done to resolve it?

2. How would you have resolved the conflict? Why?

8.4.7 Power and Influence

Leaders and managers today must be able to function effectively in diverse environments with diverse behaviors. Power and influence are characteristics that can create access to key individuals and resources in the workplace. Power and influence may sound like they have the same definition, but they are distinctly different. **Power** is the capacity to influence others by controlling valuable resources. **Influence** is the process of persuading someone to do something. Influence is triggered when effective power is implemented. For effective leadership, you cannot have one without the other.

Several tactics can be used when **Exerting Power and Influence**:

*   *Rational persuasion* involves logical arguments and information that can be backed up by facts.

*   *Inspirational appeals* make an emotional request to build enthusiasm and spirit by appealing to the values, mission, and vision of the organization.

*   *Consultation* recruits engaging minds that are willing to participate in decision making and implementation of planning.

*   *Personal appeal* goes to a specific person based on their loyalty to the organization or loyalty to you as a friend.

*   *Pressure* imposes threatening behaviors, demands, belittling, and intimidation to encourage their behavior for your benefit.

- *Coalition* involves building and using support from a group to help persuade others.
- *Exchange* offers to make a trade or share in potential incentives, rewards, or reciprocating favors.

8.4.8 Managing Negotiation

Any leader of a group or team needs a variety of skills, including decision making, communication, problem solving, team management, conflict resolution, and negotiation skills. The term negotiation is often used interchangeably with the term bargaining. In this section, we will focus on the term negotiation.

Negotiation is a process in which two or more parties exchange goods or services and attempt to agree on the exchange rate for them (Robbins & Judge, 2011). **Negotiation Agreements** lead to a settlement that disputing parties reach between themselves, especially with the help of their attorneys. However, this happens without the benefits of formal mediation.

These five steps are involved in the negotiation process: preparing and planning, defining ground rules, clarification and justification, bargaining and problem solving, and closure and implementation.

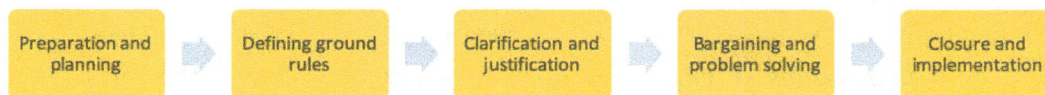

| Preparation and planning | ⟹ | Defining ground rules | ⟹ | Clarification and justification | ⟹ | Bargaining and problem solving | ⟹ | Closure and implementation |

Figure 8.9: Steps to Resolve Conflict

Source: Original Work
Attribution: Melissa Jordan
License: CC BY-SA 4.0

The Negotiation Process

Preparing and Planning. Leaders and managers must know what they need to do before starting negotiations by questioning who is involved. What are the goals? What is the nature of the conflict? What do the parties want the results to be after the negotiation? After it is gathered, this information can be used to develop a strategy. When developing the strategy, one side should determine their own while the other party does the same to develop the best alternative to a negotiated agreement (BANTA) (Robbins & Judge, 2011). BANTA will determine the lowest value acceptable for leaders in a negotiated agreement. Both sides must think carefully about what they are willing to give up. Individuals often underestimate their opponent's willingness to give up on issues and factors that are important to them.

Defining Ground Rules. Ground guidelines and/or rules are a main part of the negotiation's procedures. These guidelines and/or rules can include how much time will apply, where negotiations will take place, what issues will be included in the negotiation, and who will do the arbitration.

Clarification and Justification. Both parties need to have a clear understanding of what will be explained, amplified, clarified, and justified from the original demands. This clarification offers an opportunity for the parties to learn and understand each other's issues and why they are important.

Bargaining and Problem Solving. To bargain is to have an actual give-and-take situation. Each of the parties involved will have to give something to get something in trying to reach an agreement.

Closure and Implementation. This is the final step in the negotiation process, and it is when the agreement is finally formalized. The conflict has been resolved and procedures will be developed for necessary implementation and monitoring.

8.4.9 Improving Performance: Managing Innovation and Change

Change is a part of life, and understanding the environmental forces that lead to change is vital for any leader or manager in the workplace. A smooth transition is necessary for growth and success for all parties involved. In order to grow, increase quality performance, and be an innovative organization, change is necessary. Innovation is a new idea applied to initiating or improving a product, process, or service (Robbins & Judge, 2011). This concept is a unique change that can be derived from various sources.

Leaders and managers can create a climate of innovation by developing learning organizations. A learning organization is an organization that focuses on and welcomes a continuous capacity to adapt and change with the environment. Leaders and managers can create learning organizations through engagement. Allowing employees to organize actively, share information and ideas, and build and support job talents will assist in overcoming resistance to change. Identification of errors and correcting those errors effectively and efficiently is crucial for progress.

Characteristics of learning organizations include the following (Robbins & Judge, 2011):

- Leaders and managers have a shared understanding and agreement of the mission and vision of the organization.

- They have a willingness to discard old habits and outdated mindsets.

- They build interrelationships for organizational activities, processes, functions, and interactions in the workplace environment.

- They allow open communication at all levels without fear of retaliation, criticism, or being fired.

- Individuals integrate their personal interests with departmental interests in order to work together and achieve the organization's goals, objectives, mission, and vision.

Managing learning and innovation through performance improvements. Leaders and managers focus on several techniques and strategies to foster learning and innovation, including establishing a strategy or plan of action, redesigning existing structures, or changing the organization's culture.

Establish a plan/strategy. Leaders must be clear about the commitment needed for positive change, innovation, and continuous improvement to take place.

Redesign. Structural changes may be necessary and can cause fear, panic, and anxiety for the creative learning environment. Redesigning may cause departments to be eliminated and job tasks to be combined, moved, or entirely removed. Leaders must do all they can to assure employees that though the environment is causing stress and anxiety, it is temporary and necessary for positive change. Leaders can reduce stress in the workplace during a redesign through effective communication, employee inclusion, and offering stress management resources.

Organization culture change. In order to grow and become a creative, innovative, and learning organization, leaders will have to take risks. Leaders and managers can calm employees' fears by showing they, too are human but are willing to take chances rather than do nothing at all. An organization that has no vision, no futuristic mindset, and no intent to innovate is an organization that will cease to exist.

Stop and Apply

You are selected for an improvement team in response to this event. Consider your own clinical environment. What changes would you suggest in shortening the time before access to emergency services, CPR and possible defibrillation?

8.5 CONCLUSION

Chapter eight expanded on leadership and management's different skills by delineating the roles of leaders and managers in influencing organizational culture, performance, and change. Teams are increasingly the primary reason for organizing work, and how leaders manage, influence, and resolve conflict will determine the organization's success.

8.6 KEY POINTS

- In order for individuals to be willing to bear partial responsibility in regards to the organization's success, one must understand leadership and management's roles in influencing others.

- Communication is key when it comes to leaders and managers motivating, building, clarifying, and affirming the organization's shared values.

- Leaders and managers must understand how to get the best performance from individuals who bring their talents together for common goals to be accomplished efficiently and effectively.

- Effective conflict maagement involves defining acceptable behavior, addressing conflict proactively, understanding the involved parties' motivations, and using the conflict as an opportunity for growth.
- Negotiation is a continuous activity in groups, teams, and organizations.

8.7 KEY TERMS

Group vs. Team, Motivation, Team design, Cross-Functional Team, Self-Managed Team, Virtual Team, Effective communication process, Exertion of Influence, Conflict Resolution, Negotiation, Innovation

8.8 QUESTIONS FOR REVIEW AND DISCUSSION

1. What do you believe a mission and vision statement should contain?
2. How should organizations create team players in the workplace?
3. Why does conflict develop?
4. From your own experiences, think of a conflict and negotiation situation you have been through that didn't go well. How would you have done things differently?
5. How can organizations create a culture of innovation and change?

8.9 REFERENCES

ActiveCollab. (2017). "Types of teams." Retrieved from https://activecollab.com/blog/collaboration/types-of-teams

ASQ.ORG. Quality quotes. Retrieved from https://asq.org/quality-resources/more-on-quality-quotes

Goetsch, D. L., & Davis, S. B. (2016). *Quality management for organizational excellence: Introduction to quality*. 8th Edition. Pearson.

Goo, S. K. (2015). "The skills Americans say kids need to succeed in life." Published February 19. www.pewresearch.org/fact-tank/2015/02/19/skills-for-success/.

Institute for Health Improvement. "Case study: Code blue? Where to (AHRQ)?" Retrieved from http://www.ihi.org/education/IHIOpenSchool/resources/Pages/Activities/AHRQCaseStudyCodeBlue.aspx

Kouzes, J. M., Posner, B. Z. (2002). "The leadership challenges." 3rd ed. Jossey-Bass: CA.

Managing conflict in the workplace video. Retrieved from https://youtu.be/BweNXKahb8I

Merriam-Webster. (2016). "Conflict." Retrieved from https://www.merriam-webster.com/dictionary/conflict

Robbins, S. P., Judge, T. A. (2011). Organizational behavior, 14th ed. Prentice Hall: Boston

Spath, P. L., Kelly, D. L. (2017). *Applying quality management in healthcare: A systems approach.* 14th ed. Health Care Administration Press: Washington, DC

Walston, S. L. (2016). *Organizational behavior and theory in health care.* Health Care Administration Press: Washington, DC

YouTube. Creating culture in the workplace. Retrieved from https://www.youtube.com/watch?v=4-APGd2oT3Y

PART III

ORGANIZATIONAL BEHAVIOR AND MODELS

9 ORGANIZATIONAL THEORY AND BEHAVIOR PRACTICES IN HEALTHCARE: EXAMINING THE THREE LENSES OF THE HEALTHCARE INDUSTRY

9.1 LEARNING OBJECTIVES

- Define organizational behavior
- Illustrate how individuals and organizations interact
- Describe how attitudes and perceptions influence organizational behavior
- Recognize the importance of effective communication for healthcare leaders and managers
- Describe the benefits of applying organizational behavior at the individual, team, and organizational levels
- Describe the facets of organizational behavior that contribute to effective leadership and management responsibilities
- Identify ways to apply organizational behavior concepts to healthcare management challenges

9.2 INTRODUCTION

The study of organizational behavior and theory originated during the Industrial Revolution when early theorists, such as Max Weber, Henri Fayol, and Fredrick Taylor, examined key attributes that contributed to increased organizational performance and efficiency (as discussed previously in this text). Healthcare managers need to understand the relationship between organizational behavior and organizational theory in order to adapt to the ever shifting internal (e.g., areas of focus that managers address daily) and external (e.g., outside resources, activities, and stakeholders that directly influence the organization) healthcare demands. The purpose of this chapter is to explore how managers can apply these concepts in order to improve behavior, performance, and satisfaction. This chapter will discuss the knowledge and skills needed to successfully lead and manage individuals, groups, and teams within a healthcare organization.

Organizational behavior illustrates how the individual and organization interact. Organizational theory explains the dynamics of power relationships, how structure works, and illustrates how healthcare organizations adapt to changing economic, social, and political conditions (Buchbinder & Shanks, 2012). Organizational behavior is essential to health care managers who facilitate the delivery of medical services, which are delivered by professionals with whom the manager may not directly oversee. Additionally, the healthcare manager works in a challenging industry that is facing rising costs and increasing demand due to an aging population and rise in costly chronic conditions, in addition to shifting policies and declining financial reimbursements. The healthcare industry is shifting to a value-based system where payments are based on the value and impact of care delivered, rather than the ineffectual fee-for-service system that determines reimbursement by the quantity of tests ordered and patient visits (Brown and Crapo, 2017). The concepts within organizational behavior and theory can explain how, despite the challenges, a competent healthcare manager facilitates the effective, coordinated delivery of healthcare by professional networks and teams throughout the organization.

Organizational behavior and theory consist of examining behaviors across three levels: **individual**, **group**, and **collective behavior** across the healthcare organization and illustrates applications of each in order to improve healthcare management practices, positively influence employees, and reach organizational goals (Buchbinder & Shanks, 2012).

The Chapter Case

The managers and staff at Southern Healthcare Hospice Center are increasingly overworked as everyone takes on mounting responsibilities and longer workdays as a result of the high staff turnover. Amanda, the director of the facility, has devised a set of organizational policies. One of the policies specifically states that staff members are not allowed to sleep while on duty. A staff member made a complaint to the long-term care manager that several night-shift workers were taking naps and sleeping in beds in unoccupied patient rooms. These staff members were in violation of the night shift policy as well as neglecting their responsibilities. As you read through the various leadership and management theories, consider how a manager would address this scenario using concepts from the leadership or management theory.

*Adapted from Xu, J. (2017). Leadership theory in clinical practice. Clinical Nursing Research

---

9.3 EXAMINING ORGANIZATIONAL BEHAVIOR AT THE INDIVIDUAL LEVEL

Examining organizational behavior at the individual level links the organization to its staff by examining the interaction between the individuals and the organization. Organizational behavior explains the interaction between individuals and the organization. In order to overcome the challenges facing today's healthcare organizations, managers must be able to understand how individuals influence the overall performance of the organization. They must be able to create organizational settings that are conducive to the optimal performance of organizational employees. The environment of the organization established by the manager, in addition to manager and individual staff perceptions, beliefs, and experiences, influence workplace behaviors and actions (e.g., reactions, decision-making, learning, and organizational practices).

Individual characteristics of human interaction, such as bias based on prior experiences, stress, and emotions, can obscure organizational communication, problem solving, and decision-making. In order to understand behavior, it is essential to understand the thoughts, assumptions, and perceptions that precede actions. The **attribution theory** states people naturally seek to explain the likely cause of others' behavior. Reactions to others' behaviors depend on our perception of individuals' internal **attributes** rather than external circumstances that may be out of their control. For example, a physician who assumes negative things about a patient may mistakenly attribute the patient's health issues to risky behaviors and consequently provide subpar care. Studies show a physician's perceptions, or whether a physician likes or dislikes a patient, have implications for healthcare quality and outcomes. Research illustrates male and healthier patients are liked better by physicians than female and sickly patients (Buchbinder & Shanks, 2012). Further, the physician's positive perception is associated with providing information, longer patient visits, and positive expectations, which thereby improve patient adherence and compliance to treatment. Thus, positive physician perceptions lead to improved patient satisfaction and health outcomes (Buchbinder & Shanks, 2012).

The way a person makes sense of a situation will affect their attitude and actions. In other words, our perception of another's behavior is based on our perception of the individual and the context of the situation. Therefore, it is important to understand **expectancy,** which is how our prior knowledge and experiences shape our perception and expectations of others. Understanding how perceptions, attitudes, and personality traits influence individual behavior in the workplace helps managers establish ways to motivate employees to reach organizational goals and increase the satisfaction, dedication, and learning of staff.

Emotions also shape how individuals feel about their jobs and affect organizational behaviors. **The Affective Events Theory (AET)** posits specific organizational situations evoke different emotions for different people, and these emotions can either impede or benefit work productivity (Buchbinder & Shanks, 2012). For example, a co-worker unexpectedly bringing you lunch on a rather hectic day may invoke positive feelings and inspire you to work harder. Studies indicate positive feelings stemming from positive work experiences may inspire individuals to complete more work than they planned to. Likewise, if an individual is unfairly reprimanded by their manager, then the ensuing negative emotions may cause them to withdraw from work and even act harshly toward other co-workers. Collectively, workplace experiences shape emotions that drive individual behavior and influence their overall job satisfaction. Although positive incentives and benefits can contribute to an individual's happiness with their workplace, according to AET, job satisfaction stems from the combination of an individual's personality, collective emotional experiences at work, and values. Workplace environments that are negative and foster negative emotions can cause individuals to experience ongoing negative emotions, including job frustration and dissatisfaction.

We experience an array of emotions every day. Consider how many emotions you have experienced today alone. What made you happy today? Did you get an unexpected, uplifting text from a friend? Alternatively, did anyone cut you off on the road while driving? Were you sad? Did you receive some really bad news? Imagine trying to hide your most intense emotions for hours at work. Oftentimes, that is exactly what we are expected to do—which results in a **persona**, or a professional role, that involves acting out of feelings that we may not necessarily feel. We may be sad, angry, or afraid at work, but workplace expectations take precedence over emotions. **Cognitive dissonance** refers to misalignment amongst emotions, attitudes, beliefs, and behaviors resulting in individuals acting in ways that do not align with their feelings. An example of such is being polite to patients even when they are being extremely rude. Although acting positive can make you and others feel positive, without alleviating cognitive dissonance, individuals may experience personal conflict and stress. We will further discuss potential sources of stress and ways to manage the work-life balance in chapter fourteen. However, increasing your **emotional intelligence**, or awareness of the gap between your actual feelings and your expected professional persona, can help manage the effects of cognitive dissonance. Emotional intelligence refers to how well individuals understand their emotions as well as those of others. The following are the four key components of emotional intelligence:

- **Self-awareness:** the ability to accurately perceive, evaluate, and display appropriate emotions
- **Self-management:** the ability to positively express appropriate emotions
- **Social awareness**: the ability to understand how others feel
- **Relationship management:** the ability to support others and help individuals manage their emotions (Buchbinder & Shanks, 2012).

Emotional intelligence is an important skill for healthcare managers and should be used to motivate and inspire employees. Managers should be able to understand how their emotions and actions influence the emotions and behaviors of their employees. Managers should also be able to empathize with and relate to their employees. Individuals with strong emotional intelligence have higher self-efficacy in coping with adversity, perceiving situations as challenges rather than threats, and having higher satisfaction, which leads to reduced stress levels.

Stop and Apply

Have you ever experienced an emotional exertion while balancing work or academic responsibilities? How were you able to balance your duties while controlling your emotions? If you were a manager who noticed an employee lashing out at patients or other staff members and experiencing a seemingly "off" day, how would you handle the situation?

The way managers view their constituents can determine their management approaches and how they encourage their staff to complete organizational tasks. The success of the organization depends upon the motivation and satisfaction of its employees. Work motivation is "a set of energetic forces that originate both within as well as beyond an individual's being, to initiate work-related behavior and to determine its form, direction, intensity, and duration (Pinder, 2008). According to **Maslow's Need Hierarchy Theory**, employees have such basic physiological needs as air, food, and water as well as such needs as social interaction, self-actualization and self-fulfillment. Besides the basic necessities and resources required to complete tasks, managers also must provide motivation, support, and training in order for employees to find satisfaction in the workplace and remain motivated to complete organizational tasks. A key responsibility of managers is providing such motivation, in addition to the above-mentioned support, training, and necessary resources.

Psychologist Douglas McGregor described two disparate views regarding how managers view what motivates their employees (see also chapter six). The first assumption, referred to as Theory X, posits employees naturally do not like to work and will avoid responsibility; therefore, managers must coerce such employees to work. Theory X managers assume staff are unmotivated to work and need frequent micromanagement, rewards, or punishments to complete tasks. The second assumption suggests employees are naturally motivated to work; thus, managers allow such employees to take ownership of their work and will increase the potential of these employees by providing opportunities for growth and development. Theory Y managers will encourage a less authoritarian and more collaborative management approach.

Prior knowledge and experiences can also determine the approach used by managers. Past experiences can lead to faulty expectancies that can cause managers to misconstrue staff interactions and behaviors. For example, a manager who believes an employee has a bad attitude may treat that person in a way that provokes the expected negative behavior. Understanding that the behavior and motives of others are subject to **bias**, depend on the situation, and are interpreted through the attributes that were assigned by one individual to another are vital in ensuring that employees are treated fairly. This bias is a fault in thinking that may affect one's judgments and assumptions regarding the behavior of other individuals. For example, if someone we know who is typically diligent makes a good grade in a class, we may assume the person studied hard, thereby assigning a positive attribute. However, if a person we know who is typically lazy does well on an exam, we may assume the test was just easy. **Vroom's expectancy theory (1964)** assumes the performance of employees is based on individual factors, such as personality traits, skills, and experience. Accurately understanding these individual characteristics and providing appropriate encouragement and support will motivate employees to reach organizational goals. According to the expectancy theory, an employee's motivation is determined by the extent the individual wants to be rewarded. Understanding what motivates employees and properly rewarding them will lead to increased performance (Vroom, 1964).

The way we perceive, process, and act upon information is based on our knowledge and expectations. Similarly, the way organizational change is viewed is defined by an individual's internal view of reality. An individual's interpretation of how an organization should operate and respond to change can limit how they learn and share information. The way individuals perceive situations may be much different from the actual situation that is occurring. For example, the Southern Care Hospice Center occupancy rate has been dropping. The staff were initially convinced the location was undesirable. However, following her evaluation, the manager learned patient decisions were based not on the facility's location but on the lack of linguistic services it offered on-site. The staff's inaccurate assumption of the facility's undesirable location had to be shifted to address the language barrier in order to address actual concerns and improve the occupancy rate.

A manager has the task of working through perceptions by creating shared meaning and sensemaking in order to enable staff to fulfill the actual, not perceived, organizational goals. Managers must also be aware of their own perceptions and treat all staff fairly. Misperceptions can often be remedied through effective and ongoing communication with clear feedback mechanisms. Communication is the means by which organizational tasks are coordinated, processed, and completed by the organization's constituents. Thus, as discussed previously, effective communication is vital to the organization's success. Miscommunication can often lead to frustration, but in the healthcare industry, miscommunication can be the difference between life and death.

Taking shortcuts in judgment simplify the decision-making process by drawing conclusions without assessing the entire situation. These judgment shortcuts, however, create bias which leads to decisions that are vulnerable to the influence of previous experiences and assumptions. There are four main types of cognitive biases, or shortcuts in judgment, individuals take when reaching decisions; these include (1) prior beliefs that limit the ability to absorb additional information, (2) oversimplification of the issue or reliance on instinct that limits other possibilities that can address the issue, (3) faulty understanding of the situation and (4) overestimating one's ability to address the situation (Buchbinder, Shanks, 2012;

Das and Teng, 1999). Managers must have an understanding of the potential disruptions to communication and organizational processes as well as be aware of their own cognitive bias. Through careful reflection, transparent discussions, and incorporating comprehensive information, managers can improve organizational decision-making.

Effective communication is also necessary to establishing a strong and welcoming organizational culture. Organizational culture is the behavioral norms of individuals within the organization that can progress or impede the organization's success. A solid organizational culture is conducive to workplace productivity. Managers can achieve this atmosphere by clearly conveying and reinforcing the organization's vision to all staff. Furthermore, determining strategic direction and assigning specific job tasks in addition to individual accountability for specific roles is a part of establishing the organizational culture. Managers also establish the culture by rewarding positive performance and/or tolerating poor performance. The culture that is tolerated and/or rewarded by the manager in the workplace becomes the culture of the organization. By rewarding positive behavior, reprimanding poor performance, and simply communicating specific expectations, the culture the managers seek to establish will form in order to support organizational success and productivity.

Managers must also create common understanding among members of the organization. Awareness of how members may think and the factors that may affect organizational flow can guide managers in working to change how the members think and address the misperceptions that may exist. Managers can address faulty differences in thinking through open discussions and sharing information that will guide and motivate organizational members (see table below).

Table 9.1 The Effect of Thoughts on Behavior

Situation →	Thinking →	Behavior/Action
Organizational environment	Perceptions, intentions, beliefs, biases, cognition, knowledge	Reaction, decisions, work tasks, learning, organizational practices

Source: Buchbinder and Shanks, 2012
Attribution: Whitney Hamilton, Adapted from Buchbinder and Shanks, 2012
License: Fair Use

Moreover, according to the **need for achievement theory**, individuals with a high need for achievement will put more effort into their work than those who have a low need for achievement (McClelland, 1961). Those with a low desire for achievement should be given specific goals to work toward in order to compensate for their lack of self-motivation and to avoid falling short of organizational goals (McClelland, 1961). This concept is also reinforced by Locke's goal setting theory which posits employees who set goals are motivated to reach goals. According to the theory, achieving set goals are rewarding, and performance is best when goals are specific and challenging, the workers are capable, rewards are offered, managers are supportive and provide feedback, resources are available, and goals are internalized.

Managers should begin by hiring qualified workers who align with the organization's mission. Proper training and a system of ongoing communication with feedback from managers and employees should also be established in order to ensure employees are reaching organizational goals. Managers should also establish a system of reward and recognition in addition to providing adequate resources to complete tasks.

9.4 EXAMINING ORGANIZATIONAL BEHAVIOR AT THE GROUP LEVEL

Examining organizational behavior at the group level provides insight into the collective challenges of leadership, communication, decision-making, teamwork, power, and conflict. Managers work with everyone in the organization in order to make sense of their interactions and experiences in order to create a shared meaning that enables teamwork and collaboration within the organization, and attains overall organizational goals. In addition to logical evaluation, deliberate decision-making, and thorough planning and implementation, managers must also address group perceptions and collective sensemaking. Managers must ensure they communicate organizational tasks and goals in a way staff collectively understands. **Sensemaking** refers to how people collectively comprehend information or situations that could have several plausible interpretations. Sensemaking is a key component of communication, problem solving, decision-making, coordination, and navigating conflict and change. In order to create shared meaning and reduce ambiguity, managers must organize information in a way that guides sufficient organizational learning and actions (Weick, Sutcliff, Obstfield, 2005). Effective communication, problem solving, and decision-making depends upon the manager's ability to create shared understanding and foster collective action among the healthcare organization's members.

The problem-solving process starts with identifying organizational issues and then assessing various options to solve the problem and choosing, implementing, and evaluating the most plausible option to address the problem. Healthcare administrators must work in concert with medical providers and various sectors of the healthcare industry, including but not limited to physicians, nurses, social workers, and other operational staff when making organizational decisions. Health administrators must be able to facilitate communication between the various sectors of healthcare teams and build **team cohesiveness**. Team cohesiveness refers to the extent of interpersonal connectedness between members of a group that influences participants to accomplish established goals (Kozlowski & Bell, 2001). Team cohesiveness is critical to the healthcare sector in order to limit adverse health outcomes and improve not only patient but also employee satisfaction. Successfully integrating the disparate teams customary in healthcare requires a concerted effort to increase collaboration and communication within and across disciplinary teams. Therefore, the healthcare administrator must establish this strong culture of collaboration and communication. The healthcare administrator can lay this foundation by incorporating these four components:

- Clearly communicate organizational goals

- Clearly establish organizational partnerships and assigned roles and responsibilities

- Establish and enforce policies and procedures

- Develop and maintain strong interpersonal relationships through ongoing communication

Healthcare administrators work with medical providers to make decisions that affect how well the healthcare organization operates. The medical team and administration staff may approach the same decision differently; however, each member of the healthcare organization shares the same goal of ensuring individuals receive adequate access to quality, affordable healthcare. For example, administrators at Providence Hospital decided to test a new enhancement to improve patient care following the results of ongoing focus groups. Through the focus groups, the administrators found that although physicians were verbally providing care instructions to patients at the end of each visit, patients were likely to forget the information shortly after the visit and/or unable to convey the information to family members. Consequently, the marketing team suggested printing post-exam summaries, but this idea was met with skepticism by physicians who felt the summaries would hinder their already heavy schedules. The administrators and marketing team were able to show physicians evidence of how the summaries would lead to an increase in patient satisfaction and care compliance, thereby increasing the likelihood of patients recommending their physician to others. The healthcare administrators and marketing team presented the service enhancement in an evidence driven way the physicians could understand. Further, physicians repeatedly expressed concerns regarding the hospital's difficult and time-consuming referral process. The physicians suggested using one call center referral line in order to increase efficiency and maximize patient satisfaction. The administrators considered the physician feedback and implemented a referral line, thereby eliminating a major issue for physicians and improving patient care. In both of the aforementioned examples, opinions were received from both sides, then considered and implemented following open and effective dialogue that was spoken in a way each team understood (Shoebridge, 2015). First, a problem is identified as well as the cause of the problem, then goals are set, and options generated. The teams must work together to assess options, choose, implement, and evaluate selected solutions. Although communication between physicians and non-physicians can be difficult because each may approach situations differently, in order for health care teams to operate cohesively, communication must be a two-way dialogue with all team members feeling empowered to ask questions and express concerns. Physicians are concerned with how plans and processes will affect their ability to provide patient care while administrators seek to understand which practices will best align with the overall business goals of the healthcare organization. Even if each team is approaching the same issue from different viewpoints, establishing common ground permits and strong conduits for two-way communication are vital in regards to providing effective patient care. Building successful and open communication is important to creating team cohesion (Shoebridge, 2015).

Lee Iacocca, former CEO of Chrysler, said, "You can have brilliant ideas, but if you can't get them across, your ideas won't get you anywhere." A healthcare environment that fosters open communication and establishes clear task roles and responsibilities improves the quality of working relationships, job satisfaction, patient satisfaction, and outcomes. Managers must provide information in a timely manner that is easily understood, with clear instructions and comprehensive answers to any questions that may arise (AHRQ, 2017). As discussed in chapter 8, communication is a process of organizing and transmitting information while conveying emotions and feelings. However, various factors, known as noise, can disrupt or distort the communication process (please refer to figure 9.1). For example, a manager may think, "We need more computer paper." The manager, or sender, will translate this idea into words and ask the receptionist to get more computer paper from the storage unit. The manager may say, "Hey, please go grab some more computer paper from the storage closet." The medium of an encoded message can be through spoken words, written words, or symbols. The receiver is the person receiving the message. The receiver decodes the message by giving meaning to the words. In this example, Lisa, the receptionist, has a long to-do list. She thinks, "Surely the manager knows all the work I have to do today" and translates the message as "Pick up the computer paper once you have completed your other tasks." The meaning the receiver gives to the message may not be the intended meaning of the sender, because of noise factors. Noise can include environmental distractions, such as music or loud talking in the waiting room, or internal factors within the receiver, such as nervousness or feeling too tired to pay attention. The sender also may not accurately convey the message or may use language that could be misinterpreted. In this example above, later on during the staff meeting, the manager asks Lisa for the paper. The receptionist curtly responds, "You didn't say get the paper immediately." Miscommunication occurs all the time. However, communication's most important role is to convey a common focus. Additionally, each team member should feel empowered to ask questions and express concerns regarding procedures without fearing penalties (Shoebridge, 2015).

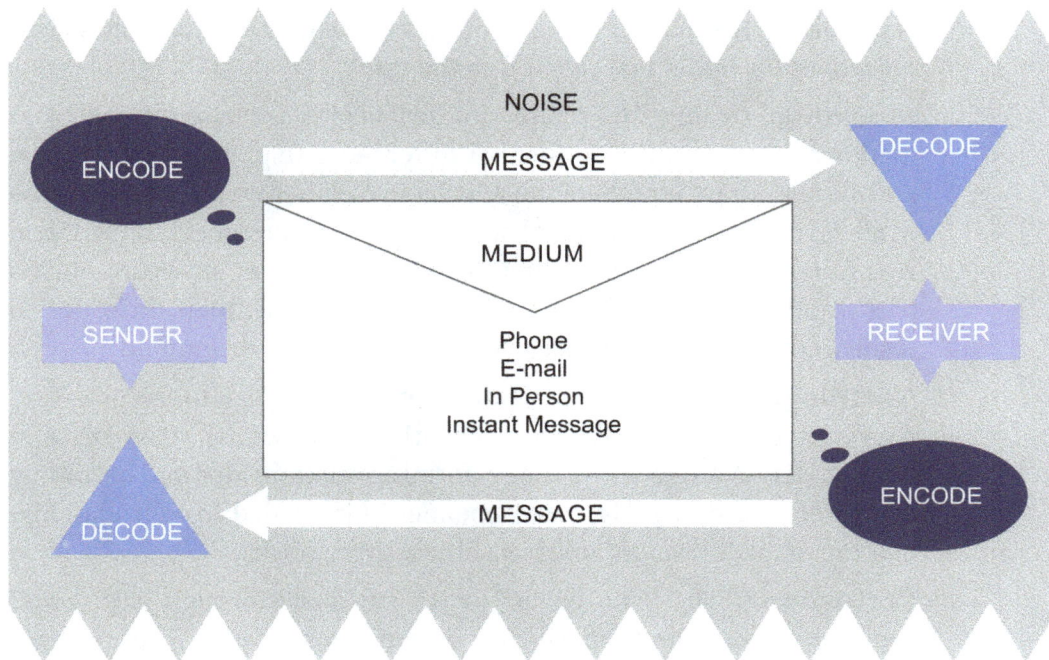

Figure 9.1: Process Model of Communication

It is important that each team member feels as though their opinions have been heard and valued. Even if certain ideas from team members seem unfeasible, it is important healthcare administrators maintain strong interpersonal relations and at least acknowledge and address team members' ideas or concerns. Maintaining an open and welcome environment for conversation is essential to building cohesion in the workplace (Shoebridge, 2015). Providing feedback to patient concerns is associated with increased employee engagement that better cultivates a culture of improved patient safety and lower workplace burnout (Health Catalysts, 2018).

Trust and enabling team members to employ their abilities is also a key factor in ensuring that groups attain organizational goals. Team building consists of group members cooperatively working together, thereby enhancing individual, interpersonal, and problem-solving skills. Managers, as well as effective groups, will leverage the knowledge, skills, and abilities of the organization's team members in order to complete tasks. Managers must clearly and effectively express organizational goals in order to enable group members to understand and accomplish each assigned job. In 1965, Bruck Tuckman introduced the five stage theory of group development, which posits that most groups change over time and develop over these five distinct phases:

1. **Forming:** During the initial phase, team members are a bit unclear regarding their roles and responsibilities, leading to mixed emotions characterized by anxiety, suspicion, curiosity, and confusion. Because of this uncertainty, team members depend heavily on leadership, and it

is important the manager clearly directs the team and establishes clear objectives for individuals as well as the team.

2. **Storming:** During this phase, conflict begins to arise among team members as a result of individual differences (e.g., values, opinions, and skills). Team members must learn to collaborate and compromise while leveraging the individual strengths among members of the team. It is important that management establishes a clear structure, builds trust, and fosters relationships between team members in order to resolve conflict and maintain a positive working environment.

3. **Norming:** Conflict among team members begins to resolve and members begin to appreciate each other's individual strengths and weaknesses. Team members begin forming relationships and becoming dedicated to group goals. Less dependence is needed from leadership, and the manager is now able to facilitate group tasks.

4. **Performing:** The team begins to achieve goals through hard work, avoiding conflict, and focusing on organizational tasks. The manager can delegate work and shift focus to other work areas.

5. **Adjourning:** This final phase refers to dissolving the team as some work projects are only meant to last for a specified period of time. Management can use this time to praise employees and teams on their performance and achievements (Tuckman, 1965).

In addition to establishing cooperative teams, effective leadership, and clear communication, managers must also leverage power to influence employees to attain organizational goals. Leaders use power as a means of influencing others. According to social psychologists French and Raven, managers drive power from these five sources (1959):

- **Reward:** the manager's ability to influence employees into complying by rewarding employees for compliance (e.g., promotions, salary increases, and bonuses). Reward power's prolonged use, however, may cause employees to become dependent on the rewards system and only be motivated to work hard when there is a reward offered. Employees may also feel manipulated and dissatisfied.

- **Coercive:** the ability of the manager to influence employees to comply through punishment (e.g., dismissals, suspensions, and demotions). Coercive power may lead to short-term compliance but also results in fear, frustration, revenge, and dissatisfaction, which can negatively impact job satisfaction and productivity.

- **Referent:** based on interpersonal relationships. This form of power stems from loyalty and an unquestioning trust in leadership. The manager does not have to conduct much micromanagement or surveillance of staff as a result of this unwavering trust and compliance.

- **Expert:** the ability of the manager to hold information employees need. This form of power requires employees to consider the manager as an expert as well as to exhibit a strong degree of trust and conformity. Similar to referent power, expert power does not require the manager to conduct much surveillance either.

- **Legitimate:** based on position and mutual agreement and is considered a delegated right to influence. This form of power may lead to resistance and dissatisfaction among employees if it is not incorporated with expert power. Legitimate power may lead to minimal compliance and employee resistance.

A new concept of power, known as **empowerment**, has begun to replace top-down notions of power and authority and has become a strategy for improving work relations. Empowerment includes members across all levels of the organization in decision-making and problem-solving. Leaders can maximize their power by enabling employees to independently achieve success. Understanding how power operates within organizations enables healthcare managers to leverage that knowledge to become more effective leaders. Managers can use power to influence employees and accomplish organizational goals by understanding which power strategies to employ and when. Strong leadership that provides stimulating work tasks that enable individuals to apply their competence, as well as grants a sense of independence, is essential to work satisfaction. **Examining the group setting** provides insight into the challenges that exist in key aspects of the organization, including leadership, teamwork, communication, decision-making, conflict, and power.

9.5 EXAMINING ORGANIZATIONAL BEHAVIOR AT ORGANIZATIONAL LEVEL

Organizational theory refers to the patterns and structures of an organization that maximize productivity and provides an understanding of how organizations function best and adapt to economic, social, and political changes. The individual actions and behaviors of the organization's members influence the effectiveness of the organization as a whole. Organizational effectiveness is an organization's ability to attain set goals and suitably function as a system while satisfying its stakeholders (Georgepoulus and Tannebaum, 1957).

According to the National Research Council, the U.S. is among the lowest in terms of life expectancy out of 10 countries with similarly high income (Papanicolas, 2018). Despite patients in the U.S. spending more on healthcare, it has an uneven return as performance and outcomes are not better as a result of the increased costs. Studies show U.S. patients are more likely to receive unnecessary, expensive tests and treatments. In contrast to other developed countries, such as Australia and Switzerland, the U.S. fares particularly low on health indicators, such as healthcare affordability, access, health outcomes, and equality between populations with high and low socioeconomic standing. (Papanicolas, 2018). Variation in life expectancy across the U.S. is also dramatic, while access to healthcare services, education, early childhood development, and work conditions vary greatly (Braveman, Gottlieb, 2014). However, the U.S. healthcare industry is undergoing essential transformation driven by value-based and patient-centered care provision and the need to control costs. Healthcare systems must adapt to ongoing technology advancements, shifting consumer demands, and reimbursement changes in order to keep up with such transformational programs.

Current societal trends, such as globalization, racial and ethnic diversity, the millennial generation, and the growing elderly population in the U.S. influence the expectations and demands of consumers. The healthcare system must keep up with these societal trends and meet the demands of current healthcare consumers by providing accommodating, personalized care, such as extended appointment hours, convenient healthcare locations, and expansive healthcare options, like telehealth services, for example (Vogenberg, Santilli, 2018). Consumers are taking advantage of personalized healthcare options that provide the level of care they desire at the time and location that is convenient. The shift to patient engagement incorporates a holistic model that personalizes healthcare and helps patients to become more accountable for their health by focusing on disease prevention and altering behaviors. Understanding the current atmosphere of the healthcare environment can help administrators develop specific goals and strategies to efficiently improve the healthcare system and adapt to health market changes, including (1) healthcare cost transparency and quality, (2) advancements in technology, (3) changes in payment models, and (4) healthcare mergers and acquisitions (Health Catalyst, 2018; Vogenberg, Santilli, 2018, Society for Health Care Strategy and Markey Development, 2020).

9.6 COST TRANSPARENCY AND HEALTHCARE QUALITY

Providing quality, yet affordable and cost comparative, healthcare is essential to healthcare organizations. Prior to January 2019, only 1 state in the U.S. required hospitals to post their prices online. Following January 1, 2019, The Center for Medicaid and Medicare Services (CMS) now requires all hospitals to post their prices online for patients to view. Preventable medical errors are also a major concern; these range from wrong procedures to excessive prescriptions to fatal surgery accidents. Studies show that when medical staff feels safe and empowered, there are fewer surgical catastrophes (Health Catalyst, 2018).

9.7 ADVANCEMENTS IN TECHNOLOGY

Continual advancements in technology impact healthcare delivery and quality. Technologies, such as telehealth, telemedicine, and mobile sensory devices that have the ability to track and monitor a patient's vitals—such as blood pressure, temperature, and movement—to produce improved treatment plans and other useful information, are transforming the way healthcare is delivered. However, a key issue with such technological advancements is ensuring patient security and privacy. In order for the effects of technological advances to be successful and long-lasting, the privacy barriers and the alignment of state and federal regulations regarding the physician-patient relationship will have to be addressed. In addition, advancing technology must demonstrate a long-term return on investment in terms of quality and cost (Vogenberg & Santilli, 2018).

9.8 CHANGES IN PAYMENT MODELS

The U.S. healthcare system is beginning to shift to a system of value-based care that incentivizes physicians to coordinate care and provide the most suitable care tailored to the actual needs of individual patients while also focusing on disease prevention. Healthcare providers and government agencies are also extending focus to preventing and alleviating the social determinants of health. The shift to a value-based system following the traditional fee-based healthcare system has changed the healthcare payment structure. CMS has five goals for value-based healthcare, including accountability, competition, quality, integrity, and beneficiary engagement. However, the economic incentives and actual impact of emerging models of value-based care are difficult to calculate (Health Catalyst, 2018).

9.9 HEALTHCARE MERGERS AND ACQUISITIONS

Companies are seeming to enter the healthcare market from far-flung industries, including Google, Apple, and even Uber. Google is hiring physicians, Apple is investing in their wellness monitoring app, and Uber is launching an app, UberHealth, to increase patient access. Mergers and acquisitions have become the norm to establishing partnerships. For example, CVS is combining stores, clinics, and enrollees with AETNA. Healthcare organizations must explore all potential avenues in order to reduce operating costs and compete in a value-based reimbursement environment. Organizations must also leverage costs through creative partnerships, including mergers, acquisitions, clinical integration efforts, operating efficiencies, and new models of collaboration. The need for cost-saving solutions that provide a strong return on investment is critical to the current health industry (Health Catalyst, 2018).

Health administrators should have a clear understanding of their goals and develop a strategic plan based on their current knowledge and the current state of the healthcare environment. Health systems must be flexible enough to adapt to changes in the industry, including shifting patient demographics, advances in technology, reimbursement changes, mergers, and acquisitions structures.

9.10 KEY ADVANTAGES OF ORGANIZATIONAL THEORY FOR HEALTHCARE LEADERS (APPLICATION)

Effective managers increase shared understanding and meaning, skillful collective communication, and problem solving among staff. Organizational theory examines three lenses of the healthcare industry, including the individual attitudes and actions that influence workplace behaviors, teams within the organization, and the effects of internal and external changes that influence the organization as a whole. In order to properly navigate internal and external changes, organizations must be effective. Organizational effectiveness refers to an organization's ability to attain goals and adequately function well as a system while meeting the needs of its stakeholders.

High-performing organizations are denoted as organizations with five distinguishable attributes:

- **compelling vision** that creates an intentionally focused culture that drives the health care organization's results

- **ongoing learning system** that constantly builds knowledge and diffuses learning throughout the organization

- **persistent focus** on patient-centered care and an insightful ability to measure the healthcare organization's results

- **well-defined innovative systems, structures, and processes** that are clearly aligned to support the healthcare organization's vision, strategic direction, and goals

  ◇ **Shared power and distributed decision making** throughout the organization that catalyzes high involvement (Blanchard & Ken Blanchard Companies, 2010).

Understanding organizational behavior and theory can increase organizational performance and effectiveness. Organizational behavior involves the attitudes and actions of individuals and groups within the organization, while organizational behavior focuses on acquiring, developing, and applying the knowledge and skills of people. Successfully navigating change requires a health care administrator who can properly integrate change, possesses strong interpersonal and communication skills, demonstrates competent leadership to leverage diversity, and the ability to direct individuals and teams toward achieving organizational goals. Healthcare administrators must develop a strategic approach to understanding how individuals and organizational factors influence the single person behaviors and values of employees as well as collective behaviors across the organization, which influence the productivity, satisfaction, and the success of the organization overall. Organizational behavior and theory can be applied across the five essential functions of management, including planning, organizing, staffing, leading, and controlling.

9.11 CONCLUSION

Given the current dynamics and everchanging state of the U.S. healthcare system, healthcare managers and leaders must apply organizational behavior and theory in order to enhance management practices, effectively navigate change, and leverage diversity within the current healthcare environment. Organizational behavior and theory consists of examining behaviors across three levels, including individual, group, and collective behaviors across the healthcare organization. Healthcare managers need to understand the relationship between organizational behavior and organizational theory in order to adapt to the ever-shifting demands of the healthcare industry.

9.12 KEY POINTS

- Organizational behavior views organizations from multiple levels internally and externally, including individual perspectives, group dynamics, and the organizational setting.

- Examining the individual setting provides insight into the thoughts, perspectives, values, and attitudes of individuals within the organization that influence workplace behaviors.

- Examining the group setting provides insight into challenges related to teamwork, communication, decision-making, power, and conflict.

- Examining the organization as a whole provides insight into how organizations interact and adapt to internal and external changes.

9.13 KEY TERMS

Organizational behavior, Organizational theory, Attribution Theory, Attributes, Expectancy, Bias, Cognitive bias, Sensemaking, Team cohesiveness, Emotional intelligence, Self-awareness, Self-management, Social awareness, Relationship management, Tuckman Theory of Group Development: forming, storming, norming, performing, adjourning, Legitimate power, Reward power, Coercive power, Expert power, Referent power, Organizational effectiveness

9.14 QUESTIONS FOR REVIEW AND DISCUSSION

1. Describe the three lenses of organizational behavior and theory. Why is an understanding of organization behavior and theory important, particularly to healthcare managers and leaders?

2. Describe the trends and recent changes in the U.S. healthcare system. How can an understanding of organizational behavior and theory help healthcare managers navigate those shifts?

3. Explain how perceptions and cognitive bias influence employee

behaviors. How do perceptions and cognitive bias influence a manager's behaviors and decision-making processes?

4. Describe specific ways a manager can create shared understanding and foster collective action among members of the healthcare organization. In what ways can you as a healthcare leader ensure clear communication in an organization?

5. Describe a dilemma where you have encountered and addressed underlying assumptions/misconceptions. Describe the situation. How did you address the misperceptions?

9.15 REFERENCES

"A Framework for High-Reliability Organizations in Healthcare." (2018). https://www.healthcatalyst.com/insights/high-reliability-organizations-in-healthcare-framework

Braveman, P., & Gottlieb, L. (2014). "The social determinants of health: it's time to consider the causes of the causes." Public health reports (Washington, D.C. : 1974), 129 Suppl 2(Suppl 2), 19–31. https://doi.org/10.1177/00333549141291S206

Brown, B., Crapo, J. (2017). "The Key to Transitioning from Fee-for-Service to Value-Based Reimbursement." https://www.healthcatalyst.com/wp-content/uploads/2014/08/The-Key-to-Transitioning-from-Fee-for-Service.pdf

Buschbinder, S. & Shanks, N. (2012). *Introduction to Healthcare Management*. Jones and Bartlett Learning.

Georgepoulus, B.S., Tannebaum, A.S. (1957). "A Study of Organizational Effectiveness." American Sociological Review. 22(5): 534-540. DOI: 10.2307/2089477

Kozlowski, S. W. J. & Bell, B. S. (2003). "Work groups and teams in organizations." In W. C. Borman, D. R. Ilgen & R. J. Klimoski (Eds.), Handbook of psychology (Vol. 12): Industrial and Organizational Psychology (333-375). New York: Wiley-Blackwell.

McClelland, D. C. (1961). *The Achieving Society*. Collier-Macmillan. New York and London.

Organizational Behaviour. "Chapter 7: Managing Stress and Emotions." Creative Commons. https://pressbooks.bccampus.ca/obcourseweir/

Papanicolas I, Woskie LR, Jha AK. "Health Care Spending in the United States and Other High-Income Countries." *JAMA*. 2018;319(10):1024–1039. doi:10.1001/jama.2018.1150)

Pinder, C. 2008. *Work Motivation in Organizational Behavior*. Psychology Press. Taylor and Frances. New York, NY.

Raven, B., French, J. (1959). "The Bases of Social Power." University of Michigan, Institute for Social Research.

Shoebridge, A. "Cohesion, Collaboration, and Communication in Healthcare." Association for Talent Development. https://www.td.org/magazines/td-magazine/cohesion-collaboration-and-communication-in-healthcare

Society for Health Care Strategy and Market Development SHSMD. "Evolving Healthcare Landscape." 2020. https://www.shsmd.org/resources/bridging-worlds2.0/evolving-healthcare-landscape

Tuckman, B. W. (1965). "Developmental sequence in small groups." *Psychological Bulletin, 63*(6), 384–399. https://doi.org/10.1037/h0022100

Vogenberg, F. R., & Santilli, J. (2018). Healthcare Trends for 2018. American health & drug benefits, 11(1), 48–54. https://www.ncbi.nlm.nih.gov/pmc/articles/PMC5902765/

Weick, K.E., Sutcliff, K.M., & Obstfeld, D. (2005). "Organizing and the Process of Sensemaking." Organization Science 16(4): 409-421. DOI: 10.1287/orsc.1050.0133

Xu, J. (2017). "Leadership theory in clinical practice." Clinical Nursing Research

10 ANALYSIS OF ORGANIZATIONAL MODELS

10.1 LEARNING OBJECTIVES

- To illustrate the meaning of organizational behavior and effectiveness
- To review the various aspects of the competing values approach to organizational behavior
- To discuss the purpose of situational analysis as it relates to organizational behavior
- To explain the role of organizational analysis on organizational behavior

10.2 INTRODUCTION

Understanding how individuals behave in a healthcare setting and how organizations perform is an important role of the manager. This knowledge lends itself to the discreet awareness of how to channel this behavior into positive service oriented and financial organizational performance. Managers bear the responsibility of ensuring the organization's mission and vision are attained. This process encompasses the institution of a strategic plan with goals and objectives geared towards achieving the plan. Once the plan is implemented, a method of evaluation must be set in place to determine if the plan is working according to its intent. There are many analysis models that can be used to assist the manager in ensuring the strategic goals and objectives are accomplished. Managers can glean a lot from acknowledging how organizations should behave to ensure their effectiveness. Organizations face many challenges related to market forces in the healthcare industry and government regulations, amid attempting to provide increased access to care, improving the quality of care delivered, and reducing the costs of delivering healthcare. Managers must be able to apprise and guide actions amidst these challenges through the initial step of understanding the meaning of organizational behavior, effectiveness, and the approaches or models/theories affecting behavior and effectiveness. Organizational behavior examines how individuals, groups, and structures within the organization function in relation to organizational effectiveness. Each of these elements influences the actions of the other. Individuals bring with them separate sets of ideals, perspectives, actions, and characteristics that should add relevance to the organization and determine how they respond to the various day-to-day activities and expectations of the organization. Managers can use this information to enhance the performance of the organization by promoting employee engagement and behavioral changes (Walston, 2017). Organizational effectiveness explores the productivity of an organization. In other words, how well does the organization meet its objectives, considering required resources such as time, money, effort, people and materials? For most healthcare organizations, effectiveness or success, again, is measured in terms of healthcare quality, patient satisfaction, and profits. This chapter emphasizes several models or frameworks that indicate how managers should think about and engage in efforts to enhance organizational performance and behavior. The following list offers a brief comparison of the competing values framework, open systems model, rational goal model, human relations model, internal process model, situational analysis, and organizational analysis.

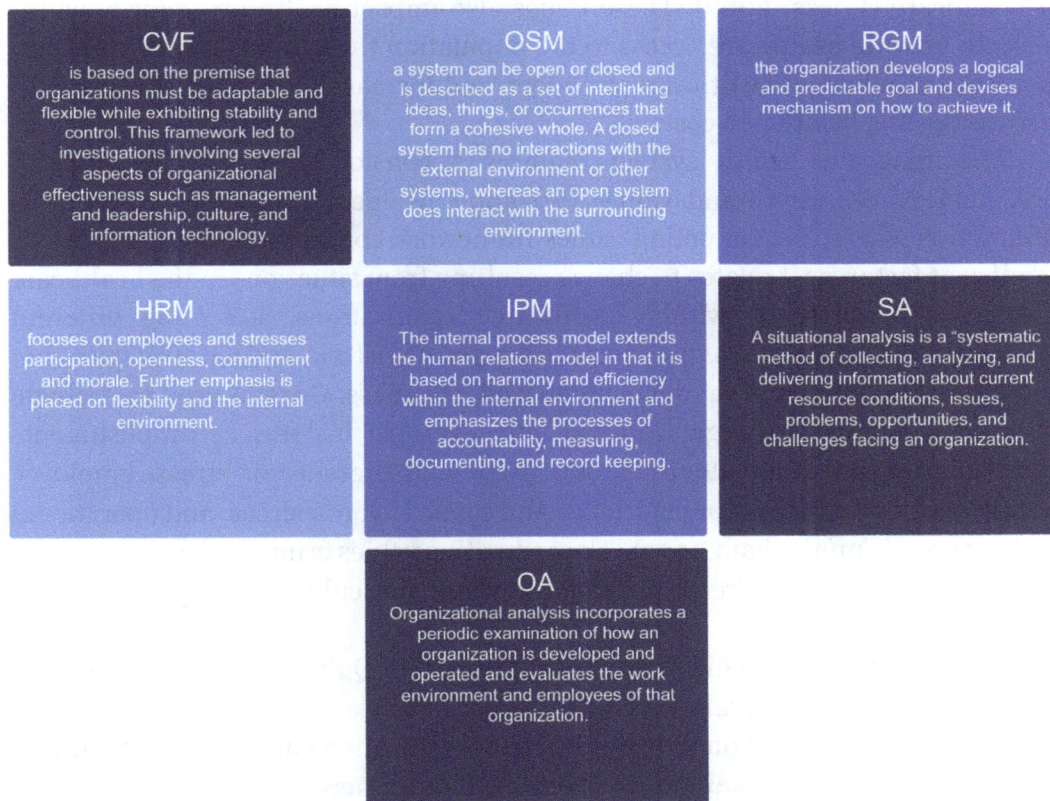

CVF
is based on the premise that organizations must be adaptable and flexible while exhibiting stability and control. This framework led to investigations involving several aspects of organizational effectiveness such as management and leadership, culture, and information technology.

OSM
a system can be open or closed and is described as a set of interlinking ideas, things, or occurrences that form a cohesive whole. A closed system has no interactions with the external environment or other systems, whereas an open system does interact with the surrounding environment.

RGM
the organization develops a logical and predictable goal and devises mechanism on how to achieve it.

HRM
focuses on employees and stresses participation, openness, commitment and morale. Further emphasis is placed on flexibility and the internal environment.

IPM
The internal process model extends the human relations model in that it is based on harmony and efficiency within the internal environment and emphasizes the processes of accountability, measuring, documenting, and record keeping.

SA
A situational analysis is a "systematic method of collecting, analyzing, and delivering information about current resource conditions, issues, problems, opportunities, and challenges facing an organization.

OA
Organizational analysis incorporates a periodic examination of how an organization is developed and operated and evaluates the work environment and employees of that organization.

Figure 10.1: Comparison of Organizational Models

Source: Original Work
Attribution: Dorothy Howell
License: CC BY-SA 4.0

10.3 COMPETING VALUES FRAMEWORK

Healthcare leaders, including the chief executive officer, chief financial officer, chief medical officer, chief nursing officer, human resources director, operations director, information management director, etc., are responsible for setting the tone or culture for the organization. They determine the kinds and types of employees and behaviors needed to achieve the organization's long-term goals. As discussed in chapter 7, organizational culture is a significant factor influencing the behavior of the organization and individuals within it. The attitudes, values, beliefs, assumptions, and behaviors of the employees affect organizational performance and effectiveness. The culture of the organization indicates how the groups within the organization think and react to various situations that arise within the organization's environment (Hartnell, Ou, & Kinicki, 2011). These situations occur in all organizations, including healthcare. Situations specific to healthcare organizations are related to technical or functional aspects of care, such as with medical errors, adverse effects or how care is delivered—all of which influence patient satisfaction. Critical factors in healthcare that affect patient satisfaction are nursing shortages, lack of communication, lack of technology, and the high cost of healthcare (Wicks, 2007). These issues also impact healthcare reform, which seeks to provide healthcare access to the population through insurance coverage, increased numbers of healthcare providers, and increase the quality of care while also decreasing healthcare costs.

Reforming the health system requires a consideration for the differing stakeholders' objectives and values (Shannon, Holden, Van Dam, 2012). This situation is where the competing values framework comes into play. Culture is a significant factor, as it relates to change resulting from situations in the healthcare system as a whole or within healthcare organizations. Resolving different organizational situations requires various types of criteria and/or strategies that will ultimately improve the organization's effectiveness. Criteria used to evaluate situations relative to organizational effectiveness include accomplishments and achievements; competence, productivity, and pressure or stress; employee competence and gratification; efficiency and capability; resources; and operational performance (Cunningham, 1977). The competing values framework is particularly appropriate for healthcare organizations where the culture is based on group values.

Two University of Michigan professors, Robert E. Quinn and Kim S. Cameron, developed the competing values framework based on measures that yielded effective organizations. It is based on the premise that organizations must be adaptable and flexible while exhibiting stability and control. This framework led to investigations involving several aspects of organizational effectiveness, such as management and leadership, culture, and information technology. From these studies, researchers were able to divide criteria for organizational effectiveness into three dimensions that were further broken down into four quadrants. The first dimension focused on internal and external environments of the organization. The internal environment centered on the employees within the organization, specifically in respect to cultivating and nurturing them and ensuring their satisfaction with the organization. These employees, who believe that the organization is committed to them, will be open to communicating and becoming actively involved in attaining organizational growth and effectiveness. The external environment focused on the organization itself. The next dimension examined the structure (stability and flexibility) of the organization. The final dimension entertained the process of how to get from "point A" (means) to "point B" (ends). It encompasses determining what strategies are required, planning and setting goals on attaining the strategies, and ensuring that outcomes are met (Quinn & Rohrbaugh, 1983).

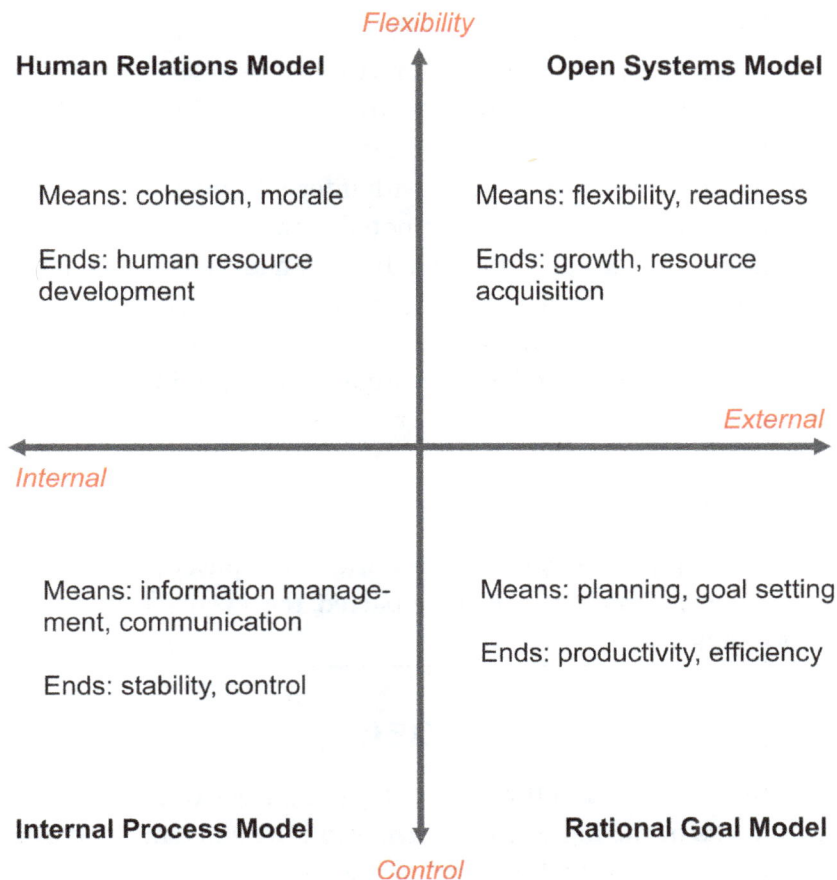

Figure 10.2: Competing Values Framework

Source: Original Work
Attribution: Corey Parson
License: CC BY-SA 4.0

Organizational leaders are responsible for determining which dimension best represents how to position their organization for growth and success and thereby improve the organization's effectiveness. In other words, the CVF assists the organization in clarifying specific growth strategies and attributes that are critical in ensuring that the organization is performing effectively. In addition, it determines the alignment between the growth strategy and what the organization can achieve in relation to accomplishing its mission and vision. The competing values approach is also useful in assessing the culture within an organization—which is necessary to effectively execute the growth strategy (Thackor, 2010). Additionally, the CVF can be used at various levels of analysis and, as such, can promote the culture required to develop successful quality improvement initiatives. This is due to the ability the CVF has to place its focus on people rather than processes and profits (Wick, 2007).

An example of how the CVF can be used in the healthcare setting was introduced by Helfrich, Li, Mohr, Meterko, and Sales (2007) who performed a study examining the underlying structure of data from a CVF instrument. Helfrich, et. al, examined cross-sectional survey data from the work environment of 168 Veterans Health Administration (VHA) facilities. Participants were non-supervisory staff members. The survey included 14 items adapted from a CVF instrument, measuring organizational culture based on four subscales: hierarchical, entrepreneurial, team, and rational. Positive results were noted with internal consistency of the subscales (α = 0.68 to 0.85). However, issues were noted with divergent properties wherein the entrepreneurial, team, and rational subscales had higher correlations across subscales than within, indicating potential problems applying conventional CVF subscales to non-supervisors. The results of the study also emphasize managerial challenges associated with the reliable examination of organizational culture in the healthcare environment.

Stop and Apply

In reviewing the competing values framework above, pick out specific elements from the framework that may have impacted the events leading up to Mr. Rodriquez's demise.

10.4 OPEN SYSTEMS MODEL

As a manager engrossed in the day-to-day operations of the organization, you must not lose focus of the big picture or ensuring the efficiency and effectiveness of the organization. Viewing the functioning of the organization as a system with inputs, throughputs, and outputs can assist the manager in achieving the organization's mission and vision. Achieving the mission and vision through effectiveness and efficiency leads to organizational success. As per the discussion on systems theory outlined in chapter 6, a system can be open or closed and is described as a set of interlinking ideas, things, or occurrences that form a cohesive whole. A closed system has no interactions with the external environment or other systems, whereas an open system interacts with the surrounding environment (Neves, 2017). Organizations that operate as closed systems typically fail. The success of the organization further depends on the ability of the organization to interact with the internal and external environment wherein it functions, which is the description of an open system (Starnes, 2000). Occurrences within the external environment that affect the organization include competitors, legal, political, sociocultural, economic, and technological factors such as state and federal laws, issues affecting population health, wellness, and safety, and the presence or absence of public or private insurance coverage. The internal environment includes employees and healthcare consumers (Starnes, 2000).

As we have previously stated, a system comprises a set of interrelated subsystems—such as tasks, control, technology, and structure—which are affected by the environment. Tasks represent the activities required for the organization to meet its mission and vision. Structure refers to how the organization is organized to support delivering products and services, such as with the various departments within the organization. Control represents how performance is measured within the organization. Technology allows the organization to operate efficiently and effectively. A breakdown in any of the individual elements affects the whole system. One way of reviewing the function of an organization is through an analysis of each of the subsystems, which provides the manager with basic knowledge on how the organization functions.

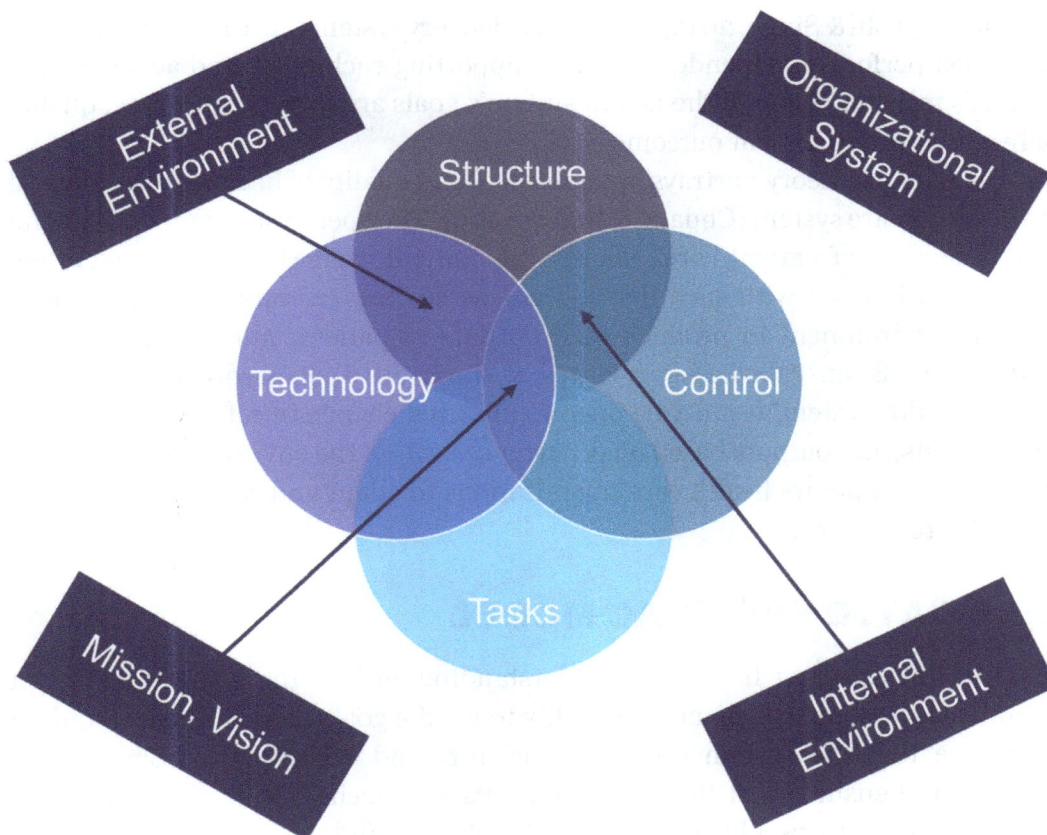

Figure 10.3: System

Source: Suchan & Dulek, 1998
Attribution: Dorothy Howell, Adapted from Suchan & Dulek, 1998
License: Fair Use

Additionally, reviewing the organization as a system yields a greater understanding of the organization's role, purpose, and function. From this view, the manager can comprehend how each subsystem interacts with each other in relation to the organization's mission and vision and to what degree the subsystems align with each other and the external environment. Organizations that operate as a system can scan the external environment to ascertain the needs of their stakeholders and use this information to adapt their operations to meet these needs. Furthermore, the scan can yield significant information on their competitors to enhance their footprint within the market and gain advantage over their competitors (Suchan & Dulek, 1998).

This description of a system indicates how healthcare delivery in the U.S. is considered a system with various subsystems. A health system consists of two or more health care organizations—such as a hospital and one or more physician groups associated with each other through shared ownership or a contracting relationship for payment and service delivery—which includes both primary and specialty care. The health system also includes community-based physicians who provide comprehensive care and are employed by a hospital (AHRQ, 2016). The health system can be highly integrated, such as with integrated delivery systems that provide coordinated health services to increase efficiency and decrease redundancy (Shi & Singh, 2015). Integrated delivery systems have many subsystems that must perform independently while supporting each other and achieving the system's mission. Some of the health system's goals are to improve safety, quality of healthcare, and patient outcomes.

The systems theory portrays patient safety and quality of healthcare as integral to the healthcare system (Chuang & Inder, 2009). The open systems model is useful in the delivery of patient care, wherein the patient, nurses, and the system are inputs that interact with such throughputs as healthcare, nursing interventions, and the environment to produce such outputs as patient, nursing, and system outcomes (O'Brien-Pallas, Meyer, Hayes, & Wang, 2010). Regardless of the size or type of health system, it must be open to allowing change in reference to inputs, throughputs, and outputs based on occurrences within the environment. The open systems model allows health care organizations to adapt and continue to provide patient care services.

10.5 RATIONAL GOAL MODEL

Once the manager has a clear understanding on how the organization must operate as a system, the manager's ability to set the goals and objectives required to ensure that the system operates efficiently and effectively becomes much simpler, and ensures that the desired outputs are reached. With this model, the organization develops a logical and predictable goal and devises a mechanism on how to achieve it. Once the goal is set, the organizational leader develops a set of objectives and activities to meet the goal. Additionally, the manager must establish and implement an evaluation tool to determine if the objectives achieved the goal within a given timeframe.

One of leadership's roles is to make decisions for the organization. Strategy is significant to healthcare because of the focus placed on value based and patient centered care. Sources, such as technology, politics, and demographics—all of which influence the access, cost, and quality of healthcare—drive change within the healthcare system. Managers must be able to address these changes. Strategic management focuses on the managers' ability to grow the organization, determine how the organization competes and cooperates with other organizations, decide how the various components of the organization relate to each other, establish which services and programs will be offered and the resources required to deliver them, and establish the culture of the organization. An organization's goals are identified by establishing the general goal, discovering means or objectives for its accomplishment, and defining a set of activities for each objective. Strategy establishes the direction the organization should take to achieve its mission and vision. Once this approach has been determined, a set of goals and a plan of action must be formulated to achieve the mission and vision.

Because the rational goal model focuses on the organization's ability to achieve its goals, it is very useful in the strategic management process. Once the plan has been implemented, the organization is evaluated by comparing the activities accomplished based on the goals and objectives outlined within the strategic plan (Walston, 2018). The rational goal model places a great deal of emphasis on control and external focus and stresses planning and goal setting as the means and productivity and efficiency as the ends (Quinn & Rohrbaugh, 1983). Productivity, accomplishment, direction and goal clarity are significant factors in organizations using the rational model. The main purpose is to increase productivity and efficiency and maximize profits. Leaders using this model assume that employees, through clear directives and simplified tasks, will be motivated to perform based on perceived financial rewards, which leads to increased productivity and profits for the organization (Yang & Shao, 1996).

10.6 HUMAN RELATIONS MODEL

The rational model describes the significance of setting and achieving goals, which cannot be completed without the use of human resources or the employees of the organization. The human relations model focuses on employees and stresses participation, openness, commitment and morale. It places further emphasis on flexibility and the internal environment. Cohesion and morale are a means to attain employee development as the end result (Quinn & Rohrbaugh, 1983). Satisfied employees working in a welcoming environment perform better. This model is concerned with developing employees through training and self-development plans and allowing them the ability to participate in the decision-making process for the organization. This theory centers on employee motivation and presumes that the employee is self-motivated to do their job. Employees want to be trained, acknowledged, supported, and empowered to complete the tasks associated with attaining the mission and vision of the organization. They desire to be treated as team-players and provided with the big picture for the organization. Therefore, the manager in this model serves as a mentor and facilitates positive work behavior. They can develop and maintain a cohesive team that engages in minimal conflict (Yang & Shao, 1996).

10.7 INTERNAL PROCESS MODEL

The human relations model focuses on people and ensuring the manager provides what is needed to assist employees in meeting the goals and objectives of the organization. The internal process model extends the human relations model in that it is based on harmony and efficiency within the internal environment and emphasizes the processes of accountability, measuring, documenting, and record keeping. Decision making is grounded in the existing rules, structures, and traditions of the organization. Information management and communications are the means to reaching stability and control. Day-to-day operations must be completed in an orderly fashion with well-informed employees, which allows them to feel a sense of continuity and security (Quinn & Rohrbaugh, 1983). The model reviews how the organization's throughput processes are transformed into the preferred outputs, which are based on the open systems view of the organization (Eydi, 2015). The manager's role is to control the internal environment, maintain structure by monitoring individual and organizational performance, and coordinate the organization's functions (Yang & Shao, 1996). In addition, the manager ensures resources are centrally located within the organization and that everyone understands the organization's policies and procedures. From this clarification, employees can see that coordinated efforts of the organization and internal practices are predictable. For example, if the manager has put a policy in place that clearly indicates the ramifications of sleeping while at work and ensured that all employees understand the policy, then any employee who is noted to be asleep will know what happens when the policy is violated.

10.8 SITUATIONAL ANALYSIS

Situational analysis takes this premise of scanning the internal and external environments a little further. A situational analysis is a "systematic method of collecting, analyzing, and delivering information about current resource conditions, issues, problems, opportunities, and challenges facing an organization" (USDA, 2005). Conducting a situational analysis involves defining the situation, bringing together a brainstorming team to gain an understanding of the situation, including its impact to the organization; developing a plan or generating strategies as a solution to the situation; determining physical, human, financial, and structural resources needed; communicating the plan to appropriate stakeholders; and implementing the plan and evaluating its effectiveness (USDA, 2005; Brnjas & Tripunoski, 2016). Situational analysis comprises a continuous scanning of the internal and external environments to determine factors, such as effectiveness of internal processes and potential negative market activities, that affect the organization's operations (Brnjas & Tripunoski, 2016).

Scanning the environment can be accomplished in several ways, including political, economic, social, technological (PEST) analysis; force field analysis; scenario analysis; or strengths, weaknesses, opportunities, and threats (SWOT) analysis. The PEST analysis looks at the following driving forces: laws, regulations, government policies, purchasing power, wealth distribution, workforce availability, financial growth, inflation, population demographics, attitudes, lifestyles, research and development, potential for innovation, incorporating advanced technology, and consumer use of technology. Force field analysis extends the PEST analysis by determining whether environment influences support or derails the organization's strategic plan. The scenario analysis proposes alternative pictures, stories, or situations that describe the effect that environmental changes can have on an organization. It allows organizational leaders to plan for the organization's future (Walston, 2018).

Scanning allows the organization to determine its current standing based on achieving their mission and vision and its strengths and weaknesses relative to its opportunities and threats (SWOT) (Vrontis & Thrassou, 2006). With this knowledge, the leader can support the mission and vision and develop strategies to aid in decision making and enhance their organization's competition in the healthcare market. The environment provides resources that allow the organization to operate and produce products and services used by consumers. Performing an external analysis assists the organization in determining threats that will be detrimental to organizational performance and opportunities that will improve that performance.

Table 10.1

SWOT ANALYSIS		
STRENGTHS (Internal)	Knowing your strengths is crucial to the success of your mission and vision.	**WEAKNESSES (Internal)**
Things you do well		Things you don't have
Attributes that set you apart from others (i.e. price, position, people, products, alliances, joint ventures, loyal customers, etc.)		Things your competitors do better than you
		Organization Culture does not align with strategic direction.
		High costs relative to competitors
Internal resources such as skilled staff	Weaknesses will need to be addressed as you move forward.	Limited resources (staffing, capital, cash flow, etc.)
Tangible assets such as property, capital, technology		Unclear selling position
OPPORTUNITIES (External)	Opportunities can be used to address weaknesses and turn them into strengths	**THREATS (External)**
New markets, How you can expand		New competitors
Minimal number of competitors	Threats need to be acknowledged to allow you to decide which ones need to be addressed. Keep in mind that you may not be able to control or eliminate them.	Governmental or other regulations
Developing need for your products or services; need for package change; industry trends		Dissatisfied customers
		Insurmountable weaknesses
		Location
Media coverage		Negative media coverage

Left margin: P O S I T I V E

Right margin: N E G A T I V E

> **Stop and Apply**
>
> Choose a local healthcare organization similar to the hospice organization where Mr. Rodriquez resided or the hospital that he was transferred to as a result of the code. Assume you are the manager of the organization; conduct a SWOT analysis on the organization based on the table above.

Several processes are needed to examine the environment. Environmental scanning is the first process that provides an avenue for the organization to discover positive and negative trends inside and outside the organization. Environmental monitoring (which is the second part of the process) provides knowledge regarding the extent of the damage or changes affecting the organization. Awareness of the competition (third part of the process) provides knowledge about the strengths and weakness of the organization's competitors. The fourth part of the process is environmental forecasting that allows leaders to predict the types of strategies required to adjust organizational operations to reach the desired outputs (Brnjas & Tripunoski, 2016). The final part of the examination process is assessment, wherein the organizational leader determines the significance of the issues and identifies influences that are required to formulate the mission, vision, and situational analysis (Ginter, Duncan, Swayne, 2015). With situational analysis, the leader is establishing motivational factors that enhance the decision-making process. It considers consequences if no decision is made and how this affects the employees of the organization (Walston, 2018).

A situational analysis is very useful to the healthcare organization in that it supports understanding the current functions and resources of the organization in addition to clarifying the facility's strengths, weaknesses, opportunities, and threats. Healthcare organizational leaders can use this information to determine which strategies are needed to propel the organization forward (USDA, 2005). In addition, this information is critical in determining the organization's ability to compete effectively in the healthcare market. Consider the following scenario. You own and manage Best Care Solutions, a company that offers in-home staffing solutions to families with elderly parents. You operate out of a rented space and remember that your lease is nearing the end of its term, so you need to renegotiate. There are many new businesses around you, a change which has increased the value of the building where you lease your business. You're worried you'll be priced out. You begin thinking about how you will remedy this problem and then come up with the following strategy. You decide to increase your online presence to alleviate some of the risk. Remaining competitive requires a proactive approach to innovative opportunities with which an organization is confronted within the healthcare market.

The following table shows the advantages and disadvantages of situational analysis (USDA, 2005):

Table 10.2: Advantages and Disadvantages of Situational Analysis	
Advantages	Disadvantages
Provides a way to study resources needed	Time consuming
Allows leaders to review needs of specific groups	Easy to introduce bias into findings
Provides a structure for data collection	Project may be influenced by changes in program priorities or public interest
Provides a method to examine both internal and external factors affecting the organization	A poorly designed communication plan can result in the ineffective delivery of messages to identified stakeholder groups
Gathers information from various stakeholders	
Develops a communication plan to deliver the findings to a large and diverse audience	

Source: Original Work
Attribution: Dorothy Howell
License: CC BY-SA 4.0

10.9 ORGANIZATIONAL ANALYSIS MODEL

There are many employee levels within an organization who are responsible for ensuring that the organization's mission and vision are accomplished. Value-based and patient centered care, again, is one of the focuses of health care organizations. The levels of healthcare employees responsible for ensuring patients receive quality care comprise dining room and custodial workers, workers in the imaging department, front line managers, and the CEO of the organization. The work accomplishments of all these employees must be coordinated to achieve the mission and vision of the organization. Organizational analysis provides an understanding of how the organization behaves. Organizational behavior is an exploration of the behavior, influence, and impact on performance that individuals, groups, and structures have on an organization. From studying this concept, the manager gains a sense of the organization's overall functioning, including activities, processes, and how behavior influences outcomes. The manager acquires an appreciation for why employees act as they do and can assist them in developing measures to alter their behavior for the betterment of the organization. An organizational model or theory describes activities, procedures, and issues that have a bearing on the structure and outcomes of the organization and how it relates to the external environment. Additionally, it allows the manager to view the organization as a whole (Walston, 2017).

Organizational analysis incorporates a periodic examination of how an organization is developed, operated, and evaluates the work environment and employees of that organization (Businessdictionary.com). This information is valuable to the healthcare manager in that it aids in identifying recent occurrences of problems or inefficiencies that will need to be addressed through developing strategies that impact the performance, survival, and success of the organization (Walston, 2017). The organizational analysis model in healthcare is related to how the structure and operations of the organization allow for efficiency and effectiveness as they benefit patient care. Delivering quality patient-centered care services requires a multidisciplinary team approach, wherein many elements are taken into consideration to accomplish the mission, vision, and values of the healthcare organization. Healthcare has limited room for error, indicating the need for a critical analysis of the behaviors and processes in the organization to improve quality, increase access, and control costs (Walston, 2017).

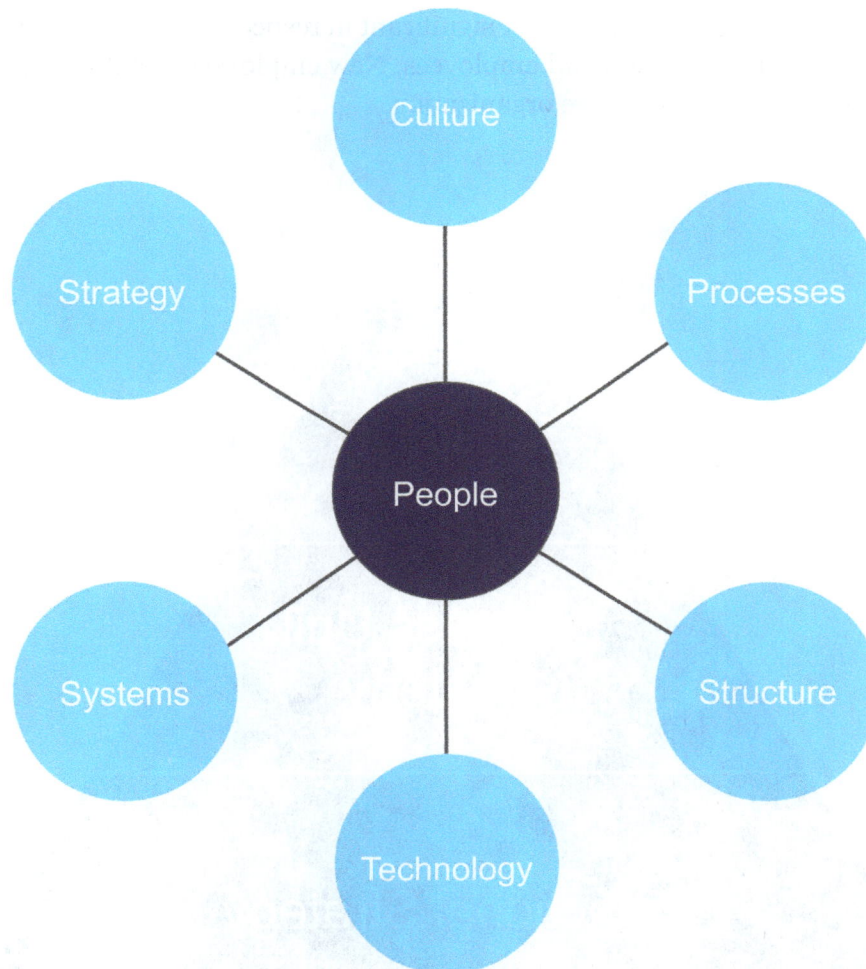

Figure 10.4: Seven Elements of the Organizational Analysis Model

Source: Nickols, 2012
Attribution: Dorothy Howell, Adapted from Nickols, 2012
License: Fair Use

Fred Nickols, Author and Managing Partner of Distance Consulting, wrote about the seven elements of the organizational analysis model. He maintains that six of the elements interact with the people element, which is the model's central focus. Without people, such as nurses, doctors, lab and x-ray technicians, and dining room and custodial staff, healthcare organizations cannot function or operate. They provide the culture, skills, expertise, values, and beliefs that make the organization successful. People also develop the structure for the organization so that the organization can pursue its mission and vision through the alignment of work performance, development of products, delivery of services, and the successful use of human and physical resources. Processes represent the flow of data and materials, and lead to accomplished work within the organization. In healthcare, the organization's employees, again, provide products and services that will improve the quality of care rendered to patients. Culture, again, refers to the attitudes, values, and beliefs of the employees who work for the organization. The culture of an organization is very significant in respect to how the organization is viewed by their customers and employees. New employees adapt to the culture that has been created within the organization.

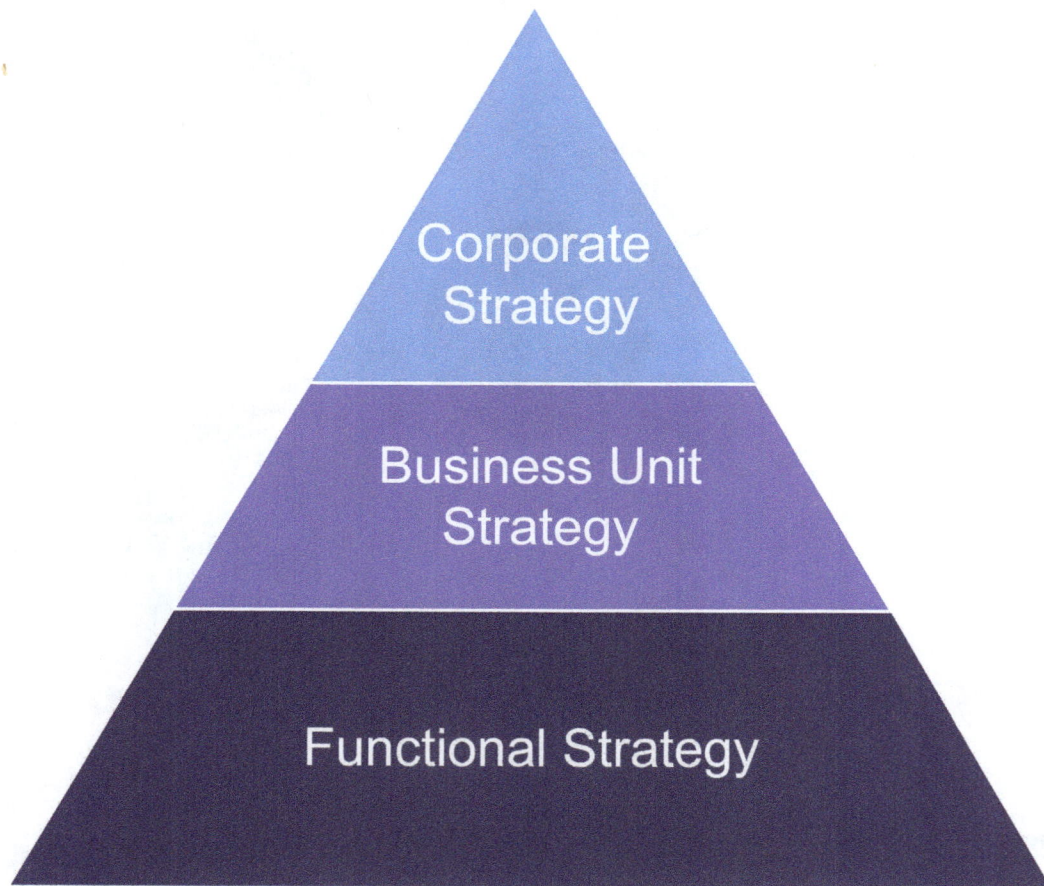

Figure 10.5: Levels of Organizational Strategy

Source: Walston, 2017
Attribution: Dorothy Howell, Adapted from Walston, 2017
License: Fair Use

Healthcare corporations require that strategies continue to meet the needs of consumers. Some of these corporations include CVS Health, which operates over

7700 pharmacies and 900 clinics, Ascension Health, which operates 131 hospitals, and HCA, which manages 184 hospitals and 2,000 care sites in 21 U.S. states and the United Kingdom. Healthcare organizations are obligated to develop and institute various strategy levels to ensure they are performing well as they compete with other organizations. Such strategies can exist at three different levels. Corporate level strategies indicate the scope and direction in which the organization is trying to go. This level of strategy often involves a board of directors, executive leaders, and stakeholders. As the top tier of the decision-making process, the corporate level oversees strategy for the entire organization, with a focus on defining the mission and big-picture goals, such as fund allocations and business deals. At this level, capital funds are raised, and the organization is deciding on the type of business they want to be in or get out of. Business level strategy focuses on only one business under the umbrella of the corporate level. Business-level strategy focuses on projects in development, and managers have the authority to develop strategies based on their directives' needs. Managers translate the directions and intent of those at the corporate level into actionable strategies for individual projects and employees. The functional level strategies provide support services at the division, department, or project level. They are ultimately driven by products and services (Walston, 2017). Functional-level strategy integrates research, marketing, production, and distribution to better connect products and services with the organization's consumers. Managers must ensure that the decisions made at each level do not negatively impact the other levels of the organization (Walston, 2017).

Table 10.3 Comparison of Strategy Levels		
Corporate Level Strategies	Business Level Strategies	Functional Level Strategies
Indicate the scope and direction that the organization is trying to go	Focus on projects in development, and managers have the authority to develop strategies based on their directives' needs	Provide support services at the division, department, or project level. They are driven by products and services

Source: Original Work
Attribution: Dorothy Howell
License: CC BY-SA 4.0

10.10 CONCLUSION

This chapter has focused on the internal and external environment and how managerial knowledge of these elements can lead to successful performance for organizations in general. This information is adaptable to the healthcare environment. Managers must be fully aware of how to review the organization through the systems approach in order to understand the purpose and function of the organization and the significance of maintaining harmony and efficiency within the workplace. The manager must be able to set goals and objectives that will help the organization achieve its mission and vision while also ensuring employees participate in decision making, open communication is engrained within the culture of the organization, and employees are trained, acknowledged, and supported as they carry out the organization's functions. Human and physical resources are significant to the day-to-day operations of the organization that influence performance. Healthcare organizations can convert its resources and capabilities into products and services to sustain its mission and vision. Conducting a situational analysis can help generate objective data based on the identification of strengths, weaknesses, opportunities, and threats. The results can be ranked, prioritized, and translated into a strategic plan that will aid in attaining a competitive edge. Applying the organizational analysis model into the organizational milieu provides insight to the manager on the significant roles that individuals play in the organization's success as they bring with them skill, expertise, values, and beliefs. Additionally, employee importance is evident as they assist the manager in mitigating the challenges experienced in today's complex healthcare structure.

10.11 KEY POINTS

- Healthcare leaders, including the chief executive officer, chief financial officer, chief medical officer, chief nursing officer, human resources director, operations director, information management director, etc., are responsible for setting the tone or culture for the organization.

- The competing values framework is based on measures that yield effective organizations, such as management and leadership, culture, and information technology.

- A system is a set of interlinking ideas, objects, or occurrences that form a cohesive whole. A system can be open or closed.

- Structure refers to how the organization is organized to support delivering products and services, such as with the various departments within the organization.

- A health system consists of two or more health care organizations, such as a hospital and one or more physician group(s) associated with each other through shared ownership or a contracting relationship for payment and service delivery, which includes both primary and specialty care.

- Productivity, accomplishment, direction, and goal clarity are significant factors in organizations using the rational model. The main purpose is to increase productivity, efficiency, and maximize profits.

- The rational model describes the significance of setting and achieving goals, which cannot be completed without using human resources, or the organization's employees.

- The human relations model focuses on employees and stresses participation, openness, commitment, and morale.

- A situational analysis is a "systematic method of collecting, analyzing, and delivering information about current resource conditions, issues, problems, opportunities, and challenges facing an organization."

- Organizational analysis provides an understanding of how the organization behaves.

10.12 KEY TERMS

Organizational behavior, organizational effectiveness, competing values approach, internal environment, external environment, open systems model, rational goal model, human relations model, internal processes model, situational analysis, SWOT analysis, organizational analysis model, culture, strategy, processes, systems, technology, structure, corporate level strategy, business level strategy, functional level strategy.

10.13 QUESTIONS FOR REVIEW AND DISCUSSION

1. Explain the significance of Organizational Behavior and Effectiveness to Organizational Approaches.

2. Describe how individuals, groups, and structures within the organization function in relation to organizational effectiveness.

3. What is the competing values approach, and what is its relationship to organizational effectiveness?

4. Describe the differences between the internal and external environment.

5. Compare and contrast the human relations model, the open systems model, the rational goal model, and the internal process model.

6. Why is a SWOT analysis useful to a healthcare manager?

7. Explain the advantages and disadvantages of a situational analysis.

8. Define the organizational analysis model.

9. Describe the seven elements of the organizational analysis model.

10. Explain the differences between corporate level, business level, and functional level strategies.

10.14 REFERENCES

Agency for Healthcare Quality (AHRQ), 2016. "Defining Health Systems." Retrieved March 30, 2020 from https://www.ahrq.gov/chsp/chsp-reports/resources-for-understanding-health-systems/defining-health-systems.html

Ashraf, G. & Kadir, S. (2012). "A Review on the Models of Organizational Effectiveness:

A Look at Cameron's Model in Higher Education." International Education Studies, 5(2). Retrieved from https://files.eric.ed.gov/fulltext/EJ1066736.pdf

Brnjas, Z., & Tripunoski, I. (2016). *Situational Analysis in the Function of Developing Company Competitive Advantage*. Retrieved from http://ebooks.ien.bg.ac. rs/1168/1/eee_brnjas_tripunoski.pdf

Buchbinder, S. & Shanks, N. (2017). *Introduction to Healthcare Management*. 3rd ed., Burlington, MA: Jones & Bartlett

Chuang, S., Inder, K. "An effectiveness analysis of healthcare systems using a systems theoretic approach." BMC Health Serv Res 9, 195 (2009). https://doi. org/10.1186/1472-6963-9-195

Connolly, Terry, Edward J. Conlon, and Stuart Jay Deutsch. 1980. "Organizational Effectiveness: A Multiple-Constituency Approach." Academy of Management Review 5 (2): 211–18. doi:10.5465/AMR.1980.4288727.

Cunningham, J. Barton. (1977). "Approaches to the Evaluation of Organizational Effectiveness." The Academy of Management Review 2, no. 3: 463-74. www.jstor.org/ stable/257702.

Cunningham, J. Barton. 1979. "The Management System: Its Functions and Processes." Management Science 25 (7): 657–70. doi:10.1287/mnsc.25.7.657.

D'souza, M. & D'souza, M. (2017). "A Study of the Success Value of the Four Approaches to Organizational Effectiveness in 18 Companies in the Indian Service and Manufacturing Industry Sectors." IOSR Journal of Business and Management (IOSR-JBM. Retrieved from http://www.iosrjournals.org/iosr-jbm/papers/Conf.17016-2017/Volume%201/11.%2077-89.pdf

Eydi, H. (2015). "Organizational Effectiveness Models: Review and

Apply in Non-Profit Sporting Organizations." American Journal of Economics, Finance and Management. 1(5). Retrieved from http://www.aiscience.org/journal/ajefm

Fajčíková, Adéla, Hana Urbancová, and Martina Fejfarová. 2018. "New Trends in the Recruitment of Employees in Czech Ict Organizations." Scientific Papers of the University of Pardubice. Series D, Faculty of Economics & Administration 25 (43): 39–49. https://ezproxy.mga.edu/login?url=http://search.ebscohost.com/login.aspx? direct=true&db=a9h&AN=132031637&site=eds-live&scope=site.

Hartnell, C. A., Ou, A. Y., & Kinicki, A. (2011). "Organizational culture and organizational effectiveness: A meta-analytic investigation of the competing values framework's theoretical suppositions." Journal of Applied Psychology, 96(4), 677–694. https:// doi.org/10.1037/a0021987.supp (Supplemental)

Helfrich, C. D., Li, Y. F., Mohr, D. C., Meterko, M., & Sales, A. E. (2007). "Assessing an organizational culture instrument based on the Competing Values Framework: exploratory and confirmatory factor analyses." Implementation science: IS, 2, 13. https://doi.org/10.1186/1748-5908-2-13

Holbeche, Linda. 2012. "Organisational Effectiveness: A Fresh Mindset." People

Management, February, 32–37. https://search.ebscohost.com/login.aspx?direct=true&AuthType=ip,shib&db=rgm&AN=71729643&site=eds-live&scope=site.

McGrath, M. (1984). "An Application of the Competing Values Approach to Organizational Analysis as a Diagnostic Tool." Academy of Management Proceedings (00650668), 254.

Millman, R.W. 1962. "A General Systems Approach to the Analysis of Managerial Functions." Academy of Management Proceedings (00650668), December, 133–38. doi:10.5465/AMBPP.1962.5068287.

National Academy of Engineering (US) and Institute of Medicine (US) Committee on Engineering and the Health Care System; Reid PP, Compton WD, Grossman JH, et al., editors. "Building a Better Delivery System: A New Engineering/Health Care Partnership." Washington (DC): National Academies Press (US); 2005. 2, A Framework for a Systems Approach to Health Care Delivery. Available from: https://www.ncbi.nlm.nih.gov/books/NBK22878/

Neves, VÍTOR. 2017. "Economics and Interdisciplinarity: An Open-Systems Approach." Brazilian Journal of Political Economy / Revista de Economia Política 37 (2): 343–62. doi:10.1590/0101-31572017v37n02a05.

Nickols, F. (2012). "The Organizational Analysis Model: A Framework for Understanding Organizations." Retrieved from https://www.nickols.us/Organizational_Analysis_Model.pdf

O'Brien-Pallas, L., Meyer, R.M., Hayes, L.J., & Wang, S. (2010). "The Patient Care Delivery Model – an open system framework: conceptualisation, literature review and analytical strategy." Journal of Clinical Nursing, 20, 1640–1650. doi: 10.1111/j.1365-2702.2010.03391.x

Organizational analysis. BusinessDictionary.com. WebFinance, Inc. http://www.businessdictionary.com/definition/organizational-analysis.html (accessed: November 19, 2019).

Pedraza, J. (2014). "What is organizational effectiveness?" Retrieved November 14, 2019 from, https://www.researchgate.net/post/What_is_organisational_effectiveness_How_an_organisation_could_achieve_it

Robert E. Quinn, & John Rohrbaugh. (1983). "A Spatial Model of Effectiveness Criteria: Towards a Competing Values Approach to Organizational Analysis." Management Science, 29(3), 363. Retrieved from https://search.ebscohost.com/login.aspx?direct=true&AuthType=ip,shib&db=edsjsr&AN=edsjsr.2631061&site=eds-live&scope=site&custid=ns235467

Shannon, E., Holden, J., & Van Dam, P. (2012). "Implementing National Health Reform – Is Organizational Culture the Key?" Australian Political Studies Association Conference. Retrieved March 29, 2020 from https://www.auspsa.org.au/sites/default/files/implementing_national_health_reform_elizabeth_shannon.pdf

Shi, L. & Singh, D. (2015). *Delivering Health Care in America: A systems Approach*. 6th ed. Jones and Bartlett Learning.

Suchan, Jim, and Ron Dulek. 1998. "From Text to Context: An Open Systems Approach to Research in Written Business Communication." Journal of Business Communication 35 (1): 87–110. doi:10.1177/002194369803500106.

Thakor, A. V. (2010). "The Competing Values Framework and Growth Strategy." Mergers & Acquisitions: The Dealermaker's Journal, 45(1), 46.

TNC, 2007. *Guidance for Step 5: Complete Situation Analysis in Conservation Action Planning Handbook.* The Nature Conservancy, Arlington, VA. Retrieved from https://www.conservationgateway.org/Documents/CAP%20Handbook%20 Chapter%205%20062007.pdf

USDA Natural Resources Conservation Service. (2005). "Using a Multidisciplinary Approach to Conduct a Situational Analysis." Retrieved from https://www.nrcs.usda. gov/Internet/FSE_DOCUMENTS/stelprdb1045578.pdf

Vrontis, D., & Thrassou, A. (2006). "Situation Analysis and Strategic Planning: An Empirical Case Study in the UK Beverage Industry." Journal of Innovative Marketing, 2(2). Retrieved from https://businessperspectives.org/images/pdf/applications/ publishing/templates/article/assets/1737/im_en_2006_02_Vrontis.pdf

Walston, S.L. (2018). *Strategic Healthcare Management: Planning and Execution.* 2nd ed. Health Administration Press (HAP). ISBN 9781567939606

Wicks, A. M., & St. Clair, L. (2007). "Competing Values in Healthcare: Balancing the (Un) Balanced Scorecard." Journal of Healthcare Management, 52(5), 309–324. https:// doi.org/10.1097/00115514-200709000-00007

Yang, O., & Shao, Y. E. (1996). "Shared leadership in self-managed teams: A competing values approach." Total Quality Management, 7(5), 521–534. https://doi. org/10.1080/09544129610621

PART IV

ORGANIZATIONAL CULTURE PERFORMANCE AND CHANGE

11 ELIMINATING HEALTH DISPARITIES IN HEALTHCARE ORGANIZATIONS THROUGH CULTURAL PROFICIENCY

11.1 LEARNING OBJECTIVES

- Define health disparity, cultural competency, linguistic competency, and cultural proficiency

- Identify U.S. demographic trends

- Describe the factors that contribute to health disparity

- Describe initiatives to foster cultural proficiency within healthcare organizations

- Discuss best practices in fostering cultural proficiency within healthcare organizations

11.2 INTRODUCTION

Chapter eleven describes culturally competent strategies that address health disparities in healthcare organizations. Health disparities are differences in the health status of specific segments of the population due to greater barriers to health. As the population of the U.S. shifts and becomes increasingly diverse, the gaps in health outcomes continue to persist among certain subpopulation groups. Culturally competent managers and leaders must recognize, understand, and address health disparity in order to adapt healthcare delivery and services to meet the unique needs of the community served as well as enhance internal workplace productivity.

> **The Chapter Case**
>
> Southern Healthcare Hospice Center is a long-term care facility that provides assistance to elderly residents. The mission of the facility is "to provide individualized, empathetic long-term care services while helping patients navigate one of the most difficult phases of their lives." The vision of the facility is to provide specialized, transformative care through providing innovative clinical and administrative strategies. The center has been in operation for over 25 years and mainly served a largely upper-class, caucasian population until recent demographic shifts. The surrounding area now consists of predominately low-income, Hispanic, Spanish-speaking residents. In addition to low income and limited health insurance, many of the Hispanic residents face additional barriers to care, including fear of their immigration status, illiteracy, and mistrust of the healthcare system stemming from culturally different health beliefs. Patients tend to seek natural healing and home remedies before seeking medical treatment. Amanda is the facility director, and she focuses on staffing, financial management, supervising resident care, community outreach, and evaluating the programs the facility provides to elderly patients and their families. The facility currently lacks linguistic services and is also not fully equipped to handle patients exhibiting dementia symptoms. As you read this chapter, consider how the director should address the potential health disparity and ensure cultural competence in the facility.

11.3 HEALTH DISPARITY OVERVIEW

Certain subpopulations, such as racial and ethnic minorities, are more likely to be uninsured, have limited access to care, experience poorer quality of care, and, as a result, experience worsened health outcomes (CDC, 2017). For instance, Blacks are more likely than whites to experience a higher prevalence of health conditions, including asthma, diabetes, and heart disease (CDC, 2017). Although health disparity is often discussed from the realm of race and ethnicity, the gap in health outcomes also occurs across other dimensions, including sexual orientation and socioeconomic status. For instance, research suggests members of the Lesbian, Gay, Bisexual, and Transgender (LGBT) community experience more chronic disease and higher prevalence of major health concerns, including HIV/AIDS, mental illness, substance use, and sexual and physical violence than do heterosexuals (Kates, Ranji, Beamesderfer, Salganicoff, & Dawson, 2018). Further, low-income individuals experience more burdens to healthcare access and quality, in addition to experiencing worsened health status, than do individuals with higher income (AHRQ, 2016; Braverman, et. al, 2010). Despite the advancements in healthcare technology and increased healthcare spending and utilization in the U.S., gaps in disease burden persists among certain subpopulations, particularly underserved and vulnerable groups.

A medically underserved population is a group experiencing economic, cultural, and/or linguistic barriers that limit access to primary medical services (Clark and Preto, 2018; HRSA, 2019). As defined by the World Health Organization, a vulnerable group is one that experiences limits on their rights in addition to higher rates of poverty and marginalization. Vulnerable groups typically consist of individuals who identify as LGBT, ethnic minorities, migrant, disabled, homeless, and isolated, especially isolated elderly, women, and children. Health disparities are preventable disproportions on the burden of disease, injury, violence, or opportunities to experience optimum health by such underserved and vulnerable populations. Health care disparities are a difference in health insurance coverage, the quality of health care, and the access and utilization of healthcare, affecting health disparity—which refers to the higher burden of disease, injury, disability, and death—experienced by groups relative to another that stem from poverty, environmental hazards, lack of healthcare access, and individual and behavioral factors, as well as inequalities in education (Orgera & Artiga, 2018; CDC, 2008).

Health equality is the distribution of the same health resources and opportunities to every individual across a population. On the other hand, **health inequality** refers to the uneven distribution of health or health resources as a result of genetic or other factors related to health access. When certain populations face a shorter life expectancy and higher rates of death and disease based on socioeconomic status and the distribution of resources, then clearly the disproportion of the burden is beyond a mere health inequality and denotes a moral injustice.

Health inequalities are the unequal health conditions (e.g., differences in breast cancer prevalence for men and women) while health inequity indicates a moral injustice and signifies the unfairness of health. Health inequities are the preventable differences in health that arise from the poor governance or social exclusion of underserved and vulnerable groups (APHA, 2020). However, **health equity** can occur when everyone has the opportunity to attain their highest health potential (CDC, 2020; Braveman, 2017).

Stop and Apply

When does health inequality become health inequity, or an issue of social injustice?

Cultural competence in healthcare provides a way to address health disparities by recognizing and understanding cultural differences, addressing bias, and adapting health care delivery and services to meet the individual social, cultural, and linguistic needs of the community served. Cultural competence can increase patient engagement, health care utilization, treatment compliance and adherence, and health status in general. Addressing cultural competence is a means to reduce stereotyping and stigmatization. For instance, disabled persons may face unique barriers to healthcare access, such as transportation to healthcare facilities and whether the exam room is physically accessible. Likewise, linguistic competence will differ for providers treating individuals with limited English proficiency than a transgender English-speaking individual (Meuter, 2015).

Differences in cultural values and preference pose additional barriers health professionals tend to overlook (Juckett, 2013). For example, cultural values, such as modesty, may be overlooked by medical providers during medical examinations due to seemingly immodest hospital gowns and the lack of same-sex providers for patients. Other cultural values, such as friendliness and respect, may be neglected when close physical proximity is perceived as being more personable in some Hispanic cultures while not properly addressing patients by their full name may indicate a lack of respect. Although all patients should be treated decorously with kindness, friendliness, and respect, different cultures may view such values differently, so it is important healthcare professionals have a basic understanding of the cultural practices and values of the community and patients they serve (Juckett, 2013). As the population grows more racially and ethnically diverse, it is imperative the health care system recognizes the need to deliver culturally competent care and services needed to improve health outcomes, reduce healthcare costs, and improve health care quality and patient satisfaction.

11.4 DIMENSIONS OF HEALTH DISPARITY: U.S. POPULATION TRENDS AND HEALTH DISPARITY

Current demographic and health market trends influence the provision of health care in the U.S. The demographic make-up of the U.S is expanding in racial and ethnic, multi-cultural, and religious diversity, contributing to the shift in existing social structures and beliefs. Additionally, the immigrant population has reached a record high as foreign-born individuals account for approximately 13.6% of the U.S. population (Pew Research Center, 2019). As shown in the figures below, by the year 2050, racial and ethnic minorities will make up a majority of the U.S. population. By 2050, the number of persons over the age of 65 will also increase. In 2012, less than 15% of the population was over the age of 65 in contrast to making up an approximated 25% of the population by year 2050. The aging U.S. population and escalating prevalence of obesity and associated chronic illnesses also directly contribute to rising health care costs. Moreover, despite the rising household income levels, the gap in income inequality among racial and ethnic groups is also widening, as African Americans, Hispanics, and American Native Indians have the lowest household incomes (U.S. Census Bureau, 2016; Pew Research Center, 2019).

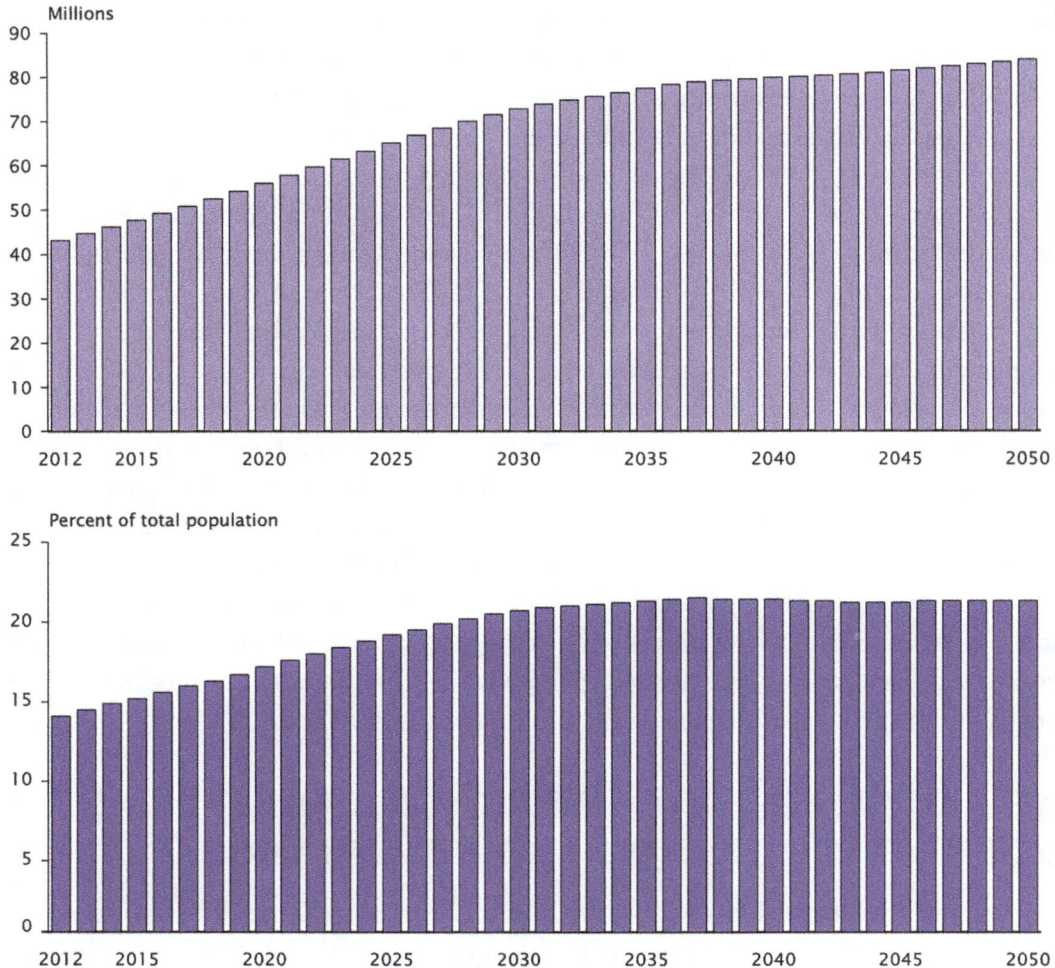

Figure 11.1: Population Aged 65 and Over for the United States 2012 to 2050

Source: Census.gov
Attribution: Jennifer M. Ortman, Victoria A. Velkoff, and Howard Hogan
License: Public Domain

Poverty is a known precursor to the disease and death prevalence that remains higher among low-income and minority populations. Likewise, the healthcare market is experiencing similar trends as a result of the shifting demographics which further adversely affect racial and ethnic minorities. Health care costs are rising, which has an impact on the ability of individuals, especially low-income persons, to afford and access healthcare. The availability and accessibility of health professionals and health resources are also unevenly distributed across the U.S., which gravely affects isolated, rural, and low-income populations (Whaley, 2015). This issue is further exacerbated if the limited available physicians have little, or completely lack, skills in cultural competence. The U.S. government has acknowledged the growing challenges associated with the demographic trends and has implemented various programs and initiatives to address the mounting challenges and widening disparity. In 2019, as a part of the section 1557 ACA provision, discrimination based on race, origin, age, and gender identity was prohibited and requires assistance services for individuals with limited English proficiency as well as individuals with disabilities in health programs, health insurance markets, and health activities receiving federal financial assistance (Musumeci, Kates, Dawson, Salganicoff, Sobel & Artiga, 2019). The ACA coverage expansion aided in providing another step towards closing the enduring disparity in health coverage for minorities and low-income individuals.

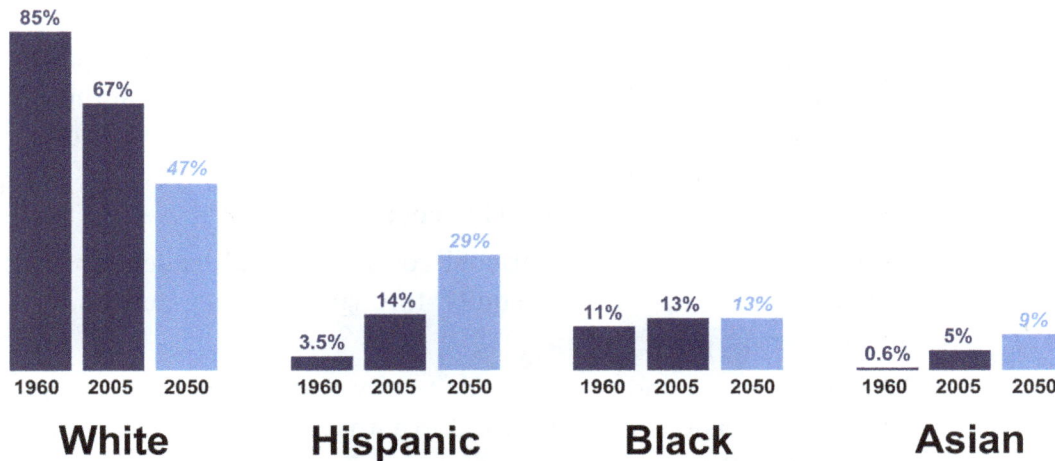

Figure 11.2: Population by Race and Ethnicity, Actual and Projected: 1960, 2005, and 2050 (% of total)

Source: Pew Research Center, 2008
Attribution: Corey Parson, Adapted from Pew Research Center, 2008
License: Fair Use

Despite medical advances and new technologies that have improved Americans' quality of life and health status, longstanding health disparities still exist between different racial and ethnic populations. Access to health services and opportunities to obtain optimal health should not be unevenly distributed based on race, ethnicity, sexual orientation or any other characteristic. Nevertheless, unjust and persistent gaps in health care and health outcomes continue to persist. In 2011, the Department of Health and Human Services (HHS) Disparities Action Plan therefore began an assessment plan to evaluate the impact of policies and programs related to health disparity. The action plan was the first federal strategic plan to address eliminating racial and ethnic health disparities and set the framework for unprecedented federal commitment to reaching this goal (Dorsey, Petersen, & Schottenfeld, 2016). The National Standards for Culturally and Linguistically Appropriate Services in Health and Health Care (the national CLAS standards) developed a framework to assist health care organizations in delivering culturally and linguistically appropriate care (see National Standards on Culturally and Linguistically Appropriate Services on next page).

National Standards on Culturally and Linguistically Appropriate Services (CLAS)

The National CLAS Standards are intended to advance health equity, improve quality, and help eliminate health care disparities by establishing a blueprint for health and health care organizations to develop.

Principal Standards:

1. Provide effective, equitable, understandable, and respectful quality care and services that are responsive to diverse cultural health beliefs and practices, preferred languages, health literacy, and other communication needs.

Governance, Leadership, and the Workforce:

2. Advance and sustain organizational governance and leadership that promotes CLAS and health equity through policy, practices, and allocated resources.

3. Recruit, promote, and support a culturally and linguistically diverse governance, leadership, and workforce that are responsive to the population in the service area.

4. Educate and train governance, leadership, and workforce in culturally and linguistically appropriate policies and practices on a continuous basis.

Communication and Language Assistance:

5. Offer language assistance to individuals who have limited English proficiency and/or other communication needs, at no cost to them, to facilitate timely access to all health care and services.

6. Inform all individuals about the available language assistance services clearly and in their preferred language, verbally and in writing.

7. Ensure the competence of individuals providing language assistance, recognizing that the use of untrained individuals and/or minors as interpreters should be avoided.

8. Provide easy-to-understand print and multimedia materials and signage in the languages commonly used by the populations in the service area.

Engagement, Continuous Improvement, and Accountability:

9. Establish culturally and linguistically appropriate goals, policies, and management accountability, and infuse them throughout the organization's planning and operations.

10. Conduct ongoing assessments of the organization's CLAS-related activities and integrate CLAS-related measures into measurement and continuous quality improvement activities.

11. Collect and maintain accurate and reliable demographic data to monitor and evaluate the impact of CLAS on health equity and outcomes and to inform service delivery.

12. Conduct regular assessments of community health assets and needs and use the results to plan and implement services that respond to the cultural and linguistic diversity of populations in the service area.

13. Partner with the community to design, implement, and evaluate policies, practices, and services to ensure cultural and linguistic appropriateness.

14. Create conflict and grievance resolution processes that are culturally and linguistically appropriate to identify, prevent, and resolve conflicts or complaints.

15. Communicate the organization's progress in implementing and sustaining CLAS to all stakeholders, constituents, and the general public.

*Taken from: U.S. Department of Health and Human Services, Office of Minority Health (2011). National Standards for Culturally and Linguistically Appropriate Services (CLAS) in Health and Health Care. Retrieved from https://thinkculturalhealth.hhs.gov/assets/pdfs/EnhancedNationalCLASStandards.pdf

11.5 DIMENSIONS OF HEALTH DISPARITY

Although racial and ethnic health disparities are often highlighted, health disparity occurs across many dimensions, including cultural and linguistic backgrounds, geographic locations, socioeconomic status, disability status, and gender and sexual orientations. Below are just a few examples of the many factors that contribute to limited access to quality healthcare.

11.5.1 Race and Ethnicity

Racial and ethnic minorities in general face disproportionate risk factors that contribute to negative health outcomes. For instance, the death rate for African Americans is generally higher than their caucasian counterparts for heart disease, cancer, asthma, diabetes, and HIV/AIDS. Non-Hispanic black infants are three times as likely than non-Hispanic white infants to die at birth from complications associated with low birth weight (HHS, 2019).

11.5.2 Language and Cultural Background

The U.S. healthcare system is largely equipped to treat English speaking patients; however, there is an increasing percentage of non-English proficient individuals. Non-English proficiency is an indicator for decreased healthcare quality and increased risk for adverse health outcomes. To exacerbate the situation, individuals from different cultures may express pain differently and may have varying perspectives on health. As a result of perceived cultural discrimination, prior negative experiences, and overall distrust in the medical community, individuals may avoid seeking needed healthcare (Thorburn, Kue, Keon, and Lo, 2012). The lack or limitation of healthcare professionals' linguistic and cultural skills may lead patients to rely on less medically knowledgeable relatives and staff, which can lead to miscommunicating health risks and patients' not complying with medical regimes or electing to not receive potentially life-saving treatments (Meuter, Gallois, Segalowitz, Ryder, & Hocking, 2015).

11.5.3 Rural v. Urban Geographic Area

Rural communities face a range of healthcare challenges in contrast to their urban counterparts, including a shortage of primary care physicians, longer travel distances to receive healthcare, and a lack of health insurance. As a result, rural Americans are more likely to suffer from heart disease, obesity, diabetes, and cancer in contrast to those living in urban areas (HHS, 2019).

11.5.4 Social Determinants (education, income, social, and economic status)

The social determinants of health are the conditions in which people live, work, and play that influence quality-of-life and health outcomes (Healthy People, 2020). Health involves not only treating disease but also addressing the root causes of disease that can often be attributed to the social determinants of health. Without being able to achieve optimal health results from the social and physical conditions that enable healthy behaviors (e.g., availability and accessibility to physical activity and healthy foods), less educated, low-income, and minority populations are therefore also less likely to have health coverage and face barriers that negatively impact their ability to access and afford care (CERD, 2008).

11.5.5 Disability Status

Over 21 million U.S. adults ages 18–64 have a disability related to serious difficulty walking or climbing stairs, hearing, seeing, or concentrating, remembering, or making decisions. Despite most adults with disabilities having the ability to participate in physical activity, most are physically inactive (CDC, 2019). Only 44% of adults with disabilities who visited a doctor in the past year were recommended to engage in physical activity by a health care professional, yet adults with disabilities were 82% more likely to be physically active if their doctor recommended it (CDC, 2019). Coincidentally, adults with disabilities are more likely to be obese, smoke, and have high blood pressure than adults without disabilities. Adults with disabilities are also more likely to have more than one chronic disease and are three times more likely to have heart disease, strokes, diabetes, or cancer than adults without disabilities (CDC, 2019).

11.5.6 Sexual Orientation

Lesbian, gay, bisexual, and transgender individuals often face challenges, such as cultural stigmas, discrimination, violence, workplace and health insurance inequality, and denial of care based on their sexual orientation or gender identity (Kates, Ranji, Beamesderfer, Salganicoff, & Dawson, 2018). Bisexual adults are almost twice as likely to be unable to obtain needed medical care due to cost compared to heterosexual adults.

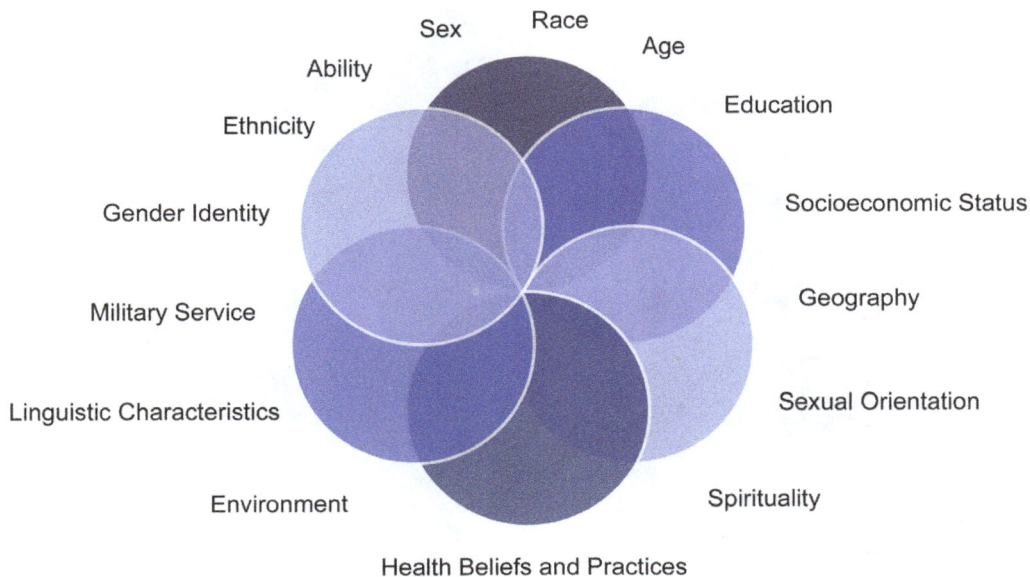

Figure 11.3: Social Determinants of Health

Source: Original Work
Attribution: Corey Parson
License: CC BY-SA 4.0

Stop and Apply

What are some of the likely health disparities and challenges faced by the community served by Southern Health Care Hospice Center?

11.6 IMPACT OF HEALTH DISPARITY ON COST, QUALITY, AND CARE

As previously mentioned in this chapter, certain subpopulations face a higher risk of being underinsured or lack insurance altogether in addition to experiencing worsened health outcomes and limited access to quality health care. Health care disparities often result from a complex relationship between the stark contrast in the social, environmental, and sociodemographic characteristics that exist among various segments of the population. These disparities occur across many dimensions, including but not limited to race and ethnicity, income, disability status, and education.

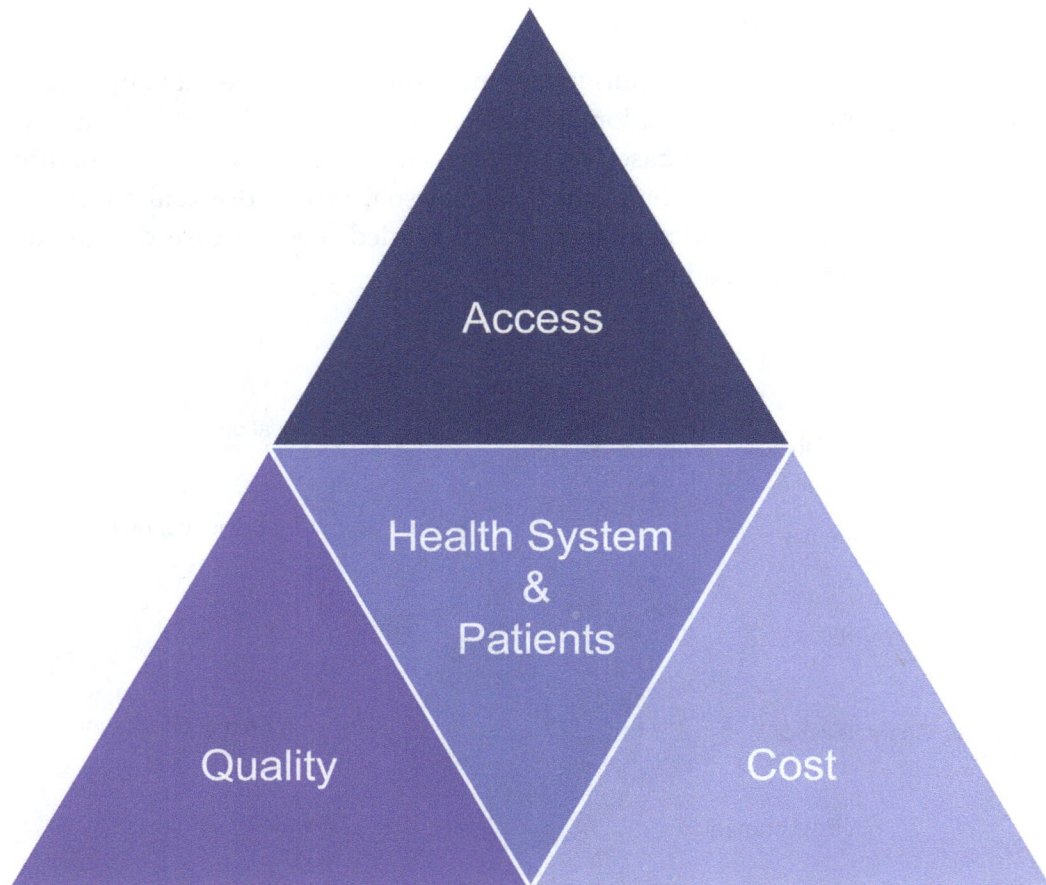

Figure 11.4: The "Iron Triangle" of Health Care: Access, Cost, Quality

Source: Berthe, 2016
Attribution: Corey Parson, Adapted from Berthe, 2016
License: Fair Use

Health and health care disparities not only affect the groups facing disparities, but also impose significant overall health care costs and reduces the health care quality for the entire U.S. population (LaVeist, Gaskin, & Richard, 2011). Health disparities cost the U.S. approximately $309 billion every year in direct costs covering the expenses required for the provision of care and indirect costs associated with the loss of work productivity and premature death. Research illustrates racial and ethnic disparity alone contributes to approximately $93 billion in direct unnecessary medical costs and $42 billion in lost productivity (Kaiser, 2012). As the population continues to diversify, the importance of addressing persistent health disparities increases (Cigna, 2016).

Stop and Apply

How would the Southern Health Care Hospice Center be affected if the facility failed to adapt to change and address their prevailing health disparities?

11.7 CHARACTERISTICS OF CULTURALLY COMPETENT HEALTHCARE LEADERS

Healthcare managers must incorporate culturally competent approaches to healthcare delivery in order to improve healthcare quality and access as well as reduce overall healthcare costs. Key culturally competent skills for health care managers include the ability to recognize issues related to health disparities and the ability to manage the dynamics related to these challenges. Healthcare managers must also value and appreciate diversity and pursue initiatives that facilitate the continual pursuit of awareness, knowledge, and skills enhancement related to cultural competence. Demographics change, culture shifts, and terminology evolves; therefore, cultural competence is an ongoing pursuit. Healthcare organizations must create a warm and welcoming environment to all patients, and all staff should have a basic understanding of cultural competence. A few examples of how healthcare organizations can strive for cultural competence include providing easy to read and bilingual medical pamphlets; culturally appropriate and diverse food options; extended visiting hours; flexible appointment scheduling; culture-specific interventions; interpretation services for patients (rather than expecting patients to rely on their families); and modest hospital gowns; as well as observing different cultural holidays; recruiting and retaining diverse staff; and permitting extra time for clinical patients with limited English proficiency (Juckett, 2013).

In addition to addressing external health disparity issues, the internal issues of workplace equality and diversity must also be addressed. Studies have found less than 1% of African Americans hold top management positions, yet they constitute 20% of hospital employees. Further, studies show African Americans are paid lower salaries, hold lower job positions, and experience lower job satisfaction than their white counterparts. The healthcare workforce should composed of diverse individuals that reflect the populations served. Healthcare managers must also insist on equality, tolerance, and respect for all individuals inside and outside the organization.

Managers should recruit and hire diverse employees, and then orient and integrate new employees. Training should incorporate education on the benefits and importance of appreciating diversity. Managers must realize and reinforce to employees that differences do exist, but difference does not indicate deficiency. Rather, diversity among employees promotes learning and growth. Exposure to the different ideas and perspectives of various cultures enables personal growth and creates well-rounded individuals. By managing diversity, the manager is able to leverage the advantages and key strengths of each employee. Diverse teams bring unique skills, knowledge, and awarenesses that contribute to enhanced productivity and creativity, especially during times of flux within the organization. When managers properly train employees and properly leverage diversity within the workplace, they are able to harmonize each employee with the other and have a greater organizational impact. A culturally competent manager has the ability to recognize and appreciate cultural diversity, address unconscious/conscious bias, and adapt health care delivery and services to meet the unique social, cultural, and language needs of the healthcare organization.

Table 11.1: Strategies to increase cultural competence in the health care organization
1. Gather demographic data, assess patient needs, and identify which patients require special services or assistance in order to ensure patient satisfaction and quality health care delivery.
2. Encourage staff to take a cultural competency assessment to increase knowledge and cross-cultural communication skills, in addition to providing staff with culturally competent resources and training.
3. Create a welcoming practice environment with culturally diverse and culturally competent staff that reflects the community served.
4. Establish linguistic services, procedures, and polices by hiring bilingual staff, providing an interpreter, and/or providing patient-friendly health education materials that are easy to read in the most common languages of the community served.
5. Work with the community, community-based organizations, and/or other healthcare organizations in order to create the best solutions to improve health

Source: CIGNA, 2016
Attribution: Whitney Hamilton, Adapted from CIGNA, 2016
License: Fair Use

Stop and Apply
What specific strategies would you suggest to Amanda and the managers to create a culturally competent facility? What barriers may exist? How would you address any reluctance to becoming a culturally competent facility?

11.8 BEST PRACTICES IN CULTURALLY COMPETENT HEALTHCARE ORGANIZATIONS

The culturally proficient healthcare organization is composed of a diverse workforce with supportive leadership that enforces policies to ensure an equitable practice, offers ongoing cultural competence education and training of all staff, provides effective multilingual services and patient-friendly materials, and collects data to track health outcomes, patient satisfaction, and community demographic information. And of utmost importance, a culturally proficient health care organization has the ability to adapt and respond to the needs of the community served (SAMSHA, 2016). By taking steps toward improving the cultural competence of the healthcare organization, health care leaders will be better equipped to provide quality care and increase patient utilization and satisfaction regardless of individual factors such as race and ethnicity, cultural and linguistic background, or gender and sexual orientation. The following examples illustrate two health systems that have incorporated culturally competent strategies to comprehensively meet the needs of their consumers.

Connecticut Latino Behavioral Health System

The Connecticut Latino Behavioral Health System integrates a comprehensive qualitative and quantitative evaluation designed to assess their program at three levels: organizational, staff, and patient/consumer. Evaluation at the organizational level includes the development and preliminary pilot implementation of a new instrument called the Cultural Competency Index. This instrument evaluates culturally responsive clinical services. Evaluation at the staff level includes pre- and post-training evaluations, satisfaction with trainings, and random tape ratings to assess for language fluency and the integration of Latino cultural values in treatment. The program has not yet evaluated the patient/consumer level; however, the future direction of the initiative is to ensure that the health system is equipped to meet changing consumer needs and systemic priorities.
(Adapted from http://www.ctlbhs.org)

Mile Square Health Center

The University of Illinois Hospital & Health Sciences System – Mile Square Health Center (MSHC) is a federally qualified health center (FQHC) that provides comprehensive health care services to a predominantly African American community in Chicago. The health center integrates behavioral health services into a primary care setting and is composed of staff with expertise in not only behavioral health but also experience working in African American communities. The program carefully matches providers and patients and utilizes culturally sensitive engagement processes, practices which have resulted in increased patient engagement. Examples of behavioral health/substance use services employed at MSHC include specialized and intensive care for patients with severe mental illness and peer counseling services led by African Americans with a personal history of substance use in order to enhance patient initiation and recovery, as well as a research project funded by the Robert Wood Johnson Foundation to provide behavioral health services to ethnic minority youth.
(Adapted from http://www.ctlbhs.org)

11.9 CONCLUSION

This chapter outlined culturally competent strategies that address health disparities in healthcare organizations. Health disparities are differences in the health status of specific subpopulations resulting from greater barriers to achieving optimal health. Culturally competent managers and leaders must recognize, understand, and address these health disparities in order to adapt healthcare delivery and services to meet the unique needs of the community served, thereby reducing overall healthcare costs and improving healthcare quality for their patients.

11.10 KEY POINTS

- A culturally competent manager has the ability to recognize and appreciate cultural diversity, address unconscious/conscious bias, and adapt health care delivery and services to meet the unique social, cultural, and language needs of a healthcare organization.

- Key strategies identified to create a culturally competent healthcare organization include empowering leadership; establishing a diverse, bilingual/bicultural staff; providing cultural and linguistic support and training to all staff; and monitoring patient demographics and outcomes.

11.11 KEY TERMS

Cultural competency, Health disparity, Vulnerable populations, Underserved populations, Health inequity, Health inequality, Linguistic competence, Cultural proficiency

11.12 QUESTIONS FOR REVIEW AND DISCUSSION

1. Define cultural competence and health disparity.
2. Describe the difference between health inequity and health inequality.
3. Describe the benefits of providing culturally competent programs within healthcare organizations.
4. As a healthcare administrator, how would you ensure cultural competence within a medical facility? What initiatives and programs would you implement?
5. Explain how cultural competence can address health disparity. What are the limitations of cultural competence to addressing health disparity?

11.13 REFERENCES

Adults with Disabilities. 2019. Centers for Disease Control. Retrieved from https: https:// www.cdc.gov/vitalsigns/disabilities/index.html

Agency for Healthcare Research and Quality, *2016 National Healthcare Quality and Disparities Report*. Rockville, MD: Agency for Healthcare Research and Quality, October 2017. https://www.ahrq.gov/sites/default/files/wysiwyg/research/findings/

nhqrdr/nhqdr16/final2016qdr-cx.pdf.

Braveman P, Arkin E, Orleans T, Proctor D, Plough A. (2017). "What is health equity? And what difference does a definition make?" Princeton (NJ): Robert Wood Johnson Foundation.

Braverman, P. et al., "Socioeconomic Disparities in Health in the United States: What the Patterns Tell Us." *American Journal of Public Health* 100(1) (April 2010):186-196.

CDC. "Community Health and Program Services (CHAPS): Health Disparities Among Racial/Ethnic Populations." Atlanta: U.S. Department of Health and Human Services; 2008.

Centers for Disease Control and Prevention. "Health Equity." CDC. 2020.

Centers for Disease Control and Prevention. NCHHSTP AtlasPlus. Updated 2017. https:// www.cdc.gov/nchhstp/atlas/index.htm. Accessed on July 7, 2018.

Clark, B., Preto, N. (2018). "Exploring the Concept of Vulnerability in Health Care." CMAJ. 2018 Mar 19; 190(11): E308–E309. doi: 10.1503/cmaj.180242

Colby, Sandra L. and Jennifer M. Ortman, *Projections of the Size and Composition of the U.S. Population: 2014 to 2060*, Current Population Reports, P25-1143, U.S. Census Bureau, Washington, DC, 2014.

Cultural Competency in Healthcare. 2016. Cigna. https://www.cigna.com/assets/docs/ about-cigna/thn-white-papers/cultural-competency-in-health-care-final.pdf

Determinants of Health. Healthy People website. https://www.healthypeople.gov/2020/ about/foundationhealth-measures/Determinants-of-Health. Updated August 23, 2018.

Dorsey R, Petersen D, Schottenfeld L. "The U.S. Department of Health and Human Services Action Plan to Reduce Racial and Ethnic Health Disparities: A Commentary on Data Needs to Monitor Progress Towards Health Equity." Health Syst Policy Res. 2016, 3:4. doi: 10.21767/2254-9137.100053

Health Equity. (2020). APHA, 2020

Health Workforce Glossary. 2019. Health Resources and Service Administration. https:// bhw.hrsa.gov/grants/resourcecenter/glossary

Henry J. Kaiser Family Foundation. "Focus on Health Care Disparities." December 2012 7. Artiga, Samantha, *The Henry J. Kaiser Family Foundation*. "Disparities in Health Care and Health Care: Five Key Questions and Answers." 12 August 2016. https:// www.kff.org/disparities-policy/issue-brief/disparities-in-health-and-health-care-five-key-questions-and-answers/

Juckett, Gregory. (2013). "Caring for Latino Patients." Am Fam Physician. 2013 Jan 1;87(1):48-54. https://www.aafp.org/afp/2013/0101/p48.html

Kates, J., Ranji, U., Beamesderfer, A., Salganicoff, A., & Dawson, L. (2018). Kaiser Family Foundation, *Health And Access to Care and Coverage for Lesbian, Gay, Bisexual, and Transgender Individuals in the U.S.*, (Washington, DC: Kaiser Family Foundation, May 2018), https://www.kff.org/disparities-policy/issue-brief/

health-and-access-to-care-and-coverage-for-lesbian-gay-bisexual-and-transgender-individuals-in-the-u-s/.

LaVeist T, Gaskin DJ, Richard P. The Economic Burden of Health Inequalities in the United States, Joint Center for Political and Economic Studies, Fact Sheet, September 2011

"Median Household Income in the Past 12 Months (in 2016 inflation-adjusted dollars)" *American Community Survey*. United States Census Bureau. 2016. Archived from the original on 17 April 2016. Retrieved 3 December 2016.

Meuter, R. F., Gallois, C., Segalowitz, N. S., Ryder, A. G., & Hocking, J. (2015). "Overcoming language barriers in healthcare: A protocol for investigating safe and effective communication when patients or clinicians use a second language." *BMC health services research, 15,* 371. doi:10.1186/s12913-015-1024-8

Musumeci, M., Kates, J., Dawson, L., Salganicoff, A., Sobel, L., Artiga, S. (2019). HHS's "Proposed Changes to Non-Discrimination Regulations Under ACA Section 1557."

https://www.kff.org/disparities-policy/issue-brief/hhss-proposed-changes-to-non-discrimination-regulations-under-aca-section-1557/

Orgera, K & Artiga, S. (2018). "Disparities in Health and Health Care: Five Kew Questions and Answers." https://www.kff.org/disparities-policy/issue-brief/disparities-in-health-and-health-care-five-key-questions-and-answers/

"Secretary's Advisory Committee on Health Promotion and Disease Prevention Objectives for 2020. Healthy People 2020: An Opportunity to Address the Societal Determinants of Health in the United States." July 26, 2010. Available from: http://www.healthypeople.gov/2010/hp2020/advisory/SocietalDeterminantsHealth.htm

Thorburn, S., Kue, J., Keon, K. L., & Lo, P. (2012). "Medical mistrust and discrimination in health care: a qualitative study of Hmong women and men." *Journal of community health, 37*(4), 822–829. https://doi.org/10.1007/s10900-011-9516-x

U.S. Department of Health and Human Services, Office of Minority Health (2011). "National Standards for Culturally and Linguistically Appropriate Services (CLAS) in Health and Health Care." Retrieved from https://thinkculturalhealth.hhs.gov/assets/pdfs/EnhancedNationalCLASStandards.pdf

"Unequal Health Outcomes in the United States." 2008. Committee on the Elimination of Racial Discrimination [CERD] Working Group on Health and Environmental Health. https://www.prrac.org/pdf/CERDhealthEnvironmentReport.pdf

U.S. Department of Health and Human Services. Infant Mortality by Race/Ethnicity. 2019. Minorityhealth.hhs.gov

(https://www.integration.samhsa.gov/@Final_Health_Report.pdf--)

Whaley, P. (2015). State Office of Rural Health. State Office of Rural Health. January 2015. Retrieved from https://dch.georgia.gov/state-office-rural-health

12 ORGANIZATIONAL CULTURE IN HEALTHCARE

12.1 LEARNING OBJECTIVES

- To discuss distinctive challenges facing healthcare organizations globally
- To analyze methods for creating and sustaining organizational culture in the workplace
- To describe strategic change and process change
- To describe a positive organizational culture
- To examine factors with cultural differences in the workplace
- To differentiate cultures that stress individualism from those that stress collectivism
- To discuss approaches that can be used for organizational cultural changes
- To analyze cultural and self-assessments and the way cultural change takes place

12.2 INTRODUCTION

Organizational culture includes attitudes, values, and work styles which, when managed properly, can lead to a highly productive workforce performance. A diverse workforce brings people from different backgrounds together. Each individual brings their own experiences and expertise to the table. The blending of these backgrounds can enhance productivity by allowing a free flow of new ideas and creativity. This chapter will explore the importance of a diverse workforce and how managers can make the most of their employees' individual knowledge and approaches in order to advance health care performance and continuously improve care quality and reach organizational goals. This chapter will focus on the case study section which involves identifying strategies for change and how to process change. This chapter will also focus on methods for creating and sustaining a healthy organizational culture, approaches for cultural change, and means of analyzing cultural and self-assessments as they relate to the case study of Mr. Rodriquez.

12.3 CREATING AND SUSTAINING CULTURE

Organizational culture is defined as "an organization's value systems and its collection of guiding principles" (Evans & Lindsay, 2014). The organization's cultural sustainability is a long-term factor of the organization's success. Many experts in the leadership field have cited that strong leadership drives culture (Evans & Lindsay, 2014; Judge & Robbins, 2011; Walston, 2016). As the organization grows and develops, the leader must continue to stay actively involved in the day-to-day operations of the organization. Being "visible" to the employees is necessary in adopting the organization's desired behaviors and personalities that are necessary for sustaining its culture. The leader's behaviors and personality are often reflected by and showcased to the employees. Leaders and managers should understand what skills are needed to manage organizational culture, which involves being able to answer the following questions (Walston, 2016):

- What makes up organizational culture?
- How is culture created?
- How can culture be maintained?
- What causes culture to change?

Rituals and routines are usually social activities that reinforce the organization's values by soliciting active participation in the organization's activities and protocols. These activities assist in building bonds and strengthening relationships within the organization. Stories are also a good start when forming an organization's culture. Stories circulate throughout the organization and typically contain narrative events about the organization's founder. They cement the past while explaining and legitimizing the organization's current practices and procedures. Symbols and structures are also meaningful to culture and can include images, events, activities, or objects. All of these features help identify, characterize, or represent an entity, an idea, or a quality of most organizations (Walston, 2016).

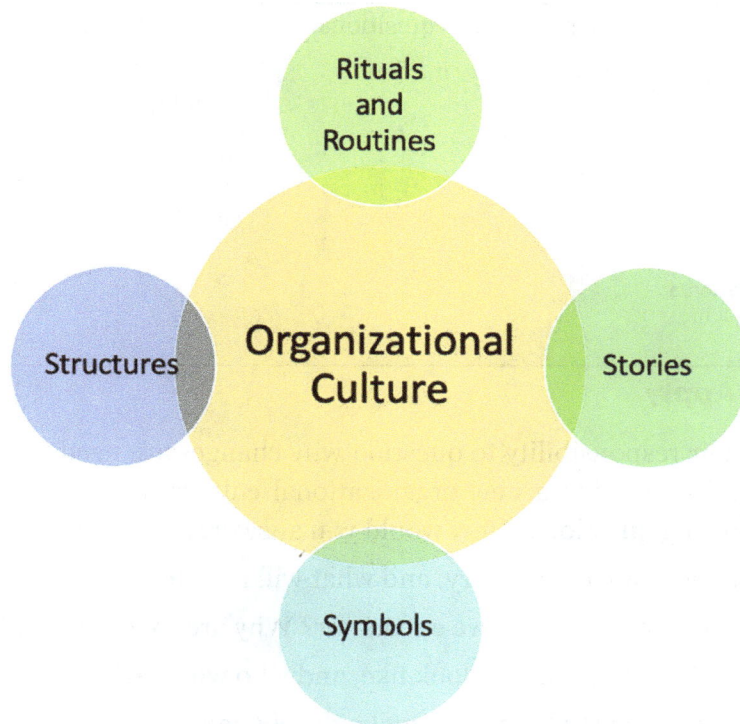

Figure 12.1: Components of an Organizational Culture

Source: Original Work
Attribution: Melissa Jordan
License: CC BY-SA 4.0

12.4 CHANGING ORGANIZATIONAL CULTURE

Understanding what changes need to be implemented and why these changes need to occur is important. If the change stems from strategic objectives, then it is a **strategic change**, and these changes are externally focused. If the change stems from operational assessments, then it is called a **process change**, and these changes are usually internal. Process change usually focuses on a particular unit, division, or function of the organization (Evans & Lindsay, 2014)

Table 12.1: Changing Organizational Culture	STRATEGIC CHANGE	PROCESS CHANGE
Theme of Change	***Shift in organizational direction***	***Adjustment of process***
Driving Force	Environmental forces—competition, technological changes, market	Internal—How can we improve or better align our processes?
Typical Antecedent	***Strategic Planning***	***Self-Assessment of Management System***
How much will the organization change?	Widespread	Usually narrow—divisional or functional

Examples	Mergers and acquisitions	Improving information systems,
	Entering new markets	Establishing hiring guidelines, and Developing improved customer satisfaction information

Source: Original Work
Attribution: Melissa Jordan
License: CC BY-SA 4.0

Stop and Apply

Regarding their responsibility to question why changes are needed in creating, changing, and sustaining a new organizational culture, the hospice manager asks the following questions (How would you answer?):

1. Is the change necessary, and what will it do for my organization?
2. What problems will we encounter? Why are we doing this?
3. What will the change look like, and who will it affect?
4. What needs to happen to make the change work?
5. What have we learned? How can we advance and/or continue to build after the change?

12.5 BARRIERS TO CHANGING AN ORGANIZATION'S CULTURE

Several barriers exist to change, and even more barriers exist when one is changing an organization's culture to transform their performance in order to lead to quality and excellence. According to Evans & Lindsay (2014), many leaders who fail to implement quality initiatives often have conflicting goals and simply do not follow through with the intended initiative. Another reason for failure is the lack of holistic system perspectives. The authors acknowledged that many approaches to implementing quality are often one-dimensional and prone to failing the overall goal. Focusing on a small area of the organization will render only small successes. When leaders concentrate on a very narrow area for change, small improvements occur rather than a large measurable improvement for the entire organization. The most significant failure encountered in most organizations is the lack of alignment and integration (Evans & Lindsay, 2014). **Alignment** refers to consistent plans, processes, information, resource decisions, actions, results, and analyses to support key organization-wide goals. Effective alignment calls for common understanding of the organization's purposes and goals. **Integration** refers to harmonizing plans, processes, information, resource decisions, actions, results, and analyses to support key organization-wide goals. Integration is successful when the individual components of a performance management system operate as a fully interconnected unit.

Stop and Apply

The hospice manager identifies the need to create a new organizational culture and is ready to implement changes for organizational performance improvement. What common barriers to change can you identify that the hospice manager may encounter? What are some examples you can use?

12.6 CULTURAL DIMENSIONS

As it relates to diversity, our world is changing, and so is our workplace. Individuals are finding that the people they work with may not have the same culture as they do, may be of a different gender, race, religion, and even ability. We have a wealth of knowledge and experience that we can put to use in the workplace by learning from one another. According to Walston (2016), we can start by understanding differences through the following dimensions: (1) Power distance, (2) Uncertainty avoidance, (3) Time orientation and (4) Individualism vs. collectivism.

Power distance— this dimension reflects on the way power is distributed and the degree to which individuals accept the inequality of power distribution. Low power equates to high power distribution and equality. High power distance results in powerful bosses, leader-only problem resolutions and a top-down direction.

Uncertainty avoidance— this dimension incorporates the degree to which members feel uncomfortable in uncertain situations and take action to avoid them. These individuals usually have inflexible codes of conduct and exhibit intolerance towards unorthodox behaviors.

Time orientation— this dimension involves the degree to which individuals are willing to defer their satisfaction and focus on achieving long-term, rather than short-term, goals or outcomes.

Individualism vs. collectivism— this aspect involves an individual's focusing their performance on personal (individual) gain rather than group benefits (collectivism). Individualism exists in a loose social framework in which responsibility is primarily only to oneself, whereas collectivism is seen in a tightly knit society whose members look after each other.

Stop and Apply

The hospice manager sees a need to identify factors with cultural differences in the workplace as they relate to service and process. What factors related to cultural differences can be identified? What are some examples you can use?

12.6.1 Effective approaches to a Positive Organizational Culture Change

A positive organizational culture emphasizes building and advancing the employees' strengths and rewards more than it punishes. It emphasizes the individual creativeness and diversity in its growth, where everyone has something to contribute to the organization. Numerous books have focused on effective approaches to organizational change. Schein (2010) suggests providing leaders with these six primary approaches to effect cultural change:

1. *Pay attention to measure and control those behaviors and outcomes important to change.* Select key indicators that signal desired changes, then monitor and reward or discipline as appropriate regarding the basis of the indicators.

2. *React to critical incidents and crises with a view of how management's behavior will affect the culture.* React consistently with valuable actions that emphasize and reinforce desired behaviors.

3. *Allocate resources towards enhancing organizational change.* Provide employees with the necessary resources to motivate and drive desired changes within the organization.

4. *Model, teach, and coach desired behaviors.* Leaders and managers should model the behaviors they want to see within their employees. Take time to teach, coach, and mentor individuals, groups, and teams.

5. *Allocate rewards and status to encourage cultural change.* Provide incentives and rewards to those who demonstrate positive cultural behaviors.

6. *Recruit, select, and promote employees who foster the desired culture, and terminate those who distract from it.* Establish hiring screening to test the best cultural fit for new employees of the organization. Be ready, willing, and able to act on those employees who decisively refuse to live by the new desired cultural values.

Stop and Apply

The hospice manager must decide which primary approach or approaches listed above would best benefit the organization's culture. What would you suggest the hospice manager use as an effective mechanism for organizational cultural change? What are the pros? What are the cons? Please explain why and give examples.

12.7 JOURNEY TOWARDS ORGANIZATIONAL CULTURE EXCELLENCE

In order for change to happen, leaders and managers must first consider which components to use in order to deal with the instability of the culture, the need for improvement, the need for innovation and creativity, and the desire for variety in employees' skills and tasks. According to Evans and Lindsay (2014), both the culture and the organizational structure must be designed to support the direction in which the organization is moving. The need for change is exemplified in the concept of a learning organization.

12.8 LEARNING ORGANIZATION

A **learning organization** is "an organization skilled in creating, acquiring, and transferring knowledge and in modifying the behavior of their employees and other contributors to their enterprises" (Evans and Lindsay, 2014).

Developing an effective learning organization depends on how well and effectively the leadership functions within the organization. Learning organizations should be able to perform these five main activities effectively:

1. *Systematic problem solving,* A learning organization should be able to effectively solve problems quickly without allowing the issues to grow into more challenges and/or obstacles. Effective leadership provides the guidance to solve problems quickly by making sound decisions with available resources and skilled employees. Effective leadership and management will move towards creative and innovative ways to solve problems.

2. *Experimentation with new approaches.* A learning organization is not afraid to take on a challenge and try something new. The fear of failure is always there, but an effective leader will model the way forward and be able to create a shared vision of where the organization will be and how to get the organization there.

3. *Learning from their own experiences and history.* Mistakes are human, and a learning organization will effectively advance towards excelling by learning from its experience and history. Leaders and managers will use experiences as a foundation to build upon, identifying what changes need to be made and understanding how they will make their organization and employees better.

4. *Learning from the experiences and best practices of others.* Learning from the experiences and best practices of others is reflected in benchmarking practices throughout learning organizations.

5. *Transferring knowledge quickly and efficiently throughout the organization.* Transferring knowledge quickly and efficiently

throughout the organization is the basic building block or foundation of knowledge management practices.

Stop and Apply

The hospice manager would like to talk with her supervisors and discuss implementing a learning organization. How should the hospice manager discuss the five main activities of a learning organization and how they can be utilized? Please give examples for five main activities that the hospice center can utilize.

12.9 CULTURAL ASSESSMENT

A cultural assessment is another type of assessment tool many organizations use to compare their organization's culture with their mission and core values. This type of assessment differs from a regular assessment because it focuses mainly on problem areas specifically dealing with the organization's culture. Leaders and managers must maintain proper alignment with the following questions (Walston, 2016):

- Can employees in the organization easily identify the core values?
- Do human resources specifically screen applicants who fit the desired company culture?
- What happens to the employees who do not fit the organizational values?
- Do leaders and managers monitor, measure, and evaluate people accountable for core values?
- Are individuals rewarded or given incentives for following core organizational values?
- Do leaders and managers model and demonstrate desired behavior towards the organization's values and norms through their actions?

Another way an organization can build learning into culture is by initiating a self-assessment indicating where the organization currently stands as it relates to best practices and continuous improvement requirements. Leaders and managers must understand that this type of assessment, along with any type of organizational change, takes time to process. Cultures must change or adapt to maintain the organization's alignment to its core values and mission in order to continue improving its services, products, and processes. A cultural assessment is just one way to uncover areas of organizational culture that do not align with core values and mission.

12.10 IMPLEMENTING A SELF-ASSESSMENT

Another way an organization can build learning into its culture is to implement self-assessments of where the organization currently stands as it relates to best practices and continuous improvement requirements. A **self-assessment** is "the holistic evaluation of processes and performance" (Evans & Lindsay, 2014). To manage self-assessment, leaders and managers should ask the following questions:

- How are we currently doing?
- What are our strengths?
- What are our weaknesses?
- Which areas need improving the most?
- What are our opportunities for improvement?
- What are our challenges for improvement?

According to Evans & Lindsay (2014), a self-assessment should address the following:

- *Management involvement and leadership.* To what extent is management involved at each organizational level?
- *Product and process design.* Do the products/services we have meet the customer's needs? Is the customer satisfied? Is the process effective and efficient for the services provided?
- *Product control.* Is a control system in place to monitor errors or defects before the problematic issues occur, rather than defect removal/replacement after the product is made or used?
- *Customer and supplier communications.* Do all employees understand who the customer is? How well do the customers communicate with the employees in order to form an effective relationship?
- *Quality improvement.* Is a quality improvement plan in place? What results have been achieved if such a plan is in place?
- *Employee participation.* Are all employees actively engaged in the organization's quality improvement?
- *Education and training.* What resources are available to ensure that everyone understands their job and the necessary skills and tasks associated with the job?
- *Quality information.* How is feedback on quality results collected and used?

Once information is gathered, leaders and managers often may not know what to do with it. Often the information may be hard to understand in terms of how to turn the data into action. Follow-up requires expertise from senior leaders to engage in action planning and tracking the implementation process. The action plan identifies certain activities necessary in addressing the quality improvement problems and issues. Once this information is identified, the action plan should be documented and communicated to inform individuals directly affected so as to gain their cooperation. Once this step is completed, the action plan should be reviewed to ensure it is addressing the key opportunities identified by the self-assessment findings (Evans & Lindsay, 2014).

Stop and Apply

The hospice manager, along with other department leaders and managers, decide to implement a self-assessment. Why would a self-assessment be valuable to the hospice manager? What issues should the self-assessment address? Please complete an example using the following points of a self-assessment:

- *Management involvement and leadership.* What extent at all levels of management is involved?

- *Product and process design.* Do the products/services meet the customers' needs? Is the customer satisfied? Is the process effective and efficient for the services produced?

- *Product control.* Is a control system in place to monitor errors or defects before the problematic issues occur, rather than defect removal/replacement after the product is made or used?

- *Customer and supplier communications.* Do all employees understand who the customers are? How well do the customers communicate with the employees in order to form an effective relationship?

- *Quality improvement.* Is a quality improvement plan in place? What results have been achieved if such a plan is in place?

- *Employee participation.* Are all employees actively engaged in the organization's quality improvement?

- *Education and training.* What resources are available to ensure that everyone understands their job and the necessary skills and tasks associated with it?

- *Quality information.* How is feedback on quality results collected and used?

12.11 CONCLUSION

Chapter twelve demonstrates how organizational culture influences the organization's performance. Leaders have a primary role in improving their organization's culture, which is a continuous and complex process. Leaders can demonstrate new behaviors by example and use primary approaches to motivate cultural change.

Topics discussed in this chapter are creating and sustaining organizational culture, barriers to changing an organization's culture, cultural dimensions, as well as effective approaches to a positive organizational culture change, journeying towards excellence in creating learning organizations, and implementing an organizational self-assessment.

12.12 KEY POINTS

- Organizational culture significantly influences whether a healthcare facility is a success or failure.

- Cultures can be classified into the dimensions of power distance, uncertainty avoidance, time orientation, and individualism versus collectivism.

- Each individual brings their own experiences and expertise to the table. The blending of these backgrounds can enhance productivity by allowing for the free flow of new ideas and creativity.

- An important aspect of a healthy culture is the presence of organizational justice. Companies that promote distributive, procedural, and interactional justice embed the concept of fairness, which leads to a positive culture.

- Both the culture and the organizational structure must be designed to support the direction in which the organization is moving, and the need for change is exemplified in the concept of a learning organization.

- Cultural assessments are just one way to uncover areas of organizational culture that do not align with core values and mission.

- Organizations can build learning into culture by implementing a self-assessment that shows where the organization currently stands as it relates to best practices and continuous improvement requirements.

12.13 KEY TERMS

Organizational culture, strategic change, process change, alignment, integration, power distance, time orientation, uncertainty avoidance, individualism vs. collectivism, learning organization, self-assessment.

12.14 QUESTIONS FOR REVIEW AND DISCUSSION

1. What are some characteristics of organizational culture?

2. Explain the difference between strategic change and process change.

3. Describe questions that organizations must ask and steps they must take on the managerial side in order to create and sustain a healthy

organizational culture.

4. Summarize in your own words a simple explanation of what senior leaders and managers need to do to accomplish creating a quality culture.

5. How would you describe the culture of your college or university?

6. What is your opinion on the future of a quality culture? Do you agree with the comments made in this chapter? Why or why not?

12.15 REFERENCES

Evans, J. R., Lindsay, W. M. (2014). *Managing for quality and performance excellence.* 9th Ed. Cengage Learning: Mason, OH

LSA Global. Ignoring corporate culture is a big mistake cartoon. Retrieved from https://lsaglobal.com/blog/ignoring-corporate-culture-big-mistake/

Robbins, S. P., Judge, T. A. (2011). *Organizational behavior.* 14th ed. Prentice Hall: Boston

Schein, E. H. (2010). *Organizational culture and leadership.* 4th ed. San Francisco: Jossey-Bass

Walston, S. L. (2016). *Organizational behavior and theory in health care.* Health Care Administration Press: Washington, DC

13 ORGANIZATIONAL PERFORMANCE

13.1 LEARNING OBJECTIVES

- To discuss the distinctive challenges facing healthcare organizations globally
- To describe performance management
- To analyze performance management through the Baldrige Criteria
- To investigate factors that lead to employee contribution
- To analyze methods of performance evaluation
- To describe tools for performance engagement, including key performance indicators
- To discuss customer engagement and workforce engagement
- To examine how organizations can contribute to performance improvements
- To analyze strategic advantages and opportunities
- To describe who the customer is in performance management
- To describe the purpose of an organization's performance assessment and list methods by which it can be done

13.2 INTRODUCTION

Organizational performance management is a necessary factor for the success of any business. Understanding performance standards and ensuring goals and objectives are effectively and efficiently met encompasses critical quality management. This chapter will explore the mechanisms used to manage performance in achieving goals, evaluating the process in meeting these goals, and encouraging constant improvement in the workplace. This chapter will focus on the section of the case study that emphasizes strategies on analyzing performance management. Factors will include recognizing methods for performance evaluation;

employee contribution; utilizing tools for performance engagement, including key performance indicators; and understanding who the customer in performance management is.

13.3 PERFORMANCE MANAGEMENT

For leaders and managers in healthcare, performance is a critical factor in the safety and health of the employees and organization itself. Management of organizational performance can be defined as "a process of establishing performance standards and evaluating performance to ensure that goals are being effectively accomplished" (Walton, 2017). Performance is also defined as "outputs and their outcomes obtained from processes, products, and customers that permit you to evaluate and compare your organization's results to performance projections, standards, past results, goals, and other organizations' results" (Baldrige, 2016).

13.4 ORGANIZATIONAL EXCELLENCE MODEL AND FRAMEWORK

One program highlighting the traits and attributes of organizational performance excellence is the Malcolm Baldrige National Quality Award (Baldrige, 2018). In the **Baldrige Excellence Framework**, the attributes of organizational performance excellence include these following criteria:

- Leadership
- Strategic planning
- Customer and market focus
- Measurement, analysis, and knowledge management
- Human resources/workforce focus
- Process management
- Business results

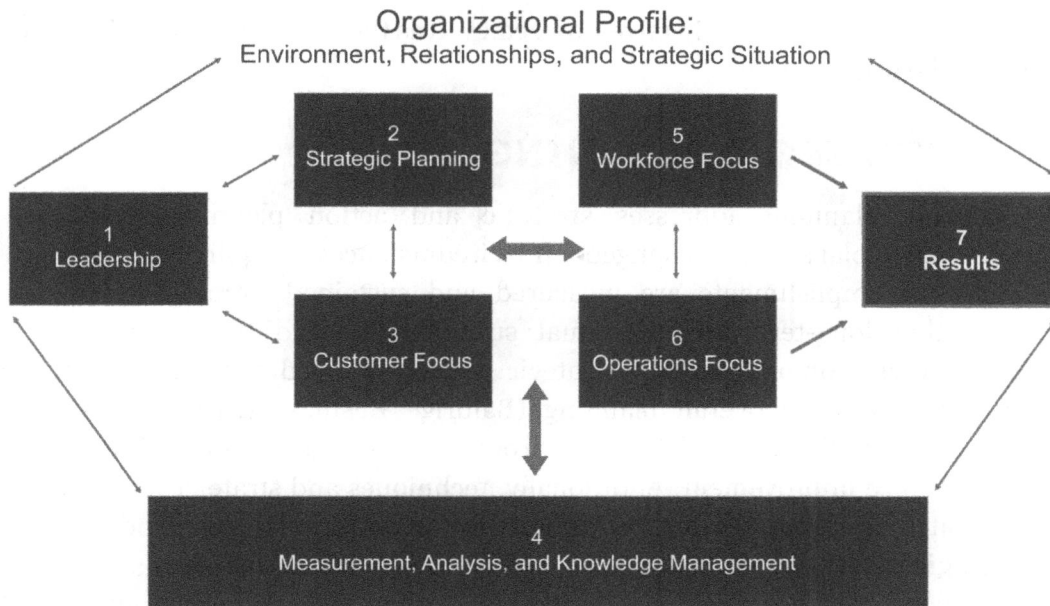

Figure 13.1: Baldrige Criteria

Source: Baldrige21
Attribution: Corey Parson, Adapted from Baldrige21
License: Fair Use

13.5 LEADERSHIP

The leadership section addresses how senior leaders guide and sustain the organization, setting organizational vision, values, and performance expectations. Attention is given to how leaders communicate with employees, develop future leaders, and create an environment that encourages ethical behavior and high performance. Leadership also includes the organization's governance system, its legal and ethical responsibilities to the public, and how the organization supports its community (Baldrige Business Excellence, 2018). The mission represents the organization's overall effectiveness in accomplishing these functions. The vision brings to fruition the organization's desired future state. Management's role is to be visionaries and futuristic thinkers who understand which segment or part of their organization's role serves in the customer, market, product offering, or workforce base.

All members of an organization need to comprehend that growth is movement towards improvement in providing excellence in products or services. Leaders of healthcare organizations have implemented balanced scorecards to measure performance management. A **balanced scorecard** is a reporting mechanism that incorporates financial and nonfinancial aspects of performance to allow a concise, comprehensive, and balanced perspective of the organization's performance results (Baldrige, 2016; Walston, 2017). Leaders must self-evaluate to make sure they are demonstrating competence in management domains, such as leadership skills and behaviors, organizational climate and culture, communicating mission and vision, and managing change effectively and efficiently. All must contribute to making sure the goals and objectives are achieved as they relate to the mission and vision of the organization.

13.6 STRATEGIC PLANNING

Strategic planning addresses strategic and action planning, deploying plans, how plans are changed if circumstances require a change, and how accomplishments are measured and sustained. Strategic planning stresses that long-term organizational sustainability and the organization's competitive environment are key strategic issues that need to be integral parts of the organization's overall planning (Baldrige Business Excellence, 2018). Knowledge regarding the healthcare environment must be considered in relation to performance improvement. Additionally, techniques and strategies need to be incorporated into processes that contribute to the organization's failure and success. A **strategic plan** incorporates tools that focus on current aims or responses that an organization articulates to address major change or improvement, competitiveness or social issues, and business advantages (Baldrige, 2016). **Strategic advantages** are those marketplace benefits that exert a decisive influence on the organization's likelihood of future success. These advantages frequently are sources of current and future competitive success relative to other providers of similar products. **Strategic challenges** are those pressures that exert a decisive influence over the organization's likelihood of future success. These challenges frequently are driven by the organization's anticipated competitive position in the future relative to other providers of similar products (Baldrige, 2016). **Strategic opportunities** are the prospects for new or changed products, services, processes, business models (including strategic alliances), or markets (Baldrige, 2016). Every organization should be aware that their performance should never be static. No matter how well their performance, services, and products may be, there is always room for improvement. Leaders and managers of healthcare organizations must understand that their organization must identify challenges related to hindering the accomplishment of their objectives and goals; they need to do so by observing possible strategic threats. A **strategic threat** is any significant aspect of the external environment that can block or derail the organization from moving to a brighter future that the strategic vision offers.

13.7 CUSTOMER FOCUS

Customer focus addresses how the organization seeks to understand the voices of customers and the marketplace, with a focus on meeting customers' expectations and requirements, delighting customers, and building loyalty. Customer focus stresses relationships as an important part of an overall listening, learning, and performance excellence strategy. The organization's customer satisfaction and dissatisfaction results provide vital information for understanding customers and the marketplace (Baldrige Business Excellence, 2018). In many cases, such results and trends provide the most meaningful information on not only the customers' views but also their marketplace behaviors, repeat business, and positive referrals—and how these views and behaviors may contribute to the organization's sustainability in the marketplace. Organizations must understand who their customers are and take this information into account on an internal and external basis. A **customer** is an actual or potential user of the organization's products, programs, or services. All employees should be familiar with their organization's mission, vision, and core competencies, especially in terms of their customers. **Core competencies** are the organization's areas of greatest expertise, those strategically important, possibly specialized capabilities that are central to fulfilling the mission or that provide an advantage in the marketplace or service environment (Baldrige, 2016). Excellence in understanding who the customer is in an organization will lead to improvement in services, products, and performance for employees, consumers, stakeholders, and the organization as a whole. Quality customer service leads to customer satisfaction, customer loyalty and customer retention. All are needed for an organization to thrive and compete in a global economy. **Customer engagement** is the organization's customers' investment in commitment to your brand and product offerings. As such, it reflects strategic success or limits in terms of the organization's mission and vision.

Stop and Apply

How well did the personnel in this case study know their patient? Can you think of a patient population (a culture, ethnicity, religious group, sexual orientation) with which you do not have much familiarity? How might this lack of knowledge impact your care? Regarding the case scenario, what could have been done to better serve Mr. Rodriguez? How could Mr. Rodriquez's risk management have been effectively assessed?

13.8 MEASUREMENT, ANALYSIS AND KNOWLEDGE MANAGEMENT

This area is the main point within the criteria for all key information about effectively measuring, analyzing, and reviewing performance and managing organizational knowledge in order to drive improvement and organizational competitiveness. It has been called the "brain center" for aligning the organization's operations and strategic objectives. Central to such use of data and information are their quality and availability. Furthermore, since information, analysis, and knowledge management might themselves be primary sources of competitive advantage and productivity growth, this area also includes such strategic considerations (Baldrige Business Excellence, 2018).

In order to understand and monitor the areas needed for improvement, they need to have clearly established goals and means of measurement. Leaders and managers can analyze areas for improvement through knowledge assets. **Knowledge assets** are the organization's accumulated intellectual resources, which include the knowledge possessed by the organization and its workforce in the form of information, ideas, learning, understanding, memory, insights, cognitive and technical skills, and capabilities. **Key indicators** are numerical information that quantifies the input, output, and performance dimensions of processes, products, programs, projects, services, and the overall organizational outcomes (Baldrige, 2016). These indicators are critical to performance management and so should incorporate periodic evaluation of these goals and objectives at appropriate time intervals. Performance projection is another measurement for analyzing performance improvement. An organization often will target its process in performance management through benchmarking. **Benchmarking** represents the processes and results that represent the best practices and best performance for similar activities, inside or outside the organization's industry. **Performance projection** provides estimates of the organization's future performance. Future performance can be examined by looking at the market's trends. **Trends** are numerical information that show the direction and rate of change for the organization's results and the consistency of its performance over time (Baldrige, 2016).

13.9 WORKFORCE FOCUS

Workforce focus addresses key *human resource* practices directed towards creating and maintaining a high-performance workplace and developing employees in order to enable them and the organization to adapt to change. This area covers human resource development and management requirements in an integrated way, e.g., alignment with the organization's strategic objectives and action plans. Human resource focus includes the work environment and the employee support climate (Baldrige Business Excellence, 2018). The organization's performance and point of contact is from the customer to the employee/workforce. Workforce focus incorporates the performance of the organization's workforce. A **workforce** comprises all people actively supervised by the organization and involved in accomplishing its work, including paid employees—e.g., permanent, part-time, temporary, on-site, and remote employees, as well as contract employees supervised by the organization—and volunteers, as appropriate. Workforce focus involves workforce capability, workforce capacity, and workforce engagement of employees. Leaders must understand that the workforce goals, objectives, and expectations must be realistic as they relate to workforce skills and task performance. Job satisfaction, job retention, employee coaching and mentoring, and training and development all play an integral role in the organization's performance. The goal is for leaders and managers to effectively and efficiently develop the workforce organization's most important internal value-creation processes.

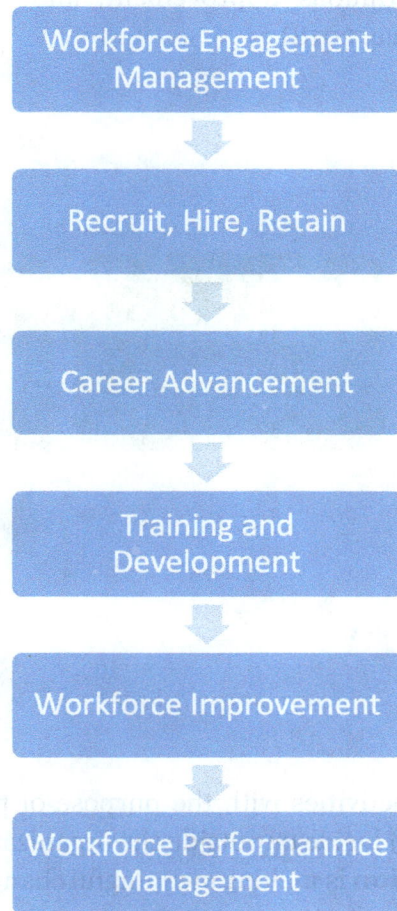

Figure 13.2: Workforce Engagement Management

Source: Original Work
Attribution: Melissa Jordan
License: CC BY-SA 4.0

Stop and Apply

The hospice manager believes in creating opportunities for the workforce to improve and grow in their job tasks for performance improvement. What are some ways the hospice manager can reinstate a human resource focus to include employees' work environment in order to support the current climate?

13.10 PROCESS MANAGEMENT

Process management is the focal point within the criteria for all key work processes. Built into this section are the central requirements for efficient and effective process management: effective design; prevention orientation; linkage to customers, suppliers, and partners, and a focus on value creation for all key stakeholders; operational and financial performance; cycle time; and evaluation, continuous improvement, and organizational learning (Baldrige Business Excellence, 2018).

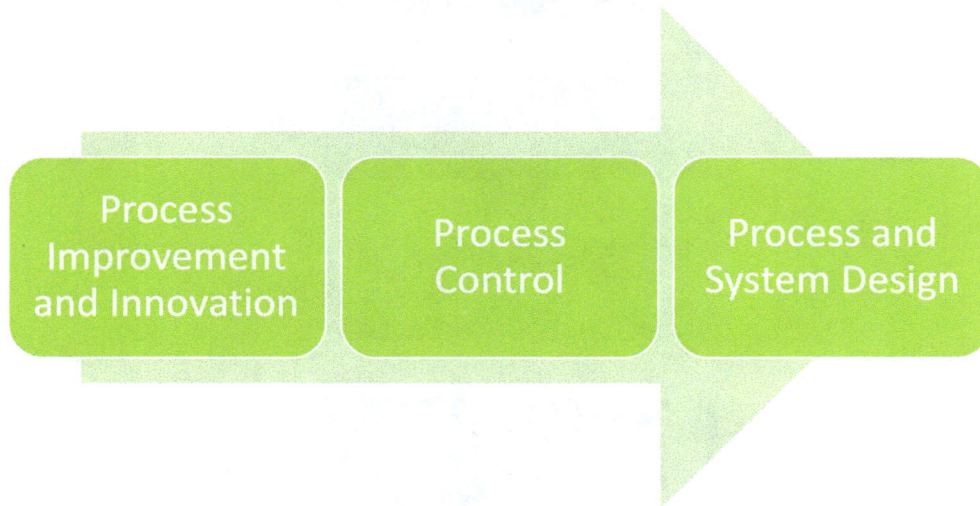

Figure 13.3: Process Management

Source: Original Work
Attribution: Melissa Jordan
License: CC BY-SA 4.0

Processes are linked activities with the purpose of producing a product or service for a customer (user) inside or outside the organization (Baldrige Business Excellence, 2018). **Innovation** is making meaningful change to improve products, processes, or organizational effectiveness and create new value for stakeholders. The outcome of innovation is a discontinuation of old processes or a breakthrough improvement (Baldrige, 2016).

Process improvement refers to the task of identifying opportunities for improvement, implementing changes, and, ideally, measuring the impact of those changes. Leaders and managers can use several tools for process improvement. For example, lean management is a familiar tool in the process improvement toolkit.

Process design is the activity of determining the workflow, equipment needs, and implementation requirements for a particular work process. Leaders and managers of healthcare organizations can use a number of tools available for performance improvement in process design, such as flowcharting, check lists, root cause analysis, force field analysis, pareto analysis, and cause and effect diagrams.

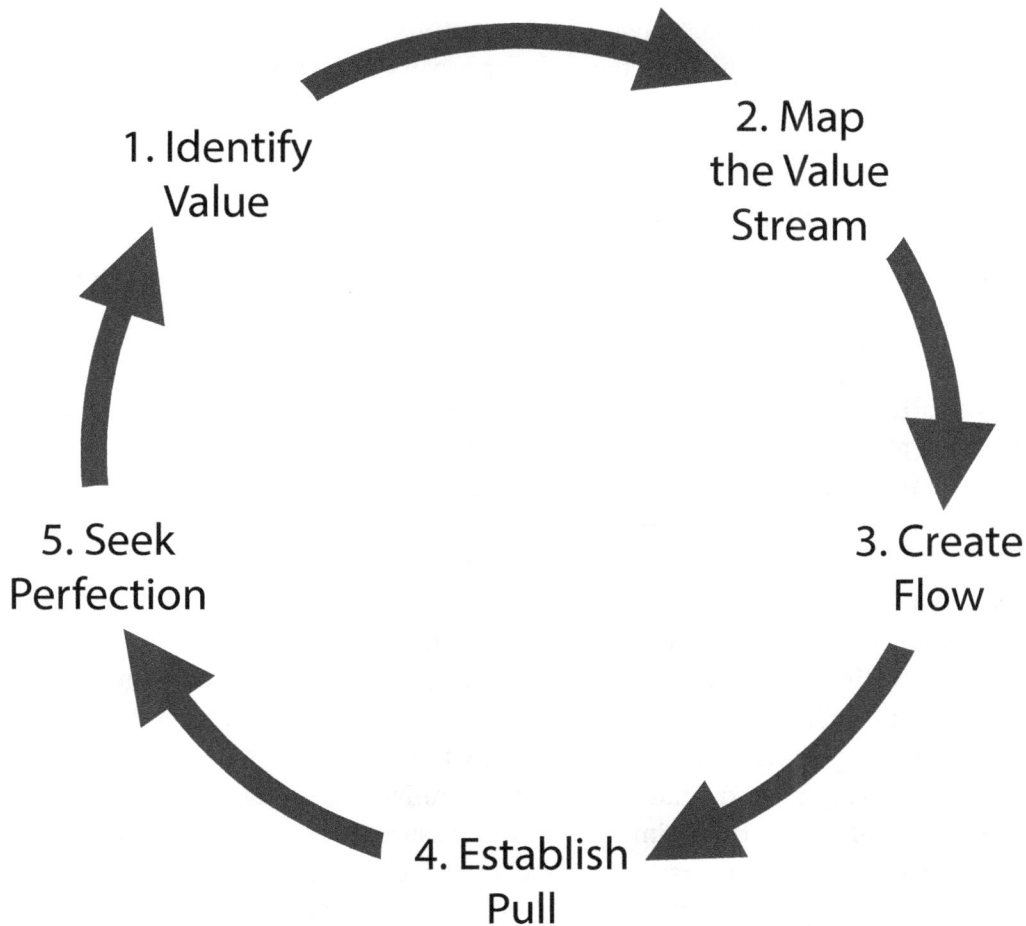

Figure 13.3: Customer Needs

Source: Lean Enterprise Institute, 2021
Attribution: Corey Parson, Adapted from Lean Enterprise Institute, 2021
License: Fair Use

The five-step thought process for guiding the implementation of lean techniques is easy to remember but not always easy to achieve (Lean.org). It involves the following:

1. *Identify Value.* Specify value from the standpoint of the end customer by product family.

2. *Map and Value Screen.* Identify all the steps in the value stream for each product family, eliminating whenever possible those steps that do not create value.

3. *Create Flow.* Make the value-creating steps occur in tight sequence so the product will flow smoothly toward the customer.

4. *Establish Pull.* As flow is introduced by letting customers pull value from the next upstream activity.

5. *Continuous Improvement.* As value is specified, value streams are identified, wasted steps are removed, and flow and pull are introduced;

begin the process again and continue it until a state of perfection is reached in which perfect value is created with no waste.

Stop and Apply

Create a "Five-Step" Process for process improvement in the case of Mr. Rodriquez.

13.11 RESULTS

Results are outputs and outcomes achieved by the organization. Leaders and managers at all levels and employees contributing either individually or as a team all have parts to play in successfully achieving performance management goals. The results category provides a results focus that encompasses the objective evaluation and the customers' evaluation of the organization's products and services, its overall financial and market performance, its leadership system and social responsibility results, and the key processes and process improvement activities (Baldrige Business Excellence, 2018). Through this focus, the criteria proposes superior value offerings, as viewed by the customers and the marketplace; superior organizational performance, as reflected in the operational, legal, ethical, and financial indicators; and maintenance of organizational and personal learning. Results provide "real-time" information (measures of progress) for evaluation and improvement of processes, products, and services, in alignment with the overall organizational strategy (Baldrige, 2016). Leaders and managers of healthcare organizations must understand how the organization performs in terms of customer satisfaction, finances, human resources, supplier and partner performance, operations, governance and social responsibility, and how the organization compares to its competitors.

Stop and Apply

How can leaders and managers understand how to get the best performance from individuals who bring their talents together for the common goal of accomplishing results efficiently and effectively?

13.12 CONCLUSION

This chapter discusses organizational performance management as a necessary factor for the success of any business. Understanding performance standards and ensuring goals and objectives are effectively and efficiently met encompass critical quality management. This chapter also explores the Baldrige Criteria for Organizational Excellence and identifies the mechanisms used to manage performance in achieving goals, evaluating processes in meeting these goals, and encouraging constant improvement in the workplace.

13.13 KEY POINTS

- Organizational performance management can be defined as a process of establishing and evaluating performance standards to ensure that goals are being effectively accomplished.

- Performance is also defined as outputs and their outcomes obtained from processes, products, and customers that permit leaders and managers to evaluate and compare the organization's results to performance projections, standards, past results, goals, and other organizational results.

- Strategic planning addresses strategic and action planning, deployment of plans, gauging how plans are changed if circumstances require a change, and how accomplishments are measured and sustained. Strategic planning stresses that long-term organizational sustainability and a competitive environment are key strategic issues that need to be integral parts of the organization's overall planning.

- The mission represents the organization's overall function towards accomplishing these functions. The vision supports the organization's desired future state.

- Management's role is to be visionaries and futuristic thinkers and to understand which segment or part of their organization's role plays in the customer, market, product offering, or workforce base.

- The Baldrige Excellence Framework—the attributes of organizational performance excellence—include the following criteria: (1) leadership, (2) strategic planning, (3) customer and market focus, (4) measurement, analysis, and knowledge management, (5) human resources/workforce focus, (6) process management, and (7) business results.

- Organizational performance management is a necessary factor for the success of any business. Understanding performance standards and ensuring goals and objectives are effectively and efficiently met encompass critical quality management.

13.14 KEY TERMS

Baldrige Excellence Framework, Baldrige Criteria, Performance, Performance Management, Core Competencies, Customer Focus, Customer Service, Teamwork, Continuous Improvement, Workforce Focus, Key Indicators, Knowledge Assets, Benchmark, Balanced Scorecard, Strategic Plan, Trends, Performance Projection, Process, Strategic Plan, Strategic Advantages, Strategic Opportunities, Strategic Threat, Customer Engagement, Process Management.

13.15 QUESTIONS FOR REVIEW AND DISCUSSION

1. One aspect of patient-centered care is fostering a culturally sensitive and diverse clinical environment that makes patients feel more welcome. What are some ways in which this goal may be accomplished?

2. In order to provide good care for a culturally diverse patient population, it is important to gain some understanding of their ways of being (their belief systems, their traditions, their feelings towards western medicine, etc.). Can you think of a particular patient population in your area that may have unique beliefs about health and illness that would be important to understand?

3. How well do you know your patients? Can you think of a patient population (a culture, ethnicity, religious group, sexual orientation) with which you do not have much familiarity? How might this lack of knowledge impact your care?

4. What are some ways in which you could be better educated in regards to the beliefs and traditions of the patient population in your area? How might that intervention benefit the patients?

5. Discuss a time when you had a bad experience with either a customer or customer service representative. What could have been done differently? How could the performance be improved?

6. Discuss staff morale at your organization. Do people feel joy in work? Do they feel burned out? What factors influenced your answer?

13.16 REFERENCES

ASQ.ORG. Quality quotes. Retrieved from, https://asq.org/quality-resources/more-on-quality-quotes

Baldrige Business Excellence. Baldrige Criteria. Retrieved from http://www.baldrige21.com/

Baldrige, M. (2016). Baldrige key terms. Retrieved from https://www.nist.gov/baldrige/self-assessing/baldrige-key-terms#performance

Business Dictionary. Process design. Retrieved from http://www.businessdictionary.com/definition/process-design.html

Goetsch, D. L., & Davis, S. B. (2016). *Quality management for organizational excellence: Introduction to quality*. 8th Edition. Pearson.

HR Bartender. "Employee Engagement." Retrieved from https://www.hrbartender.com/2018/employee-engagement/minimize-employee-distractions/

Institute for Health Improvement. Cause and effect diagram. Retrieved from http://www.ihi.org/education/IHIOpenSchool/resources/Pages/AudioandVideo/Whiteboard16.aspx

Institute for Health Improvement. "Four steps leaders can take to increase joy in work." Retrieved from http://www.ihi.org/education/IHIOpenSchool/resources/Pages/AudioandVideo/Jessica-Perlo-Four-Steps-Leaders-Can-Take-to-Increase-Joy-in-Work.aspx

Institute for Health Improvement. "The crowded clinic." Retrieved from http://www.ihi.org/education/IHIOpenSchool/resources/Pages/Activities/TheCrowdedClinic.aspx

Lean.org. Principles of Lean. Retrieved from https://www.lean.org/WhatsLean/Principles.cfm

Walston, S. L. (2016). *Organizational behavior and theory in health care.* Health Care Administration Press: Washington, DC

14 MANAGING ORGANIZATIONAL CHANGE

14.1 LEARNING OBJECTIVES

- To analyze distinctive challenges facing healthcare organizations globally
- To examine ways of creating a culture of change in the workplace
- To discuss global challenges to change
- To analyze the effects of workforce, technology, economic shock, competition, social trends, and world politics changes in the workplace
- To describe stress associated with workplace changes and identify sources/stressors
- To investigate individual and organizational approaches to managing stress through creating a healthy work-life balance

14.2 INTRODUCTION

Chapter fourteen provides strategies for managing organizational change. From managing individuals and understanding group dynamics to managing conflict and initiating change, organizational alterations affect everyone in an organization. This chapter will focus on the case study section regarding the different challenges healthcare hospice employees encountered with Mr. Rodriquez. These challenges included locating pertinent departments, prevention of using faulty equipment on patients, challenges focusing on change in the hospice center and around the world, and management of stress in the workplace by identification of sources/stressors.

According to the Cambridge Dictionary (2019), **organizational change** is "a process in which a large company or organization changes its working methods or aims, for example in order to develop and deal with new situations or markets." **Change** is the act or instance of making something different from what it originally was. Realizing that change is inevitable, organizations must understand how to manage change in order to improve, and that evaluating where improvements need to be made in itself involves change. Many people have stated one must adapt to change or die because no company today is in a stable environment. Leaders and managers will find themselves implementing changes that are necessary for growth and improvement. They may have to act as change agents. A **change agent** is a person inside or outside the organization who will assist in the transformation by focusing on continuous improvement, effectiveness, process, and development.

14.3 UNDERSTANDING FORCES OF CHANGE

Forces of change are internal or external forces that can disturb an organizational system. These forces include the nature of the workforce, technology, economic shocks, competition, social trends, and world politics. These challenges can directly or indirectly affect the quality of healthcare services and products (Robbins & Judge, 2011).

Nature of the workforce includes the demographics of a population, like aging, cultural diversity, and increased immigration.

Technology includes social networking sites, online resources, telemedicine, efficiency and easy usage, and growth of computers.

Economic shocks include the global recession, financial funding, and employment.

Competition includes regulation of commerce, other healthcare agencies offering the same or better services, mergers and consolidations.

Social trends include increased awareness of the environment, sustainability, increased knowledge on how information is shared due to the information available through social networking, and streamlined operations.

World politics include relationships with other countries, changes in opinions due to violence and wars, as well as scrutiny and level of trust in the financial sectors.

14.4 OVERCOMING RESISTANCE TO CHANGE

Change is natural and often a necessity for individual, team, and organizational growth. Leaders and managers will be met with individuals who welcome the change and individuals who resist it. Leaders and managers must implement a change management strategy in which the mission, vision, and goals are shared by others. This plan can be accomplished through open communication, participation, building a learning organization, recruiting advocates of change by building support, and operating in a fair manner. Communication and awareness of changes can help ease the tension for those the change will affect. This strategy is just one way leaders and managers can clear up misunderstandings, false information, and create a less stressful environment.

Stop and Apply

The hospice manager decides to immediately call a department meeting to focus on improving the quality of care given to Mr. Rodriquez and address employee concerns. As the manager of the hospice center and an acting change agent, what are the forces of change that can be identified in the case study at the beginning of this textbook? In what ways could the manager of the hospice center overcome resistance to change(s)?

14.5 APPROACHES TO MANAGING ORGANIZATIONAL CHANGE

Leaders and managers can utilize several approaches for effective organizational change. This chapter will discuss Lewin's Three-Step Change Model (1951) and Kotter's Eight-Step Plan for Implementing Change (2007).

14.5.1 Lewin's Three-Step Change Model

Kurt Lewin developed **Lewin's three-step process for implementing change** (1951), which included the following steps: unfreezing, changing, and refreezing.

Unfreezing identifies the status quo or the problem/issue's current level of acceptance that is hindering the organization from moving forward. During this stage, old behaviors are identified, processes are evaluated, and people and structures are examined to show how necessary the change is in order to create improvements or advantages for the organization. During this step, communication is crucial so that employees are informed and educated about the impending changes to come.

Changing is the next step. This step is often referred to as "moving" or "transitioning" to the new situation or status. Leaders and managers must identify that this is the stage where individuals will have difficulty moving forward. Change affects people differently, especially if they must learn new behaviors, processes, or ways of thinking. Again, communication, awareness, education, and support are vital to easing a stressful transition period. Leaders and managers must understand that, for the sake of the organization as a whole, change must be carefully planned and implemented.

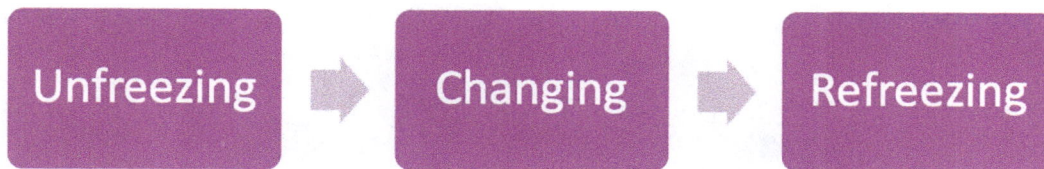

Figure 14.1: Lewin's Change Model

Source: Original Work
Attribution: Melissa Jordan
License: CC BY-SA 4.0

Refreezing is reinforcing the change and solidifying the new condition of change. The changes are accepted and refrozen as the new status quo, and leaders and managers must model the way to make sure employees do not revert to old, ineffective habits. These changes must be solidified into the organization's culture to make sure the change is actively present.

Stop and Apply

After a few meetings with department heads and employees of the hospice center, the hospice manager decides to apply Lewin's Three-Step Change Model to the problem area of miscommunication between employees during a code.

- How would the hospice manager 'unfreeze' the current level of acceptance for miscommunication between employees in the case study?

- How would the hospice manager implement "changing" the current level of acceptance for miscommunication between employees?

- How would the hospice manager 'refreeze' the new changes implemented so employees would not revert to old, ineffective ways and habits?

14.5.2 Kotter's Eight-Step Plan for Implementing Change

John Kotter developed **Kotter's Eight Steps to Implementing Change** (2007) and the strategies used to overcome such problems. He built on Lewin's three-step model by adding more detail on how to implement change in an organization. Kotter reviewed common mistakes and issues when initiating change in the workplace. He explained how these mistakes can prolong and/or hinder change and eventually impede in achieving the organization's mission, vision, and upholding core values.

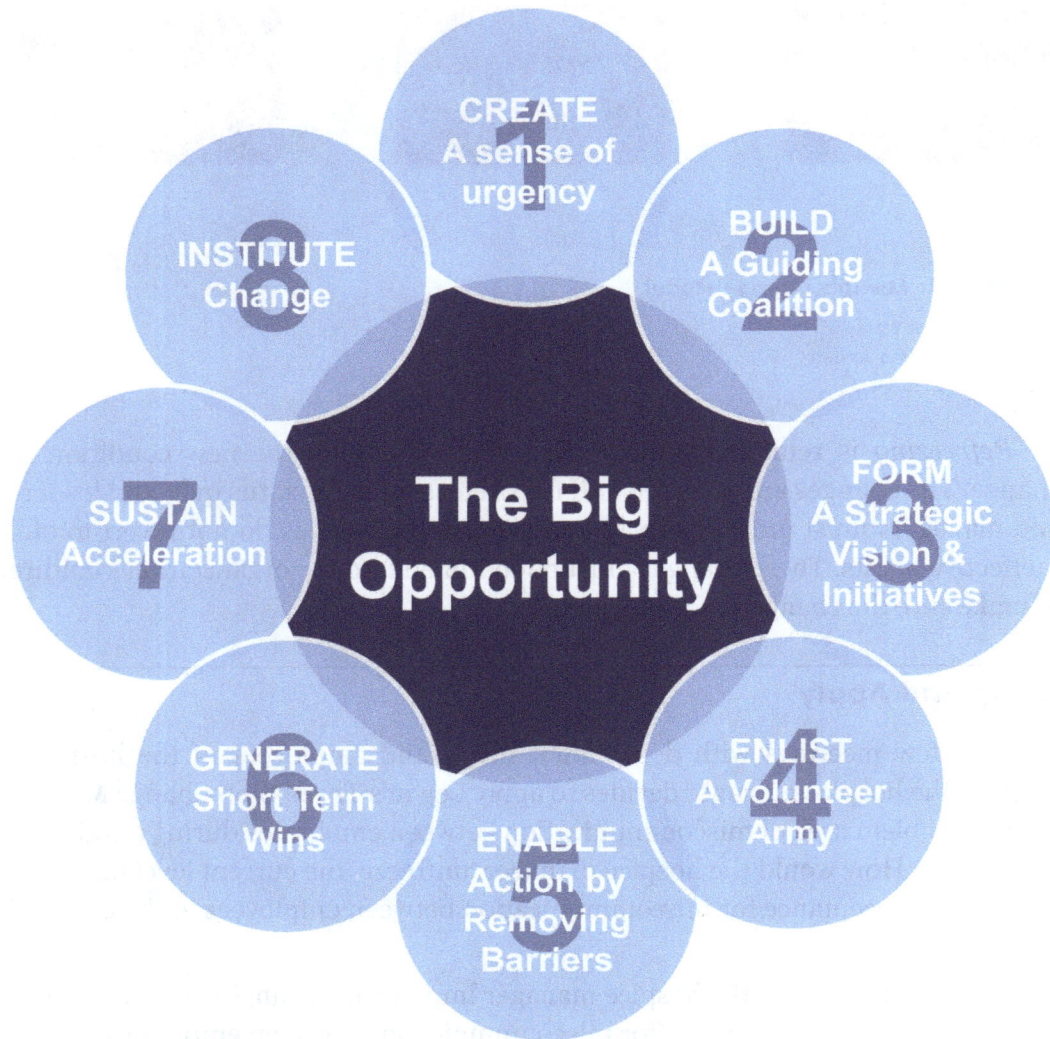

Figure 14.2: Kotter's Change Model

Source: Original Work
Attribution: Corey Parson
License: CC BY-SA 4.0

These steps included the following:

1. *Create a sense of urgency.* Leaders and managers should act quickly when identifying problem areas that need changing for improving services and products. During this phase, investigation is pertinent in identifying why change is necessary.

2. *Build a guiding coalition.* Power is needed to lead different individuals towards a common and shared goal.

3. *Form a strategic vision and initiatives.* Leaders and managers must build the foundation of change upon the vision of where they want to see the most improvement. Forming a vision and creating initiatives will assist in employees gaining full understanding of why the change

is necessary and how they plan to implement the change in moving forward.

4. *Enlist an army*. Building an army of like-minded people will help leaders and managers in the recruitment of leading and managing change.

5. *Enable action by removing barriers*. This step is crucial in the role of leading. Building a team of people that can empower others to act on and communicate the vision, and initiatives assists in removing barriers; it encourages creative and innovative thinking.

6. *Generate short term wins*. Change requires effective planning in order to create small "wins" for the organization as a whole. Leaders and managers must understand that change can be difficult but necessary, and how effectively and efficiently that change is made depends on how well it was planned for.

7. *Sustain acceleration*. Keep the changes' movements active and alive. If necessary, consolidate and collaborate on the improvements needed, re-evaluate the changes, and make the necessary modifications or adjustments as necessary.

8. *Institute changes*. Leaders and managers must model the way. Positively reinforce the changes by demonstrating positive behaviors and acknowledging organizational success.

Stop and Apply

The hospice manager decides new life saving equipment with appropriate labels and stickers is needed at the hospice center. All employees involved with patient care must be trained on this new equipment and how to identify the labels and stickers. Immediately, employees resist learning how to operate the new equipment when they are familiar with operating the equipment they have used for years. The hospice manager decides to implement Kotter's Eight-Step Plan for Implementing Change. How should she proceed with this change?

14.6 MANAGING ORGANIZATIONAL CHANGE THROUGH INNOVATION

According to Merriam-Webster (2019), **creativity** is "the ability to create," and **innovation** is defined as "the introduction of something new or a new idea, method, or device."

Creativity is affected by changing an environment through knowledge, leadership, and the organization's culture. However, creativity alone is not enough to transform ideas into quality products and services, effective and efficient processes, and quality improvements. Innovation creates a unique style of change in the workplace by allowing new ideas to be initiated for improvements of products, processes, or services. Leaders and managers can stimulate change through innovation techniques.

According to Walston (2016), certain activities can influence and encourage creativity and innovation in the workplace. These activities focus on three areas: Employees' Culture, Jobs, and Leaders and Rewards.

Table 14.1: Activities that encourage innovation	
	Activities that encourage innovation
Employees Culture	• Hire employees with creative and innovative characteristics. • Create a diverse pool of employees throughout the organization. • Provide the necessary training and development of resources. • Create an innovative 'mindset' throughout the workplace.
Jobs	• Allow time for employees to hone creativity and innovation skills. • Design jobs inventiveness, resourcefulness, significance, and variety. • Make time for employees to form a true relationship with customers/patients.
Leaders and Rewards	• Mission, vision, and core values should be clear. • Acknowledge and reward creativity and innovation. • Apply a participative leadership style.

Source: Original Work
Attribution: Melissa Jordan
License: CC BY-SA 4.0

Stop and Apply

The hospice manager is pleased with the positivity and changes thus far in improving the medical processes, products, and services of the hospice center. Now the manager would like to create a culture for creativity and innovation for the employees and their jobs.

- Which activities would you choose to encourage innovation, and how would you use them in this case study scenario?

- Why are you choosing these activities and in what way do they benefit the hospice center?

14.7 EFFECTIVE CHANGE WITH STRESS MANAGEMENT AND WORK-LIFE BALANCE

According to Robbins & Judge (2011), **stress** is "a dynamic condition in which an individual is confronted with an opportunity, a demand, or a resource related to what the individual desires and for which the outcome is perceived to be both uncertain and important." Change in general can bring emotions of fear, anxiety, and panic. Stress can cause low productivity, poor ability to complete tasks, poor job performance, and insecurities in abilities, low self-esteem, and even a hostile environment. Leaders and managers must recognize the causes of stress and offer possible resources and solutions on how to deal with it in the workplace.

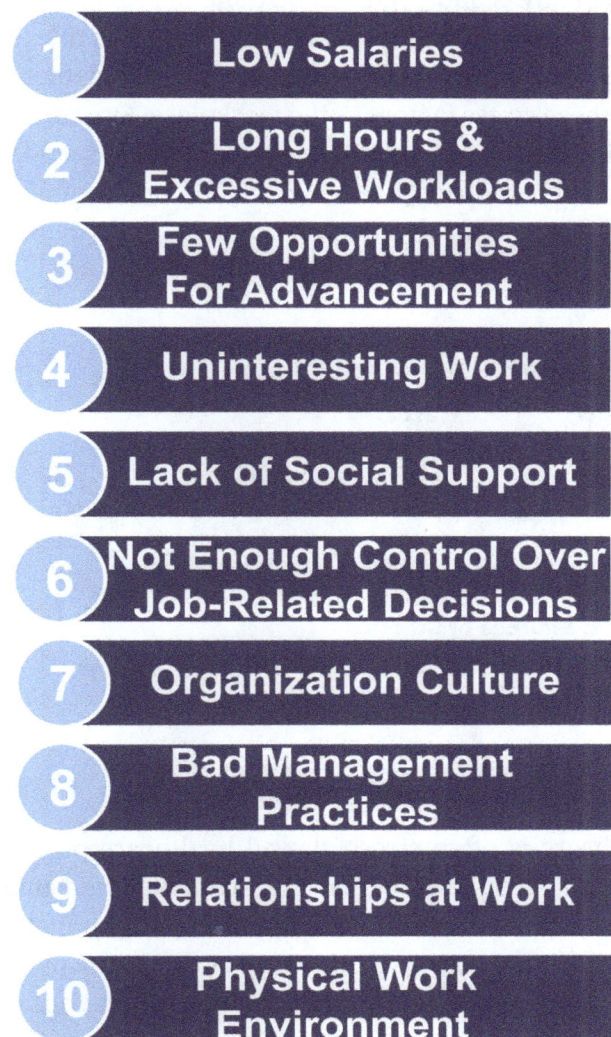

1. Low Salaries
2. Long Hours & Excessive Workloads
3. Few Opportunities For Advancement
4. Uninteresting Work
5. Lack of Social Support
6. Not Enough Control Over Job-Related Decisions
7. Organization Culture
8. Bad Management Practices
9. Relationships at Work
10. Physical Work Environment

Figure 14.3: Top 10 Workplace Stressors

Source: Original Work
Attribution: Corey Parson
License: CC BY-SA 4.0

14.7.1 Potential Sources of Stress

Recognizing what causes stress is the first step in understanding how to move forward towards organizational improvement. A **stressor** is a condition which keeps an employee from reaching their goals or creates an obstacle associated with workload, tasks, and time urgency (Robbins & Judge, 2011). Three categories are identified as potential sources of stress: environmental factors, organizational factors, and personal factors.

14.7.2 Approaches to Managing Stress in the Workplace

As stated above, leaders and managers must evaluate and manage the causes and consequences of stress and what can be done to reduce it in the organization. Many workplace factors cause stress, particularly, task and role demand. These are often controlled by management, which means that management has the ability to modify or change these stress factors in the workplace. Organizational approaches can include training and development, realistic job tasks and settings, realistic time management and workloads, a redesign of jobs, open communication through employee discussions and involvement in change, and organizational wellness programs.

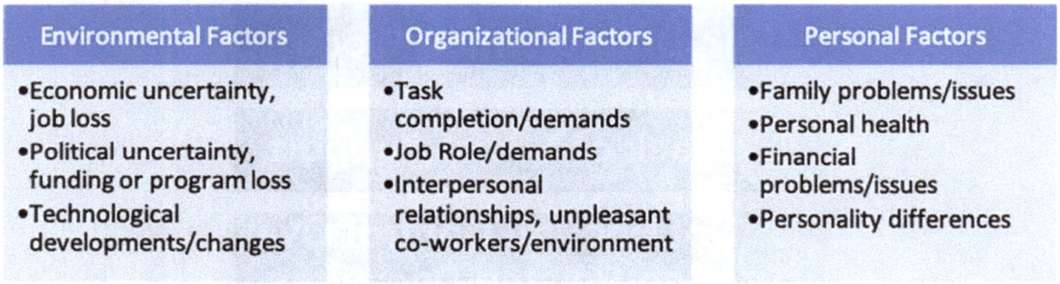

Environmental Factors	Organizational Factors	Personal Factors
•Economic uncertainty, job loss •Political uncertainty, funding or program loss •Technological developments/changes	•Task completion/demands •Job Role/demands •Interpersonal relationships, unpleasant co-workers/environment	•Family problems/issues •Personal health •Financial problems/issues •Personality differences

Figure 14.4: Potential Sources of Stress

Source: Original Work
Attribution: Melissa Jordan
License: CC BY-SA 4.0

14.7.3 Creating Work-Life Balance

Work in healthcare is often stressful, and healthcare professionals are often burned out early into their healthcare careers. Leaders and managers can assist employees in managing their stress to create stability in producing a healthy work-life balance. **Work-life balance** is a term used to describe a person's work and life roles. It also describes the balanced state of equality demands on an individual's personal and professional life. Leaders and managers can create a stable and realistic work-life balance for employees through flexible work arrangements, paid or unpaid time off for mental rejuvenation, remote or work from home job positions, and creating job positions in which job responsibilities can be shared with other employees.

Stop and Apply

The hospice manager identifies that the employees of the hospice center are under immense stress from the changes implemented. This has created an environment heavy with anxiety and panic. The hospice manager wants to implement one more change in managing and creating a healthy work-life balance for all. What would you suggest in decreasing work stress to have an effective work-life balance?

14.8 CONCLUSION

The need for change is necessary for organizational improvement, and leaders and managers are the primary change agents. Their ability to model the way, create a shared vision, demonstrate acceptance with new behaviors towards the change, and develop a new organizational culture that generates acceptance to change move the organization towards improvements of services, products, and processes.

14.9 KEY POINTS

- Change is natural and often a necessity to individual, team, and organizational growth.

- Forces of change are internal or external forces that can disturb an organizational system. These forces include the nature of the workforce, technology, economic shocks, competition, social trends, and world politics.

- Kurt Lewin developed Lewin's three-step process for implementing change which included these steps: unfreezing, changing, and refreezing.

- John Kotter built on Lewin's three-step model by being more detailed about how to implement change in an organization and reviewing common mistakes and issues when initiating change in the workplace.

- Innovation creates a unique style of change in the workplace by allowing new ideas to be initiated for improving products, processes, or services. Leaders and managers can stimulate change through innovation techniques.

- Leaders and managers can create a stable and realistic work-life balance for employees through flexible work arrangements, paid or unpaid time off for mental rejuvenation, remote or work from home job positions, and creating job positions in which job responsibilities can be shared with other employees.

14.10 KEY TERMS

Organizational Change, Change Agent, Forces of Change, Lewin's Three-Step Process for Implementing Change, Kotter's Eight-Step Plan for Implementing Change, Creativity, Work-Life Balance

14.11 QUESTIONS FOR REVIEW AND DISCUSSION

1. What forces stimulate change?

2. How can managers create a culture for change?

3. Think about a problem you need to solve through change. How would you apply Lewin's Three-Step Method or Kotter's Eight-Step Model for Implementing Change?

4. What is the difference between innovation and creativity? Can an organization have innovation without creativity?

5. Think about your work-life balance. What are some areas of stress in your work-life, and which discussed approach would you use to decrease or eliminate it in order to create a healthy work-life balance?

14.12 REFERENCES

Cambridge Dictionary (2019). Organizational change definition. Retrieved from https://dictionary.cambridge.org/dictionary/english/organizational-change

Elliot, T. (2014). Time to innovate cartoon. Retrieved from https://timoelliott.com/blog/2014/07/cartoon-the-perils-of-business-innovation.html

Kotter, J.P. (2007). "Leading change: Why transformational efforts fail." *Harvard Business Review* 85, 96-103.

Kouzes, J. M., Posner, B. Z. (2002). *The leadership challenges*. 3rd ed. Jossey-Bass: CA.

Lewin K (1951) *Field Theory in Social Science: Selected Theoretical Papers* (ed. Cartwright D). New York: Harper & Row.

Merriam-Webster (2019). Innovation definition. Retrieved from https://www.merriam-webster.com/dictionary/innovation

Robbins, S. P., Judge, T. A. (2011). *Organizational behavior*. 14th ed. Prentice Hall: Boston

15 ORGANIZATIONAL CHALLENGES FROM A GLOBAL PERSPECTIVE

15.1 LEARNING OBJECTIVES

- To examine distinctive challenges facing healthcare organizations globally
- To describe how to overcome challenges through best practices from a global perspective
- To describe contributing factors to health care professional workforce shortages
- To analyze recent trends and opportunities from a global perspective for health care organizations
- To examine the key trends that are evolving in health care organizations
- To investigate areas within your own career and organization with future strategic positions in health care
- To analyze strategies that can solve problems that have an impact on the quality and appropriateness of diagnostics and therapeutic procedures that have a heavy impact on cost at the hospice center
- To discuss how to evaluate the components of a long-term care strategy

15.2 INTRODUCTION

Health care organizations will face many challenges as the world continues to evolve over time. Understanding key operations management during these challenging times will further drive operational excellence through addressing increased visibility and resources for patients, creating integrated service delivery systems, developing greater collaborations with payers and vendors, developing a process for additional education for health care administrators, and having a strategic focus on value in all parts of a health care organization. This chapter presents global organizational challenges, such as aging populations, health care accessibility, health care provider shortages, technology, and reformed and value-based health care systems. It will focus on overcoming challenges through best practices, dealing with healthcare professional workforce challenges, identifying strategies that can assist in decision making and solving problems, and determining the impact of quality and appropriateness of diagnostic and therapeutic procedures affecting cost at the hospice center in this particular case study.

15.3 HEALTHCARE PROVIDERS AND SHORTAGES

The U.S. has made great strides in providing quality care to individuals through continuous improvements in products, services, and processes. The U.S. health care industry is the largest employer in the nation, and employs at least 13% of the total labor force in the U.S., according to the Bureau of Labor Statistics (2014). For three unique reasons, the health care segment of the U.S. economy will continue to grow because of the overall growth in the U.S. population. These reasons for this population growth are (1) mainly immigration; (2) the aging population, which increases as baby boomers continue to turn 65 years and older through 2029; and (3) increased life expectation. According to Merriam-Webster, a **Baby Boomer** is a person born in the U.S. following the end of World War II (usually considered to be the years from 1946 to 1964).

This growth in the U.S. population has driven the demand for highly skilled and competent health service professionals. Health care professionals follow demographic trends, including continued improvements in research and technology, disease and illness trends, and the constant changes related to health insurance coverages and service delivery. An effective health system can function only with highly qualified health workers upholding the highest attainable standard of health. This attainment will only be achieved through the availability, accessibility, acceptability, and quality of those health care professionals. From a global perspective, the World Health Organization (WHO) (2019) has estimated that 18 million additional health workers will be needed by 2030 in low and lower-middle income countries.

The largest array of health care professionals needed ranges from various roles in health care practice settings in which they are generally employed, and the critical issues concerning their professions. Our world of health care is facing an imbalance of primary and specialty services, misdistribution of practitioners, and impending health care professional shortages.

According to Shi & Singh (2017), health professionals are among the most educated and diverse of all workforce groups. The majority of these health professionals (39%) are employed by hospitals (U.S. Bureau of Labor Statistics, 2014).

15.3.1 Physicians and Surgeons

Physicians are individuals who play a key role in the health care of an individual by evaluating a patient's condition by the signs, symptoms, and test results, and prescribing treatment along with the possibility of medication therapy. Physicians and surgeons diagnose and treat injuries or illnesses. Physicians examine patients; take medical histories; prescribe medications; and order, perform, and interpret diagnostic tests. They often counsel patients on diet, hygiene, and preventive healthcare. Surgeons operate on patients to treat injuries, such as broken bones; diseases, such as cancerous tumors; and deformities, such as cleft palates. Many physicians and surgeons work long, irregular, and overnight hours. Physicians and surgeons may travel between their offices and hospitals to care for their patients. While on call, a physician may need to address a patient's concerns over the phone or make an emergency visit to a hospital or nursing home.

All states require physicians to be licensed before they can practice medicine, and the licensure requirements may vary from state to state. Some physician licensure requirements include graduation from an accredited medical school that awards a Doctor of Medicine or Doctor of Osteopathic Medicine, successful completion of a licensing examination administered by either the National Board of Medical Examiners or the National Board of Osteopath Medical Examiners, and completion of a supervised internship/residency program (Shi & Singh, 2017).

Many physicians and surgeons work in physicians' offices. Others work in hospitals, in academia, or for the government. Increasingly, physicians are working in group practices, healthcare organizations, or hospitals, where they share a large number of patients with other doctors. The group setting allows them more time off and lets them coordinate care for their patients; however, it gives them less independence than solo practitioners have. Surgeons and anesthesiologists usually work in sterile environments while performing surgery and may stand for long periods (BLS, 2019).

Forthcoming Shortages for Physicians

The growing and aging population is expected to drive overall growth in the demand for physician services. As the older population grows and rates of chronic illnesses increase, consumers will seek high levels of care that use the latest technologies, diagnostic tests, and therapies. Demand for physicians and surgeons is expected to increase, despite factors that can temper growth. New technologies, such as improved information technologies or remote monitoring, are expected to allow physicians to treat more patients in the same amount of time. If adopted, new technologies can reduce the number of physicians who would be needed to complete the same tasks. Demand for physicians' services is sensitive to changes in healthcare reimbursement policies. Consumers may seek fewer physician services if changes to health coverage result in higher out-of-pocket costs for them (BLS, 2019).

A projected shortfall of between 46,100 and 90,400 physicians is foreseen by 2025. Projected shortfalls in primary care will range from between 12,500 and 31,100 by 2025 and between 28,200 and 63,700 in various physician specialties (Shi & Singh, 2017). The Affordable Care Act (ACA) expanded medical coverage, which has likely increased the demand for physicians. The ACA is addressing the shortages by seeking to modify federal Medicare payments for medical residency training and to authorize more funding for medical residency training programs. The ACA has established the National Health Care Workforce Commission, which is tasked with developing a national workforce strategy (Shi & Singh, 2017).

Geographic Misdistribution

Many physicians choose to work in metropolitan and suburban areas rather than rural or inner-city areas because the standard of living, professional growth, salary, professional integration, access to modern facilities, and advancements in technology are more favorable. Often, the actual delivery of services depends on the individual's ability to pay, and many people living in rural and inner cities areas do not have that ability (i.e., money or medical insurance). This predicament often leaves rural and inner city areas with severe provider shortages.

If the physician is a primary physician, then the higher income earned by specialists can lead to an imbalance between primary and specialist healthcare providers. According to Shi & Singh (2017), specialists have more predictable work hours as well as high job prestige and status, which may have influenced their career decisions as medical students.

Many academic institutions, hospitals, and other health care organizations are combating the primary physician shortage by offering incentives to recruit physicians to their areas. From offering a salary bonus upon hiring to paying off any student loans to those working in a rural or inner-city area, many health care organizations have now become creative in how they recruit highly skilled medical physicians to their health care systems.

15.3.2 Nurses

Nurses are the largest group of all the health care professionals. **Nurses** are the primary caregivers to individuals who are ill and/or injured, and they address their physical, mental, and emotional health as a whole. A nurse's educational program consists of completing an approved nursing program and successfully completing a national examination for licensure requirements. There are two types of nurses: (1) Registered Nurses (RN) who must complete an associate degree (AND), a diploma program, or a Bachelor of Science in nursing (BSN) degree, and (2) Licensed Practical Nurses (LPN), or LVN in some states, who must complete a state approved program in practical nursing and take a national written examination. Many practical nursing programs include one year of education with both classroom and supervised clinical practice.

Registered nurses typically do the following job tasks (BLS, 2019):

- Assess patients' conditions

- Record patients' medical histories and symptoms and observe patients and record their observations

- Administer patients' medicines and treatments

- Set up plans for patients' care or contribute information to existing plans

- Consult and collaborate with doctors and other healthcare professionals

- Operate and monitor medical equipment and help perform diagnostic tests and analyze the results

- Teach patients and their families how to manage illnesses or injuries

- Explain what to do at home after treatment

Because patients in hospitals and nursing care facilities need round-the-clock care, nurses in these settings usually work in shifts, covering all 24 hours. They may work nights, weekends, and holidays. They may be on call, which means that they are on duty and must be available to work on short notice. Nurses who work in offices, schools, and other places that do not provide 24-hour care are more likely to work regular business hours. Patient-to-nurse staffing ratios have increased over the years due to much sicker patients. Diseases are becoming harder to diagnose or treat as well as much more resistant to antibiotics.

According to the Bureau of Labor Statistics (2019), employment of registered nurses is projected to grow 12% from 2018 to 2028, much faster than the average for all occupations. The RN workforce is expected to grow from 2.9 million in 2016 to 3.4 million in 2026, an increase of 438,100 or 15%. This growth will occur for a number of reasons, including

- Demand for healthcare services will increase because of the aging population, given that older people typically have more medical problems than younger people. Nurses will also be needed to educate and care for patients with various chronic conditions, such as arthritis, dementia, diabetes, and obesity.

- The financial pressure on hospitals to discharge patients as soon as possible may result in more people being admitted to long-term care facilities and outpatient care centers as well as a greater need for healthcare at home. Job growth is expected in facilities that provide long-term rehabilitation for stroke and head injury patients and in facilities that treat people with Alzheimer's disease. In addition, because many older people prefer to be treated at home or in residential care facilities, registered nurses will be in demand in those settings.

- Growth is also expected to be faster than average in outpatient care centers, where patients do not stay overnight, such as those which provide same-day chemotherapy, rehabilitation, and surgery. In addition, an increased number of procedures, as well as more sophisticated procedures previously done only in hospitals, are being performed in ambulatory care settings and physicians' offices.

Critical Factors Contributing to Nursing Shortages

The Bureau of Labor Statistics projects the need for an additional 203,700 new RNs each year through 2026 to fill newly created positions and to replace retiring nurses. Experts forecast the RN shortage to be most intense in the southern and western United States (BLS, 2019). Critical factors contributing to the nursing shortages are as follows:

- Aging Population. According to the U.S. Census Bureau, by 2050, the number of U.S. residents age 65 and over is projected to be 83.7 million, almost double its estimated population of 43.1 million in 2012. With larger numbers of older adults, there will be an increased need for geriatric care, including care for individuals with chronic diseases and comorbidities.

- Insufficient Number of Faculty at Nursing Schools. Nursing schools across the U.S. are struggling to expand capacity to meet the rising demand for care, given the national move towards healthcare reform. U.S. nursing schools turned away more than 75,000 qualified applicants from baccalaureate and graduate nursing programs in 2018 due to insufficient numbers of faculty, clinical sites, classroom space, and clinical preceptors, as well as budget constraints. Almost two-thirds of the nursing schools responding to the survey pointed to a shortage of faculty and/or clinical preceptors as a reason for not accepting all qualified applicants into their programs (AACN, 2019).

- Stress and Work-Life Balance. In the July 2017 issue of *BMJ Quality & Safety*, the international journal of healthcare improvement, Dr. Linda Aiken and her colleagues released findings from their study of acute care hospitals in Belgium, England, Finland, Ireland, Spain, and Switzerland; it found that a greater numbet of professional nurses at the bedside is associated with better outcomes for patients and nurses. Reducing nursing skill mix by adding assistive personnel without professional nurse qualifications may contribute to preventable deaths, erode care quality, and contribute to nurse shortages.

- *Nurses Leaving the Workforce*. The Health Resources and Services Administration projects that more than 1 million registered nurses will reach retirement age within the next 10 to 15 years. *According to* healthcare economist David Auerbach (2015) of ScienceDaily, findings released from a study found that almost 40% of RNs are over the age of 50: "The number of nurses leaving the workforce each year has been growing steadily from around 40,000 in 2010 to nearly 80,000 by 2020. Meanwhile, the dramatic growth in nursing school enrollment over the last 15 years has begun to level off."

15.3.3 Allied Health Professionals

Allied health care providers consist of many job specific individuals who receive special training, and their clinical interventions complement and enhance the services provided by physicians and nurses. Employment of healthcare occupations is projected to grow 14% from 2018 to 2028—much faster than the average for all occupations—adding about 1.9 million new jobs. Healthcare occupations are projected to add more jobs than any of the other occupational groups. This projected growth is mainly due to an aging population, leading to greater demand for healthcare services (BLS, 2019). Allied health includes several unique areas and constitutes approximately 60% of the U.S. health care workforce. An allied health professional is someone who has received a certificate: associate's, bachelor's, or master's degree. Individuals with a doctoral level or post-baccalaureate training in a science related to health care have the responsibility to deliver specific health services (Shi & Singh, 2017).

According to the American Medical Association's Committee on Allied Health education and Accreditation (CAHEA), an **allied health practitioner** is defined as

> a large cluster of health care related professions and personnel whose functions include assisting, facilitating, or complementing the work of physicians and other specialists in the health care system, and who choose to be identified as allied health personnel.

A Report on Allied Health Personnel (U.S. Department of Health, Education, and Welfare) noted that the federal government adopted the latter view. It attempted to winnow out, from 3.5 million health care workers, those in fields that came under the federal purview of allied health. Its criteria excluded health care workers who (1) were treated separately by legislation other than the allied health authorization; (2) had general (rather than health-specific) expertise that could be applicable to other industries; and (3) performed functions that required little or no formal training in health care subject matter. In addition to physicians, nurses, dentists, optometrists, podiatrists, pharmacists, veterinarians, and other independent health practitioners, the authors of the report excluded

- professional public health personnel
- biomedical research personnel
- natural and social scientists working in the health field
- nursing auxiliaries, and

- occupations requiring no formal training (U.S. Department of Health, Education, and Welfare, 1979).

According to Shi & Singh (2017), allied health professionals typically fall into these two categories: (1) technicians and assistants, and (2) technologists and therapists.

- Technicians and assistants. Training and education are usually less than 2 years of post-secondary education, and they are trained to do job specific procedures. These individuals receive supervision from technologists and therapists who ensure continuous quality therapy is being delivered to the patient.

- Technologists and therapists. Training and education are more advanced for these practitioners and involves skills that are focused on patient evaluation, diagnosis, and developing and implementing a treatment plan. Some of these professions include physical therapists, respiratory therapists, occupational therapists, radiologic therapists, dieticians, social workers, and speech language pathologists.

Health care professionals in the U.S., again, are the largest portion of our labor force. Physicians, nurses, and allied health professionals must overcome challenges of the aging population, limited access to health care, and the uninsured.

Stop and Apply

The employers of health care facilities constitute a large group of stakeholders because they are the entity that pays the most cost and must be proactive in determining what those costs should be in order to function at a level of organizational performance excellence.

Health care personnel mentioned to the hospice health care leaders and managers that some of the problems/issues the organization is having with employees stemmed from stress, working too much over-time due to the staffing shortage, and difficulties managing work-life balance.

1. As the hospice manager, what can be done to combat these foreseen challenges regarding health care provider shortages?

2. What can be done by the medical profession to help alleviate the stress, to recruit, and to retain more nurses and allied health professionals?

3. The delivery of health care in the quality and appropriateness of medical care weighed heavily in the case of Mr. Rodriquez. What can be done to solve problems that have an impact on the quality and appropriateness of diagnostics and therapeutic procedures that have a heavy impact on cost at the hospice center?

15.4 AGING POPULATION

The year 2030 marks an important historical point in U.S. history. By 2030, all baby boomers will be older than 65 and thereby expand the size of the older population so that 1 in every 5 residents will be at retirement age. The U.S. Census projects that, for the first time in history, older people (aging baby boomers) will outnumber children. By 2034, there will be 77.0 million (previously 78.0) people 65 years and older, compared to 76.5 million (previously 76.7 million) under the age of 18 (U.S. Census, 2019).

The projected increased number of older individuals with chronic physical illnesses and disorders, physical ailments, and mental and cognitive disorders raises a significant concern about the capabilities of the U.S. health care system. The aging population in the U.S. poses a severe challenge to health care systems, especially in the long-term care industry. Nursing homes, home-care centers, skilled nursing centers, aging in place health care systems, assisted living facilities, and other adult care facilities will be adversely affected by problems of delivering and maintaining quality care in the future.

15.4.1 Long Term Care Facilities for the Aging Population

The aging population is the fastest growing portion of the population and comprises the major consumers of long-term care services. It is vital that health care systems create a diverse variety of long-term care services that can be available at institutional, community-based, and home-based settings.

According to the Centers for Disease Control (2016), long-term care services include a broad range of health, personal care, and supportive services that meet the needs of frail older people and other adults whose capacity for self-care is limited due to a chronic illness; injury; physical, cognitive, or mental disability; or other health-related conditions. Long term care began as early as the late 1800s to socially address the unhealthy living conditions of immigrants residing in urban tenements (Young & Kroth, 2018). Individuals living in such close quarters created a breeding ground for diseases, such as tuberculosis, typhoid, and smallpox. Nursing agencies addressed the call to care for the sick in their homes. Their job role quickly evolved into including preventative education regarding hygiene, cleanliness, nutrition, and social welfare interventions (Young & Kroth, 2018).

As of 2016 in the U.S., there were an estimated 4,600 adult day services centers, 12,200 home health agencies, 4,300 hospices, 15,600 nursing homes, and 28,900 residential care communities (CDC, 2016). Today, long term care facilities provide a variety of services, like social work services, mental health counseling, therapeutic services, pharmacy or pharmacist services, and dementia care units (CDC, 2016).

The majority of long-term care service users were aged 65 and over, with 94.6% being hospice patients, 93.4% residential care residents, 83.5% nursing home residents, 81.9% home health patients, and 62.5% participants in adult day services centers. Among nursing home residents, 81.4% of short-stay residents and 85.1% of long-stay residents were aged 65 and over (CDC, 2016).

As the years passed, agencies and institutions were created to implement safe, healthy, clean, and dignified modes of long-term care service. **Long Term Care Facilities** (LTCFs) are institutions, such as nursing homes, skilled nursing facilities (SNFs), and assisted-living facilities, that provide health care to people who are unable to manage independently in the community. The location of where this long-term care service is provided categorizes the long-term care facility. There are two categories as follows (Young & Kroth, 2018):

1. *Institution-based services*—Long term care services provided within an institution, such as a nursing home, hospital within a patient care or rehabilitation facility, or inpatient hospice.

2. *Community-based services*—Organizations that coordinate, manage, and deliver long term care services, such as adult day care programs, residential group homes, or care in the patient's home.

15.4.2 Location and Cost of LTCFs

The supply of providers in the five long-term care service sectors vary in their geographic distribution. The largest share of adult day services centers (32.2%), home health agencies (45.6%), hospices (39.4%), and nursing homes (34.8%) was in the South, while the largest share of residential care communities (40.8%) was in the West (CDC, 2016). The cost of annual national expenditures for care in long term facilities continues to increase year after year. In 2014 alone, nursing care facilities and continuing care communities totaled $155.6 billion, with Medicare and Medicaid being paid the largest portion—55%, and 45% were funded by out-of-pocket, private insurance, or other third-party health insurances (Young & Kroth, 2018).

15.4.3 Types of Long-Term Care Facilities

Skilled Nursing Facilities—A facility that is Medicare and Medicaid certified and is defined as "a facility, or distinct part of one, primarily engaged in providing skilled nursing care and related services for people requiring medical or nursing care, or rehabilitation services" (Young & Kroth, 2018).

Assisted Living—A program that provides and/or arranges for daily meals, personal and other supportive services, health care, and 24-hour oversight to persons residing in a group residential facility who need assistance with the activities of daily living (CDC, 2016; Young & Kroth, 2018).

Home Care—A community-based health care organization providing for individuals in their own residences. This health care can be either short-term or long-term. Health care professionals providing care include nurses, home health aides, physical therapists, occupational therapists, speech-language pathologists, social workers, mental health workers, and personal care aides (CDC, 2016; Young & Kroth, 2018).

Hospice Care—A program of care for the terminally ill. The term palliative care is often used synonymously with hospice are.

Adult Day Care—An organization that provides a supervised program of social activities and custodial care (social model), medical and rehabilitative care through skilled nursing (medical model), or specialized services for patients with cognitive or mental disorders/diseases like Alzheimer's and other forms of dementia (CDC, 2016; Young & Kroth, 2018).

Aging in Place—A health care system that brings together a variety of health and other supportive services to enable older, frail adults to live independently in their own residences for as long as is safely possible (Young & Kroth, 2018).

15.4.4 Challenges in the Future of Long-Term Care

Because of the increasing growth of the aging population in the U.S., health systems face a need for more options in providing quality services. Health care workers in long term care facilities are traditionally paid less and given less status than other health care professionals. This is creating a crisis in recruiting and retaining skilled long-term care facility employees.

Several factors contributing to the employment crisis include the following (CDC, 2016; Young & Kroth, 2018):

- Growing need for services
- Funding
- Wages and benefits constrained by reimbursement policies
- Competition among employers for qualified employees
- High employee turnover
- Increased employee absenteeism
- Decreased job engagement
- Low employee morale
- A lack of social supports for workers, including childcare and transportation
- A lack of opportunities for education and career mobility
- Poor work-life balance

15.4.5 Components of a National Long-Term Care Strategy

Long term care industries are developing solutions to address these crises in meeting the needs—currently and in the future—for the aging population by developing a strategy that incorporates these four primary components: (1) education and awareness, (2) caregiving, (3) healthy aging, and (4) long-term care financing.

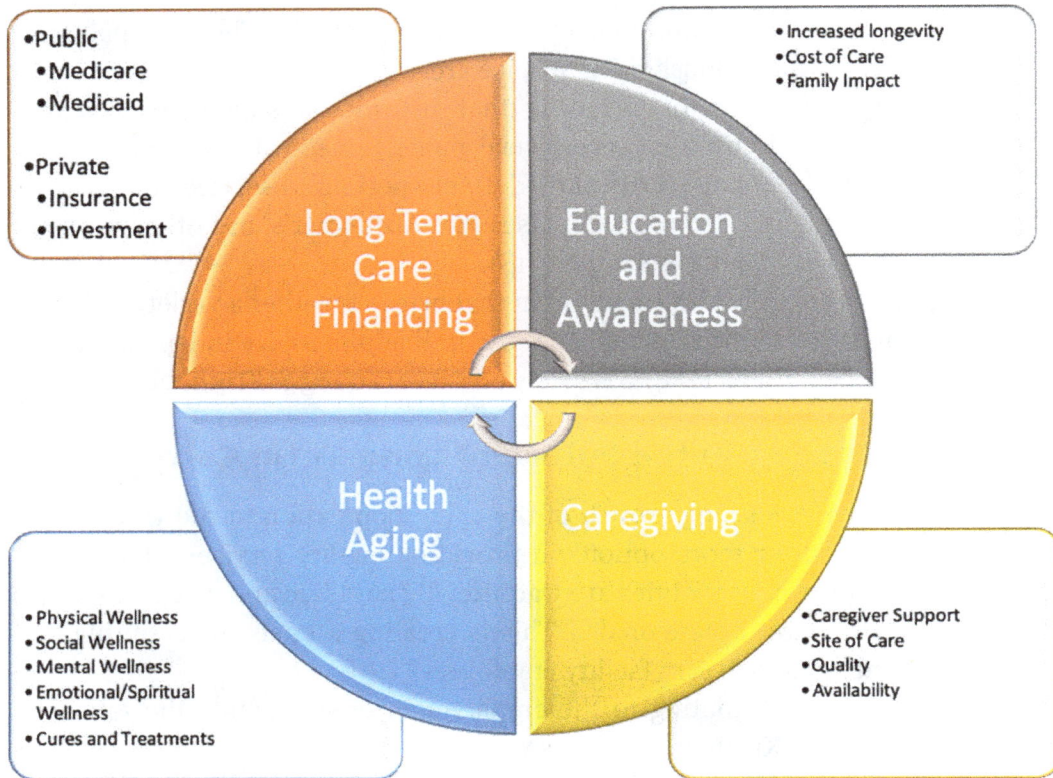

Figure 15.1: Long Term Care Strategy

Source: Original Work
Attribution: Melissa Jordan
License: CC BY-SA 4.0

Stop and Apply

The hospice manager is understanding the foreseen challenges that are facing long term care facilities in the future. How should the manager develop a strategy that incorporates the following four primary components in addressing these issues at the hospice center?

1. Education and awareness
2. Caregiving
3. Healthy aging
4. Long-term care financing

15.5 FUTURE CHALLENGES IN HEALTHCARE

15.5.1 Continuing Challenges and Technological Innovations

The growing cost of health care is contributing to the increasing need for technology. Important advances have been made in health and medical science due to technology. Technological advances have made improvements in the quality of life by providing advancements in medications, treatments, primary and preventive services, as well as in how we allocate financial resources for ambulatory clinic patients and other community populations. Technology has also allowed health care to provide outreach services and treatments to rural areas that previously may not have had access.

Several questions should be asked when choosing the need to assess the value of technological advances; these include the following (Young & Kroth, 2018):

1. How does the new technology benefit the organization?
2. How does the new technology benefit the patient?
3. How does the new technology benefit the employees?
4. Is the new technology worth the cost?
5. Are the new methods better than previous methods, and can they replace them effectively and efficiently?
6. Is the treatment plan enhanced and is quality improved?
7. Is the outcome from the disease/disorder better, or has the mortality rate improved?

Medicine in the 21st century increasingly depends on technology. Unlike in many other areas, the cost of medical technology is not declining, and its increasing use contributes to spiraling healthcare costs. Technologically advanced diagnostic equipment and treatment require expensive medical equipment, computerizations, and extremely skilled personnel.

According to Young & Kroth (2018), information technology has been adopted by many health systems over the years, and this development only increases the high cost of health care. Electronic Health Records (EHRs) began to develop in hospitals in the 1970s and 1980s. Commercial EHRs began to appear soon after in the 1990s and focused on offering a better quality of care and lower cost for hospitals and smaller physician groups. Today, this type of technology is now adopted through many health care systems across the U.S., and most hospitals now have many information technology departments with managers who work closely with one or more health information technology vendors to keep their systems operational. In order to achieve the overall goals of implementing health information systems in the workplace, managing the exploding cost will continue to be problematic.

15.5.2 Quality and Costs

In order to perform at a level of excellence, no leader or manager can tackle this issue alone. It takes the entire organization's efforts to achieve performance excellence in quality. Techniques and strategies must include training and development for employees, implementing change and addressing resistors to change, service satisfaction, teamwork, effective communication, identifying an effective organization culture focused on improving, accountability of effective leadership, identifying factors that hinder advancement, process improvements, and documentation of outcome criteria.

15.5.3 Change in Population

It has already been noted that our population is aging at an astounding rate, but increasing numbers of diversity and minority populations must not be left out of the discussions on future challenges for quality health care. Minority groups and Hispanics will become larger portions of the U.S. elderly population, and these changes will have a significant effect on mortality rates, chronic conditions, service presences, and access to medical care (Young & Kroth, 2018). According to the U.S. Census Bureau (2015), by 2060, Hispanic people will compose 28.6% of the total population, with 119 million Hispanic individuals residing in the U.S. Minority groups and Hispanics will become larger portions of the elderly population, and these changes will have a significant effect on mortality rates, chronic conditions, service presences, and access to medical care (Young & Kroth, 2018).

15.5.4 Reformed and Value Based Health Care Systems

In order to improve in all areas of health care, the U.S. health care system must focus on becoming a value-based system. Value based health care systems must include

- Patient engagement, with patients as active participants in health care decisions
- Outcome definitions and measurements, which create transparency for providers and patients
- Coordinated care among all involved providers, including community partnerships and participants
- Strong governance earmarked by providers and management involvement

Contracts that commit providers to an outcome-oriented approach to patient care.

Stop and Apply

Please answer the following questions from the hospice manager's point of view:

1. How should the new technology at the hospice center be chosen?
2. Is new technology needed?
3. When will the need to set stricter standards of health care competence be available to implement?
4. How can value based strategies be implemented at the hospice center?
5. How can the hospice center meet the needs of the growing minority population (Hispanic)?

15.6 CONCLUSION

Unforeseen challenges will continue to be on the horizon for health care systems, but preparation is the key. Leaders and managers can be certain that hard work is ahead, but success can be accomplished by implementing effective strategies, modeling the way as effective leaders, using updated techniques, and providing the resources, training, and development needed for employees, securing funding, effectively decreasing cost, welcoming innovation, commitment, and addressing the oncoming needs of our aging population.

15.7 KEY POINTS

- The U.S. health care industry is the largest employer in the nation.

- The health care segment of the U.S. economy will continue to grow because of the overall growth in the U.S. population for these three unique reasons: (1) immigration; (2) the aging population, as baby boomers continue to turn 65 years and older through 2029; and (3) increased life expectancies.

- Physicians are individuals who play a key role in the health care of an individual by evaluating a patient's condition by their signs, symptoms, and test results, and prescribing treatment along with the possibility of medication therapy. Health care professionals in the U.S. are the largest portion of our labor force. Physicians, nurses, and allied health professionals must overcome challenges of the aging population, limited access to health care, and the uninsured.

- As the older population grows and rates of chronic illnesses increase, consumers will seek high levels of care that use the latest technologies, diagnostic tests, and therapies.

- Demand for physicians and surgeons is expected to increase, despite factors that can temper growth. New technologies, such as improved information technologies or remote monitoring, are expected to allow physicians to treat more patients in the same amount of time. If adopted, new technologies can reduce the number of physicians who would be needed to complete the same tasks.

- Nurses are the largest group of all the health care professionals and are the primary caregivers to individuals who are ill and/or injured, and nurses address their physical, mental, and emotional health as a whole.

- Critical factors contributing to nursing shortages are the aging population, insufficient number of faculty at nursing schools, stress and work-life balance, and the number of nurses leaving the workforce through retirement.

- Allied health care providers comprise many job specific individuals who receive special training, and their clinical interventions complement and enhance the services provided by physicians and nurses.
- Allied health professionals fall into these two categories: (1) technicians and assistants and 2) technologists and therapists.
- The aging population in the U.S. poses a severe challenge to health care systems, especially in the long-term care industry.

15.8 KEY TERMS

Physicians, surgeons, nurses, allied health practitioner, baby boomers, technicians and assistants, technologists and therapists, long term care facility (LTCF), aging in place system, skilled nursing facility (SNF), assisted living facility, home care, hospice care, respite care, adult day care, value-based health systems

15.9 QUESTIONS FOR REVIEW AND DISCUSSION

1. What do you believe is the biggest challenge for physicians, nurses, and allied health professionals?

2. What can health care systems do to combat these foreseen health care provider shortages?

3. What can be done by the medical profession to help alleviate the shortage and recruit more nurses?

4. What are the best strategies to address workforce shortages?

5. What can health care organizations do to recruit and retain health care professionals?

6. At the state and federal level, what are the efforts being utilized to enhance access to basic health care?

7. What is the current state of preparation at your health care organization for the challenges discussed in this chapter? What strategies are in place to address these future challenges?

15.10 REFERENCES

Aiken L. H, Sloane D, Griffiths P., Rafferty, A. M., Bruyneel, L., HcHugh, M., Maier, C. B., Moreno-Casbas, T., Ball, J. E., Ausserhofer, D., and Sermeus, W. (2017). "Nursing skill mix in European hospitals: cross-sectional study of the association with mortality, patient ratings, and quality of care." BMJ Quality & Safety; 26:559-568.

American Association of Colleges of Nursing. Fact sheet: Nursing shortage. Retrieved from https://www.aacnnursing.org/Portals/42/News/Factsheets/Nursing-Shortage-Factsheet.pdf

Bureau of Labor Statistics, U.S. Department of Labor, *Occupational Outlook Handbook*, Physicians and Surgeons, on the Internet at https://www.bls.gov/ooh/healthcare/physicians-and-surgeons.htm (visited *October 23, 2019*).

Bureau of Labor Statistics, U.S. Department of Labor, *Occupational Outlook Handbook*, Registered Nurses, on the Internet at https://www.bls.gov/ooh/healthcare/registered-nurses.htm (visited *October 30, 2019*).

Centers of Disease Control and Prevention (CDC). (2016). Long-term care providers and Services users in the United States, 2015-2016: An analytical and epidemiological studies. Retrieved from https://www.cdc.gov/nchs/data/series/sr_03/sr03_43-508.pdf

Merriam Webster Dictionary. Baby boomer. Retrieved from https://www.merriam-webster.com/dictionary/baby%20boomer

Montana State University. (2015, September 21). "Shortage of nurses not as dire as predicted, but challenges remain to meet America's needs." *ScienceDaily*. Retrieved November 4, 2019 from www.sciencedaily.com/releases/2015/09/150921153457.htm

Shi, L. & Singh, D. A. (2017). *Essentials of the U.S. health care systems*. 4th Ed. Jones and Bartlett: Burlington, MA.

U.S. Bureau of Labor Statistics. Occupational employment statistics surveys. Retrieved from www.bls.gov.

U.S. Bureau of Labor Statistics. Labor force statistics from the current population survey. Retrieved from www.bls.gov/csp/cpsaat18.htm.

U.S. Census Bureau (2014). "An aging nation: The older population in the United States." Retrieved from https://www.census.gov/library/publications/2014/demo/p25-1140.html

U.S. Census Bureau. (2019). "Older people projected to outnumber children for the first time in U.S. history." Retrieved from https://www.census.gov/newsroom/press-releases/2018/cb18-41-population-projections.html

U.S. Department of Health, Education, and Welfare. 1979. *A Report on Allied Health Personnel*. Washington, D.C.: U.S. Government Printing Office.

U.S. Department of Labor, Bureau of Labor Statistics. "Current population survey: employment and earnings." Retrieved from www.bls.gov/cps/cpsa2009.pdf

World Health Organization. Health workforce. Retrieved from https://www.who.int/health-topics/health-workforce#tab=tab_1

Young, K. M. & Kroth, P. J. (2018). *Health care USA: Understanding its organization and delivery*. Jones and Bartlett: Burlington, MA.